Bariatric Surgery

What Every Provider Needs to Know

EDITORS

R. ARMOUR FORSE, MD, CM, PHD, FRCS(C), FACS, FCCM, FASMBS
Chief Academic Officer and Executive Vice President
Doctors Hospital at Renaissance
President Health Sciences Institute at Renaissance
Clinical Professor of Surgery
University of Texas Rio Grande Valley
Edinburg, Texas

CAROLINE M. APOVIAN, MD
Professor of Medicine and Pediatrics
Boston University School of Medicine
Director, Center for Nutrition and Weight Management
Section of Endocrinology, Diabetes and Nutrition
Boston Medical Center
Boston, Massachusetts

SLACK
INCORPORATED

www.Healio.com/books

ISBN: 978-1-61711-056-6

Cover illustrations by Kyisook Hong.

The procedures and practices described in this publication should be implemented in a manner consistent with the professional standards set for the circumstances that apply in each specific situation. Every effort has been made to confirm the accuracy of the information presented and to correctly relate generally accepted practices. The authors, editors, and publisher cannot accept responsibility for errors or exclusions or for the outcome of the material presented herein. There is no expressed or implied warranty of this book or information imparted by it. Care has been taken to ensure that drug selection and dosages are in accordance with currently accepted/recommended practice. Off-label uses of drugs may be discussed. Due to continuing research, changes in government policy and regulations, and various effects of drug reactions and interactions, it is recommended that the reader carefully review all materials and literature provided for each drug, especially those that are new or not frequently used. Some drugs or devices in this publication have clearance for use in a restricted research setting by the Food and Drug and Administration or FDA. Each professional should determine the FDA status of any drug or device prior to use in their practice.

Any review or mention of specific companies or products is not intended as an endorsement by the author or publisher.

SLACK Incorporated uses a review process to evaluate submitted material. Prior to publication, educators or clinicians provide important feedback on the content that we publish. We welcome feedback on this work.

Published by: SLACK Incorporated
6900 Grove Road
Thorofare, NJ 08086 USA
Telephone: 856-848-1000
Fax: 856-848-6091
www.Healio.com/books

Contact SLACK Incorporated for more information about other books in this field or about the availability of our books from distributors outside the United States.

Library of Congress Cataloging-in-Publication Data

Bariatric surgery (Forse)
Bariatric surgery : what every provider needs to know / [edited by] R. Armour Forse, Caroline M. Apovian.
p. ; cm.
Includes bibliographical references and index.
ISBN 978-1-61711-056-6 (alk. paper)
I. Forse, R. Armour, editor. II. Apovian, Caroline M., editor. III. Title.
[DNLM: 1. Bariatric Surgery. WI 900]
RD540.5
617.4'3--dc23
2015033712

Printed in the United States of America.

Last digit is print number: 10 9 8 7 6 5 4 3 2 1

Dedication

I dedicate this book to the patients who trusted me with their health care,
my students and residents who taught me as I taught them,
and to my supportive wife, Susan, who helped and encouraged me throughout this project.

—*RAF*

To all those struggling with obesity,
hopefully this textbook will help providers be caring and compassionate.
To our spouses for putting up with our strange behavior after clinic.

—*CMA*

Contents

Acknowledgments

I want to acknowledge the chapter authors for helping us to complete this project with their expertise and informative chapters. I also acknowledge the hard and persistent work of SLACK Incorporated's staff, particularly Carrie Kotlar, whose dedication to this project made it happen.

—RAF

I would like to thank Carrie Kotlar for her tireless efforts in getting this textbook published and for pushing all of us to write our best. I also thank the authors for their expertise and for giving their time to help health care providers. Lastly, I would like to thank Ashley Bourland for her assistance in the preparation of this textbook.

—CMA

About the Editors

R. Armour Forse, MD, CM, PhD, FRCS(C), FACS, FCCM, FASMBS is currently the Chief Academic Officer at Doctors Hospital at Renaissance, and President of Health Sciences Institute at Renaissance, where he oversees the educational and research programs for the health care system. He is also Clinical Professor of Surgery at the University of Texas Rio Grande Valley, and was previously Professor of Surgery and the Associate Chair of Surgery for Education in the Department of Surgery at Creighton University School of Medicine. He received his undergraduate, medical, and post-doctorate degrees from McGill University in Montreal, Quebec, Canada, and completed his surgical residency at the Royal Victoria Hospital in Montreal. He completed a Medical Research Council of Canada research fellowship in surgical metabolism at Columbia University College of Physicians and Surgeons and The Rockefeller Institute in New York. He has been in active surgical and bariatric practice for more than 30 years, including being an Assistant Professor of Surgery at McGill University, an Associate Professor of Surgery at Harvard Medical School, and the Laszlo Nando Tauber Professor of Surgery at Boston University School of Medicine. Here he worked with Dr. Caroline Apovian to build the Nutrition and Weight Management Center at Boston Medical Center where Dr. Apovian is the current director. Dr. Forse serves on the editorial boards of *Obesity Surgery* and *Surgery for Obesity and Related Diseases*. He is a prolific researcher and publisher with 15 patents, 59 research grants and more than 450 publications including abstracts, chapters, books, and papers.

Caroline M. Apovian, MD is Director of the Nutrition and Weight Management Center at Boston Medical Center and Professor of Medicine at Boston University School of Medicine. She is a nationally and internationally recognized authority on nutrition and has been in the field of obesity and nutrition since 1990. She was on the expert panel for updating the *2013 AHA/ACC/TOS Guideline for the Management of Overweight and Obesity in Adults: A Report of the American College of Cardiology/American Heart Association Task Force on Practice Guidelines and The Obesity Society*, which were published in *Circulation, Obesity,* and the *Journal of the American College of Cardiology.* She was also the Chair of the 2015 Endocrine Society guidelines on the *Pharmacologic Management of Obesity*. In 2015, she was elected as Vice President of The Obesity Society.

Contributing Authors

Nadia N. Ahmad, MD, MPH (Chapter 3)
Director
Obesity Medicine Institute
Dubai, United Arab Emirates

Venkata M. Alla, MD (Chapter 20)
Division of Cardiology
Creighton University School of Medicine
Omaha, Nebraska

Dustin M. Bermudez, MD (Chapter 1)
Fellow in Minimally Invasive Surgery
Department of Surgery
Brody School of Medicine
East Carolina University
Greenville, North Carolina

Stacy A. Brethauer, MD (Chapter 7)
Associate Professor of Surgery
Cleveland Clinic Lerner College of Medicine
Cleveland, Ohio

W. Scott Butsch, MD, MSc (Chapter 3)
Instructor in Medicine
Harvard Medical School
Assistant in Medicine
Massachusetts General Hospital Weight Center
Obesity Metabolism and Nutrition Institute
Massachusetts General Hospital
Boston, Massachusetts

Judy Y. R. Chen, MD, FACS (Chapter 17)
Staff Surgeon
Swedish Weight Loss Services
Swedish Medical Center
Seattle, Washington

Elizabeth Colsen, MD (Chapter 5)
University of Minnesota
Minneapolis, Minnesota

Yaniv Cozacov, MD (Chapter 16)
Research Fellow
The Bariatric and Metabolic Institute
Digestive Disease Institute
Cleveland Clinic Florida
Weston, Florida

Attila Csordas, MD (Chapter 24)
Creighton University
Omaha, Nebraska

Ashley Cuellar, MD (Chapter 18)
Gastroenterology Fellow
Division of Gastroenterology/Hepatology
Indiana University School of Medicine
Indianapolis, Indiana

Emily R. Cunningham, BA (Chapter 1)
Research Coordinator
Department of Surgery
Brody School of Medicine
East Carolina University
Greenville, North Carolina

Dennis Esterbrooks, MD (Chapter 20)
Division of Cardiology
Creighton University School of Medicine
Omaha, Nebraska

Kelli E. Friedman, PhD (Chapter 26)
Assistant Professor
Departments of Surgery and Psychiatry and Behavioral Sciences
Duke University Medical Center
Director of Psychological Services
Duke Center for Metabolic and Weight Loss Surgery
Durham, North Carolina

Daniel M. Herron, MD (Chapter 11)
The Barry Salky Professor of Surgery
Icahn School of Medicine at Mount Sinai
New York, New York

Kathleen B. Hrovat, MS, RD, LD (Chapter 13)
Surgical Weight Loss Program for Teens
Cincinnati Children's Hospital Medical Center
Cincinnati, Ohio

Mustafa Hussain, MD (Chapter 9)
Assistant Professor of Surgery
Medical Director of Bariatric Program
Minimally Invasive Gastrointestinal and Bariatric Surgery
University of Chicago Medical Center
Chicago, Illinois

Sayeed Ikramuddin, MD (Chapter 5)
University of Minnesota
Minneapolis, Minnesota

Thomas H. Inge, MD, PhD (Chapter 13)
Cincinnati Children's Hospital Medical Center
Cincinnati, Ohio

Daniel B. Jones, MD, MS, FACS (Chapter 10)
Professor of Surgery
Harvard Medical School
Vice Chair of Surgery
Office of Technology and Innovation
Chief
Minimally Invasive Surgical Services
Director of the Bariatric Program
Beth Israel Deaconess Medical Center
Boston, Massachusetts

Stephanie B. Jones, MD (Chapter 12)
Associate Professor of Anesthesia
Harvard Medical School
Vice Chair for Education
Department of Anesthesia, Critical Care and Pain Medicine
Beth Israel Deaconess Medical Center
Boston, Massachusetts

Sangeeta Rao Kashyap, MD (Chapter 19)
Associate Professor of Medicine
Department of Endocrinology, Diabetes and Metabolism
Cleveland Clinic Lerner College of Medicine of Case Western Reserve University
Cleveland, Ohio

Lalita Khaodhiar, MD (Chapter 21)
Assistant Professor of Medicine
Boston University School of Medicine
Boston, Massachusetts

Eugene Kim, MD (Chapter 12)
Instructor of Anesthesia
Harvard Medical School
Department of Anesthesia, Critical Care and Pain Medicine
Beth Israel Deaconess Medical Center
Boston, Massachusetts

Linda Kollar, RN, MSN, CBN (Chapter 13)
Cincinnati Children's Hospital Medical Center
Cincinnati, Ohio

Nitin Kumar, MD (Chapter 23)
Brigham and Women's Hospital
Boston, Massachusetts

Tommy H. Lee, MD (Chapter 25)
Associate Professor
Creighton University
Omaha, Nebraska

Daniel B. Leslie, MD (Chapter 5)
Assistant Professor
Director of Bariatric Surgery
Department of Surgery
University of Minnesota
Minneapolis, Minnesota

Natalia Leva, MD (Chapter 8)
University of California—San Francisco
San Francisco, California

Emanuele Lo Menzo, MD, PhD (Chapter 16)
Director
Surgical Research
The Bariatric and Metabolic Institute
Digestive Disease Institute
Cleveland Clinic Florida
Weston, Florida
Affiliate Associate Professor
Florida Atlantic University
College of Medicine
Boca Raton, Florida
Clinical Associate Professor
Florida International University
College of Medicine
Miami, Florida

Karen C. McCowen, MB, MRCPI (Chapter 21)
University of California—San Diego
San Diego, California

Lee E. Morrow, MD, MSc (Chapter 22)
Veterans Affairs Medical Center
Nebraska and Western Iowa
Creighton University Medical Center
Omaha, Nebraska

John Magaña Morton, MD, MPH, FACS, FASMBS (Chapter 8)
Chief
Bariatric and Minimally Invasive Surgery
President
American Society for Metabolic and Bariatric Surgery 2014-2015
Stanford School of Medicine
Stanford, California

Kalyana Nandipati, MD (Chapter 25)
Department of Surgery
Creighton University Medical Center
Omaha, Nebraska

Jaisa Olasky, MD (Chapter 10)
Minimally Invasive General Surgeon
Mount Auburn Hospital
Cambridge, Massachusetts
Clinical Instructor
Harvard Medical School
Boston, Massachusetts

Pradeep K. Pallati, MBBS, FACS (Chapter 18)
Assistant Professor of Surgery
Creighton University School of Medicine
Omaha, Nebraska

Alfons Pomp, MD, FACS, FRCSC (Chapter 9)
Leon C. Hirsch Professor
Vice Chairman
Department of Surgery
Chief
GI Metabolic and Bariatric Surgery
Weill Cornell Medical College
New York Presbyterian Hospital
New York, New York

Walter J. Pories, MD, FACS (Chapter 1)
Professor of Surgery, Biochemistry and Kinesiology
Department of Surgery
Brody School of Medicine
East Carolina University
Greenville, North Carolina

Amanda Powell, MD (Chapter 18)
Assistant Professor of Medicine
Tufts University School of Medicine
Boston, Massachusetts
Director of Medical Weight Loss
Lahey Hospital
Burlington, Massachusetts

Christine Ren Fielding, MD (Chapter 6)
Professor of Surgery
NYU School of Medicine
New York, New York

Raul J. Rosenthal, MD (Chapter 16)
Chief of Staff
Chairman
Department of General Surgery
Director
The Bariatric and Metabolic Institute
Cleveland Clinic Florida
Weston, Florida
Professor of Surgery
Herbert Wertheim College of Medicine at Florida International University
Miami, Florida

Francesco Rubino, MD (Chapter 15)
Chair
Bariatric and Metabolic Surgery
King's College London
London, United Kingdom

Philip R. Schauer, MD (Chapter 7)
Professor of Surgery
Cleveland Clinic Lerner College of Medicine
Cleveland, Ohio

Johanna Schubert, MD (Chapter 24)
Creighton University
Omaha, Nebraska

Scott A. Shikora, MD, FACS (Chapter 17)
Associate Professor of Surgery
Harvard Medical School
Director
Center for Metabolic and Bariatric Surgery
Brigham and Women's Hospital
Boston, Massachusetts

Alpana Shukla, MD, MRCP(UK) (Chapter 15)
Assistant Professor of Research in Medicine
Comprehensive Weight Control Center
Division of Endocrinology, Diabetes and Metabolism
Weill Cornell Medical College
New York, New York

Stephanie Sogg, PhD (Chapter 26)
Staff Psychologist
Massachusetts General Hospital Weight Center
Assistant Professor
Harvard Medical School
Boston, Massachusetts

Ashwin Soni, MD, BSc (Chapter 15)
Section of Gastrointestinal Metabolic Surgery
Department of Surgery
Weill Cornell Medical College
New York Presbyterian Hospital
New York, New York
Catholic University
Rome, Italy

Wendy Jo Svetanoff, MD (Chapter 2)
Creighton University School of Medicine
Omaha, Nebraska

Charles E. Thompson III, MD (Chapter 16)
Long Island Laparoscopic Doctors
East Setauket, New York

Christopher C. Thompson, MD, MSc, FACG, FASGE (Chapter 23)
Director of Therapeutic Endoscopy
Brigham and Women's Hospital
Associate Professor of Medicine
Harvard Medical School
Boston, Massachusetts

Oliver A. Varban, MD, FACS (Chapter 14)
Director
Adult Bariatric Surgery Program
University of Michigan Health System
Ann Arbor, Michigan

Bruce M. Wolfe, MD, FACS, FASMBS (Chapter 4)
Professor of Surgery
Oregon Health & Science University
Portland, Oregon

Andrew S. Wu, MD (Chapter 11)
General, Laparoscopic and Bariatric Surgeon
Catholic Medical Center: Surgical Care Group
Manchester, New Hampshire

Preface

This book was written in response to what we learned from our previous book. Many nonsurgical health care professionals commented about the number of bariatric patients they had treated who had undergone bariatric surgery. With the estimated number of bariatric procedures increasing, the number of these patients is also increasing. The physicians were often faced with simple questions they could not answer, and resources such as bariatric clinics provided limited access. Many textbooks were more directed to the surgeon than the other physicians. Having a simple, direct source of information that was not predominantly surgical was helpful, and they found these answers in our book. In addition, we learned that many allied health professionals also found the book helpful, as did students in all areas of health care. So we decided to edit this book to provide health care workers relatively easy, helpful, and current information in caring for bariatric surgical patients. The authors were asked to keep the book relatively simple, straightforward, and easy to use. We know that the areas of bariatric surgery and bariatric medicine are still evolving and that books can quickly fall behind; the chapters in this book were written to be sure that the important general principles are there, the ones that are relatively constant. At the same time we have made sure that current trends in the surgery and the medical treatment, such as medication dosing, are current. To help with the access for this information, we have selected chapters by common areas of question. There is certainly nothing more challenging than getting a patient through bariatric surgery with all the related risks, medical comorbidities, and psychological stresses. An additional challenge is providing complex medical treatment in a patient who month after month undergoes significant physiological and psychological changes as a result of the surgery. In the end, there is also nothing more rewarding than seeing a patient lose weight, lose medical and psychological problems, and gain his or her life back. We hope that this book helps you meet the challenges and brings you the patient successes that we have both enjoyed.

—R. Armour Forse, MD, CM, PhD, FRCS(C), FACS, FCCM, FASMBS
—Caroline M. Apovian, MD

Foreword

That bariatric surgery is a group effort is reflected in the editorial team of surgeon R. Armour Forse and physician Caroline Apovian, both with distinguished careers in the emerging field of obesity medicine. Each has assembled an A-list of colleagues from multiple disciplines to create a textbook that will serve as a bulwark against less than optimal performance of weight loss surgery. Their work is essential to make strong headway against pandemic obesity.

One of the most refractory medical conditions in the United States and around the world, obesity is the major focus of basic, clinical, and translational research. Lifestyle change, the current first-line treatment strategy, has notoriously high recidivism rates and interindividual variability. To rein in the terribly high human and economic costs of obesity, it is imperative to gain deeper insights into how surgery works and develop new ways to treat and manage the disease.

Currently, the science of food intake regulation in humans has yet to be fully elucidated. Research in this area is critical. It involves the study of complex integration across homeostasis, reward, and cognition systems.[1-3] This work is part of ongoing efforts to develop innovative surgical procedures, and perhaps most importantly, to identify the critical mechanisms that have made bariatric surgery the single most effective treatment for severe obesity and obesity-associated type 2 diabetes.[4,5]

Bariatric surgery alters the function of the gastrointestinal tract along with the dynamics of physiology and pathophysiology in ways that are essential to improve quality of life, combat disease, and resolve metabolic disorders.[6] To understand the genetic, molecular, and behavioral mechanisms that underlie these benefits, researchers have forged new approaches to scientific discovery.

Their latest research findings will be showcased in London in Fall 2015 at the Third World Congress on Interventional Therapies for Type 2 Diabetes and the Second Diabetes Surgery Summit (DSS-II). Here, world-renowned scientists will spend 2 days presenting the best new evidence on the mechanisms of action of bariatric/metabolic surgery and discuss novel interventional therapies for type 2 diabetes. In doing so, they will expand treatment options for patients with obesity and set the stage for future advances in scientific knowledge.

Many of the same internationally known experts at the Congress have contributed chapters to the textbook, *Bariatric Surgery: What Every Provider Needs to Know*, making it a definitive source of information on adult and adolescent obesity as well as the safe and effective practice of bariatric surgery. The book consists of 26 chapters that present a comprehensive introduction to obesity and an approach to treatment, followed by sections on innovations in surgical procedures and medical issues surrounding bariatric surgery.

Two recent studies focus on 5-year outcomes of weight loss surgery. The first compared results in patients who underwent laparoscopic gastric bypass or biliopancreatic diversion[6]; the other investigated the metabolic effects of laparoscopic sleeve gastrectomy.[7]

The former was a randomized controlled trial on the outcomes of each procedure compared to medical treatment of type 2 diabetes in people with a body mass index (BMI) of 35 or greater. The researchers found that regardless of weight loss, the surgery patients had healthier cholesterol levels, reduced cardiovascular risk, less medication use, and better control of their diabetes.

This is not the first time that surgery has proven superior to medical care in the management of diabetes in people with obesity. However, it is the first controlled study with long-term outcomes to add a measure of certainty to evidence that bariatric surgery is a good option for those with both conditions.[8]

The other report is an observational study that provides some of the best data yet on sleeve gastrectomy. It shows that 5 years after the procedure, some patients regained weight and some experienced a relapse in type 2 diabetes.[7]

On average, patients lost 77% of their excess weight after 1 year. Weight regain pushed that number down to 56% at 5 years. Complete diabetes remission rates went from 51% to 20% at the same time. These findings are consistent with other analyses showing that "sleeves" are not quite as effective as gastric bypass, but have lower complication rates.

Despite the drop in diabetes remission over time, the preponderance of literature indicates that weight loss surgery is one of the most effective treatment options for people with severe obesity and its complications. However, the complexities of surgery and its low utilization have spurred a drive to identify the mechanisms that underlie the success of current procedures. These discoveries can then be used as springboards to develop a variety of more accessible treatments. For example, less invasive devices combined with pharmaceutical agents could potentially improve the health of hundreds of thousands, if not millions, of people with obesity.

One of the mechanisms receiving a great deal of attention relates to the role of food reward and cognition—2 variables that are dramatically altered by certain bariatric procedures. The use of new technologies, such as functional magnetic resonance imaging (fMRI), has enhanced insight into these functions in ways that might lead to safer surgery and new directions for medications that will reset optimal homeostatic body weight.[9,10]

Caloric restriction is a subject of intense study, too, particularly as it relates to improved insulin sensitivity. Johnson et al[11] recently found that it lowers insulin-stimulated thioredoxin-interacting protein (TXNIP) levels and enhances nonoxidative glucose disposal, evidence that TXNIP plays a role in mediating the improvement in peripheral insulin sensitivity after caloric restriction.

Metabolic syndrome is another area of interest.[6] Key risk factors cluster in ways that promote obesity and insulin resistance, yet the power of each to predict future odds of developing both conditions varies. In addition, the impact of insulin resistance on metabolic profiles is affected by gender and race, suggesting that gender- and race-specific algorithms for judging the likelihood of obesity may be warranted.[12]

Data indicate that all components of metabolic syndrome are more sensitive and specific indicators for obesity than BMI; that fasting and 2-hour postprandial glucose, waist circumference, and blood pressure can safely, economically, and effectively measure risk.

Cardiometabolic disease staging (CMDS)[12] also suggests that higher risk for future diabetes differs among Black and White men and women. Waist circumference has the highest predictive power in Black men. The key measure in Black women is 2-hour glucose; in White men and women, it is fasting glucose.[12]

Blood pressure in metabolic syndrome has higher predictive power for diabetes in men than women. High-density lipoprotein (HDL) cholesterol, a trivial predictor in Black women, is important in Black men. While other algorithms include blood pressure in metabolic syndrome, the underlying mechanisms that link hypertension and insulin resistance have yet to be fully understood. For example, it is unclear whether high blood pressure contributes to the development of insulin resistance and subsequent type 2 diabetes, or just reflects shared humoral and pathophysiological changes.

Low HDL cholesterol, which promotes cellular cholesterol efflux and has direct antioxidative and anti-inflammatory properties, is also an important risk factor for type 2 diabetes. However, identifying the mechanisms that contribute to observed differences in its effects on White and Black men and women will require further investigation.

Current goals in bariatric surgery/obesity medicine include the pursuit of neurocognitive approaches that promote weight loss through lifestyle changes, the development of new surgical procedures that achieve desired medical and metabolic outcomes, and the opening of doors to the less radical treatment of obesity through combinations of behavioral changes and drug therapy.

Dramatic increases in population-wide obesity have led to a global public health crisis that demands the best that those of us in the fields of science and medicine can offer to study the disease, understand it, and alleviate the pain and suffering of those afflicted by it.

Bariatric Surgery: What Every Provider Needs to Know is a resource that can help us achieve those objectives. An elegant combination of deep investigation into science and practical advice, it is the rare book that belongs in the office of every surgeon, physician, and allied health professional. A unique resource that can be used to prepare for certification in the field of obesity medicine, it can also enhance knowledge of weight loss surgery and aid the fight against uncontrolled growth of global obesity.

—*George L. Blackburn, MD, PhD, MS, FACS*
S. Daniel Abraham Professor of Nutrition
Associate Director, Division of Nutrition
Harvard Medical School
Director, Center for the Study of Nutrition Medicine
Department of Surgery
Beth Israel Deaconess Medical Center
Boston, Massachusetts

References

1. Blackburn GL. Innovations in weight loss surgery. *Bariatric Times.* 2015;12:14-16.
2. Blackburn GL. The 2008 Edward E. Mason Founders lecture: interdisciplinary teams in the development of "best practice" obesity surgery. *Surg Obes Relat Dis.* 2008;4:679-684.
3. Foltz JL, Belay B, Blackburn GL. Improving the weight of the nation by engaging the medical setting in obesity prevention and control. *J Law Med Ethics.* 2013;41(Suppl 2):19-26.
4. Mingrone G, Panunzi S, De Gaetano A, et al. Bariatric surgery versus conventional medical therapy for type 2 diabetes. *N Engl J Med.* 2012;366:1577-1585.
5. Schauer PR, Kashyap SR, Wolski K, et al. Bariatric surgery versus intensive medical therapy in obese patients with diabetes. *N Engl J Med.* 2012;366:1567-1576.
6. Mingrone G, Panuzi S, De Gaetano A, et al. Bariatric-metabolic surgery versus conventional medical treatment in obese patients with type 2 diabetes: 5 year follow-up of an open label, single-centre, randomised controlled trial. *Lancet.* 2015;386:964-973.
7. Golomb I, Ben David M, Glass A, Kolitz T, Keidar A. Long-term metabolic effects of laparoscopic sleeve gastrectomy. *JAMA Surg.* 2015 Aug 5. [Epub ahead of print]
8. Carlin AM, Zeni TM, English WJ, et al. The comparative effectiveness of sleeve gastrectomy, gastric bypass, and adjustable gastric banding procedures for the treatment of morbid obesity. *Ann Surg.* 2013;257:791-797.
9. Shin AC, Berthoud HR. Obesity surgery: happy with less or eternally hungry? *Trends Endocrinol Metab.* 2013;24:101-108.
10. Madsbad S, Dirksen C, Holst JJ. Mechanisms of changes in glucose metabolism and bodyweight after bariatric surgery. *Lancet Diabetes Endocrinol.* 2014;2:152-164.
11. Johnson ML, Distelmaier K, Lanza IR, et al. Mechanism by which caloric restriction improves insulin sensitivity in sedentary obese adults. *Diabetes.* 2015 Aug 31. [Epub ahead of print]
12. Guo F, Garvey WT. Development of a weighted cardiometabolic disease staging (CMDS) system for the prediction of future diabetes. *J Clin Endocrinol Metab.* 2015:jc20152691.

I

General

1

The Obesity Epidemic

Walter J. Pories, MD, FACS; Dustin M. Bermudez, MD; and Emily R. Cunningham, BA

Imagine the response if this nation was confronted with the news that the prevalence of a deadly disease had doubled in the past decade and that in 2013, 1 of every 3 Americans was afflicted. Further imagine that the causes are unknown and the approaches to prevention and the recommended medical treatments are almost universally ineffective. Finally, consider the response when the only effective treatment required major surgery.

We are in the midst of just such an epidemic. Figure 1-1 documents the startling obesity trends in the United States in the 20 years from 1990 to 2010. According to the Centers for Disease Control and Prevention (CDC), today more than one-third of US adults (35.7%) are obese, with even higher age-adjusted rates in non-Hispanic Blacks (49.5%), Mexican Americans (40.4%), and all Hispanics (39.1%) when compared with non-Hispanic Whites (34.3%).[1]

It is a costly and deadly epidemic. In 2008, medical costs associated with obesity were estimated at $147 billion; the medical costs for people who are obese were $1,429 higher annually than those of normal weight. As noted below, obesity also significantly increases mortality rates due to its comorbidities. The degree to which morbidity and mortality rise with being obese coupled with a skyrocketing prevalence of obesity have led to concerns that the next generation may, for the first time in history, not live longer than its predecessors.

This obesity epidemic is not confined to the United States. According to the World Health Organization (WHO), obesity has more than doubled across the globe since 1980. In 2008, more than 1.4 billion adults, 20 years and older, were overweight. Of these, more than 200 million men and nearly 300 million women were obese. Even more disturbing is the finding that more than 40 million children under the age of 5 were overweight in 2010.

In addition to the economic costs and decrease in health, there are other costs of obesity, personal and social, that play a major role in the quality of life of individuals, families, and communities. Individuals with obesity, especially the severely obese, often confront bias in schools, in society, and in the workplace. They are frequently the target of ridicule even in their early years in school. Some estimates even suggest that 25% of severely obese women were sexually abused. People with obesity have difficulty finding jobs, and when they find employment, they all too often have high levels of absenteeism, poor performance at work, and high health care costs. Similarly,

Forse RA, Apovian CM, eds.
Bariatric Surgery: What Every Provider Needs to Know (pp 3-13).

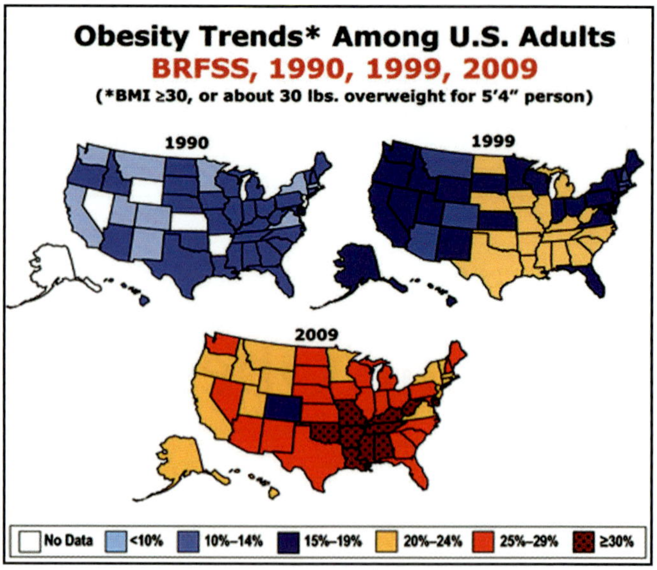

Figure 1-1. Increasing obesity trends among adults in the United States from 1990 to 2010. (Reprinted with permission from the Centers for Disease Control and Prevention, Behavioral Risk Factor Surveillance System.)

within their families, the levels of conflict regarding relationships, parenting, and sexuality are high.

There is an obesity epidemic that is quickly spreading across the United States and the world. While there may be early signs that the prevalence is leveling off, there is certainly no evidence that we are making progress in diagnosing the causes, treating the repercussions of obesity and its comorbidities, and, ultimately, preventing its development in the first place.

Diagnosing Obesity: Not as Easy as It Seems

It would appear that the diagnosis of obesity should be easy: just weigh the patient and compare that weight to a "normal" chart. However, even in 1943, it became apparent that body weight, while easy to measure, was a sharply limited measure. A single weight for each height was not a useful marker because weights vary between men and women. In addition, some individuals who were considered "overweight" or "obese" by standard tables were actually fit and lean. In response to these evident limitations, the Metropolitan Life Insurance Company devised 2 "normal" charts, one for males and another for females, with separate scales for small, medium, and large "frame" individuals.[2] Thus, for a woman 5'8" in height, the "normal" ranges varied in the following manner:

- Small frame: 126 to 139 lb
- Medium frame: 136 to 150 lb
- Large frame: 146 to 167 lb

This led to the curious conclusion that "normal" for a woman of this height could vary from 126 to 167 lb, a range of 41 lb!

This failure of weight alone to serve as a reliable measure led to the adoption of the body mass index ($BMI = kg/m^2$) as an index of obesity. The BMI is a useful and simple tool to categorize patients' obesity but is far from ideal when trying to characterize an anthropometric measurement such as weight and trying to truly define "obesity."

In general, a $BMI \geq 35$ is required for access to bariatric surgery from the standpoint of most insurance carriers. If the patient has a BMI of 34 but is burdened with diabetes that cannot be controlled, severe hyperlipidemias, and dangerously high blood pressure levels, he or she may not be eligible for surgery. In addition to the ethical questions about the use of a single indicator to determine whether a patient is eligible for the only effective therapy, the BMI is not an appropriate measure because it does not reflect adiposity.

First, the BMI is a unigender scale. It discriminates against males because it fails to reflect the evident differences in adiposity between males and females. For example, in a group studied by Jackson et al,[3] males with a BMI of 35 had a percent body fat mass of 35% while females, at the same BMI, had a percent body fat mass of 46%. Second, the BMI discriminates against Asians and Blacks. Katz et al[4] reported that at a similar BMI of 27.5, for example, while 26% White females had a prevalence of hypertension, 34% of Blacks and 44% of Chinese Asians had the disease. Similarly at the same BMI, 12% of Whites had diabetes while 15% of Blacks and 17% of Chinese Asians were so afflicted. Third, the BMI discriminates against older individuals whose weight often decreases along with increased lipid deposition in muscle and other tissues.

Finally, the BMI also fails to allow for fitness. One of our study participants at East Carolina University was a 20-year-old student with a height of 5'8" who weighed 308 lb and presented with a BMI of 47.0—clearly a candidate for bariatric surgery according to the current health insurance guidelines. He would be hard to convince. He was our fastest running back, and his body composition studies revealed that only 7% was fat. As it stands today, a young, unfit White woman has ready access to bariatric surgery while a Black woman who may be far more ill with uncontrolled diabetes and crippling osteoarthritis of her weightbearing joints will be denied the only effective treatment for her metabolic syndrome. Recently, in recognition of this concern, the Food and Drug Administration (FDA) lowered the BMI required for adjustable gastric bands to 30. It is a good start but still does not fully address the myriad of patients who may benefit from bariatric surgery but are denied based upon an imperfect and somewhat arbitrary measure of obesity.

Other Measures of Obesity

In the search for better indicators of adiposity, other measures of body composition have been proposed, tried, and abandoned.[5] Measures of skinfolds, such as the Durnin–Womersley and the Jackson–Pollock methods,[6] appeared attractive at first, but they proved to be dependent on the types of calipers used and variations in application techniques. The results often varied with the age, gender, and muscularity of the participants. More importantly, these measures provide estimates of body density rather than body fat percentage and, even more important, focused on subcutaneous fat and ignored the physiologically more relevant visceral fat deposits. Others, including the US military,[7] combined the BMI with height and circumference methods that measured abdominal, waist, hip, and neck circumferences, an approach that proved to be especially unfortunate during the First Gulf War.[8] Large, well-muscled men and women were not accepted for recruitment or "boarded out of service" even though these were often the most desirable individuals for battle. Sophisticated approaches involving ingenious technology are now also available, but again, these have not gained broad clinical acceptance.

Near-infrared interactance,[9] a technique in which a v-beam of infrared light is transmitted into the biceps, reflected from the underlying muscle, and absorbed by fat, offers a method that is safe, noninvasive, rapid, and easy to use. Dual-energy X-ray absorptiometry[10] estimates body fat percentage through the comparison of 2 types of X-ray scans in which one detects all tissues and the other does not detect fat. Other methodologies involve dilution with isotopically labeled water,[11] measures of body volume by water displacement[12] or air plethysmography,[13] and in vivo neutron activation.[14] Bioelectrical impedance analysis scales[15] offer an approach that is affordable and easy to use in a clinical setting although somewhat less accurate. The resistance reflects body composition with a high level of reliability in a normal-weight participant but loses accuracy with severe obesity.[16] Other, less direct indicators of the effects of obesity include tests for inflammation such as the "new high-sensitivity" C-reactive protein assays that discriminate

Table 1-1
World Health Organization Classification of Obesity

< 18.5	Underweight
18.5 to 24.9	Normal weight
25.0 to 29.9	Overweight
30.0 to 34.9	Class I obesity
35.0 to 39.9	Class II obesity
≥40.0	Class III obesity

Reprinted from *The international classification of adult underweight, overweight and obesity according to BMI*, World Health Organization. http://apps.who.int/bmi/index.jsp?introPage=intro_3.html. Accessed December 1, 2015.

the level of risk between individuals with low, moderate, and high risk of future heart attack and stroke. Evidence also indicates that individuals with high C-reactive protein levels are at increased risk of developing diabetes.[17] Fasting plasma glucose and insulin levels to calculate homeostasis model assessment of insulin resistance can also serve as excellent surrogate indexes of the insulin resistance so characteristic of severe obesity. "Excess weight" and "excess weight loss" have, intermittently, also been used as indicators of obesity and the efficacy of surgery. The problem, of course, is the lack of a universal "normal" or "ideal" weight baseline for the calculation. Of all of these measures, sagittal height[18] (ie, the height of the abdomen measured from the level of the examining table) is probably the most useful and reliable tool, easily recorded in even the most simply equipped offices. Curiously, even though the metric requires only a ruler, it is not used widely nor has it been explored adequately as a guideline for bariatric surgery. The tragedy of the unfortunate adoption of the BMI as the key indicator for bariatric surgery is that patients who could benefit greatly from the surgery, especially Blacks, are denied access. There is some hope; in 2012, the FDA approved the use of adjustable gastric bands for patients with a BMI ≥ 30. It is not enough, however, to disparage one metric without offering a better solution. Obviously, there are better methods for the measurement of adiposity, such as underwater weighing, but these are not feasible in clinical practice. So far, the best suggestion is to adopt the sagittal abdominal diameter, easy to measure on a recumbent patient, matched with the BMI, a combination that is an accurate enough indicator of adiposity and disease to predict incident diabetes.[19]

The Classification of Obesity

Table 1-1 summarizes the WHO classification of obesity, a widely adopted scale that deserves reexamination. Flegal et al,[20] based on a sample of more than 2.88 million individuals with more than 270,000 deaths, confirmed significantly increased all-cause mortality hazard ratios relative to normal weight (ie, as a BMI of 18.5 to 24.9). However, mortality was significantly lower among those who were overweight compared to normal-weight individuals. The findings were consistent even after adjusting for smoking and preexisting disease.[21] Given these findings, should the "normal weight" be changed to 25.0 to 29.9? Furthermore, there is a significant fraction of our population with BMIs over 40, rising to values of 80 to 90 quite frequently in the practices of bariatric surgeons. Accordingly, it might be wise to add at least a Class IV for the superobese who exceed BMI values of 50.

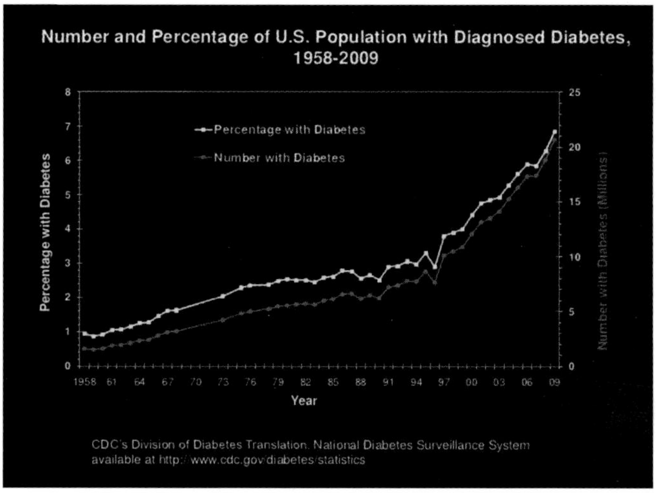

Figure 1-2. Data from the Centers for Disease Control and Prevention depicting the number and percentage of the US population with diagnosed diabetes from 1950 to 2009. (Reprinted with permission from the Centers for Disease Control and Prevention.)

The Real Problem Is Not Adiposity; It Is the Comorbidities

The level of adiposity is only part of the problem of obesity. There are a number of patients, especially Black women, who fall within the Class I to III levels of obesity who have glucose, lipid, and blood pressure levels all within normal limits. Much more serious are the comorbidities—the diseases associated with obesity, including type 2 diabetes mellitus, hypertension, hyperlipidemias, nonalcoholic hepatic steatosis, gastroesophageal reflux disease, polycystic ovary syndrome, degenerative arthritis of weightbearing joints, cardiopulmonary failure, urinary stress incontinence, pseudotumor cerebri, and increased prevalence of cancers of the breast, colon, pancreas, ovary, and prostate, among others. Figure 1-2 documents the number and percentage of the US population with diagnosed diabetes from 1958 through 2009. Note the sharp rise starting in 1996, more than doubling the prevalence of the disease in less than a decade. The reported costs of each of these diseases emphasize the public health and public policy implications of rises in obesity. In 2007, according to the CDC,[22] the total cost of treating type 2 diabetes in the United States was $174 billion, of which $116 billion were direct medical costs and another $58 billion were indirect (ie, due to disability, work loss, premature mortality, and other associated factors). According to the Novo Nordisk database,[23] in 2010, 32.3 million Americans were living with diabetes with a total medical and societal cost of $299.3 billion dollars. About 90% of these individuals were overweight or obese.

Socioeconomic Effects

Perhaps the most serious of the comorbidities of obesity are the socioeconomic effects. Overweight and obese, and especially the severely obese, often reflect poor psychological health with low self-esteem, impaired social interactions, distortions of body image, and high levels of anxiety and depression. The severity of these socioeconomic effects becomes much clearer in the clinics where we care for these patients with their stories of sexual and emotional abuse in childhood and adolescence, poor performance in school, struggling marriages, ridicule by peers in school, difficulty finding employment, bias in the workplace, difficulties in performing jobs they have, and high absenteeism rates due to failing health. The costs of these effects are difficult to measure.

Table 1-2

Some of the Potential Causes for the Obesity Epidemic

• Decreased activity	• Deprivation of sleep
• Easy access to food	• Endocrine disruptors
• Decreased cost of food	• Increased age at parenthood
• Less smoking	• Epigenetic effects, especially in pregnancy
• Medications, especially for emotional illness	• Greater fecundity in populations with obesity
• Microbiome changes	• Increase in home and work temperatures
• Food additives	• Fertilizers, herbicides, pesticides
• Marketing to children and adolescents	• High intake of sweetened drinks, especially with fructose
• Genetic disorders such as Prader-Willi syndrome	• Imbalance of hormones such as leptin, ghrelin

The Metabolic Syndrome

Obesity (BMI $\geq$ 30) is so often associated with other diseases that a metabolic syndrome has been defined by the International Diabetes Federation with raised triglycerides (> 150 mg/dL), reduced high-density lipoprotein cholesterol (< 40 mg/dL), hypertension with > 130 mm Hg systolic and > 85 mm Hg diastolic, and raised fasting plasma glucose > 100 mg/dL. This frequent association suggests there may be some common causes.

The Causes of Obesity

The obvious answer to what is the cause of obesity is that food intake exceeds energy expenditure, but this simplistic response fails to address the potential causes of that imbalance. For the most thorough and scholarly discussions of this subject, the reader is advised to review the contributions of David B. Allison, PhD, Professor of Nutrition Sciences and Biostatistics at the University of Alabama at Birmingham, whose work will be cited liberally in this next section. In addition, the reader should explore Dr. Allison's website at www.ssg.uab.edu/wiki/x/fInu, where he provides a comprehensive listing of the various citations in the literature regarding obesity.

Table 1-2 lists multiple causes that have been cited to explain the increase in obesity. There is little research that provides solid evidence for these potential myriad of causes of obesity except for the effects of medication. There is little question that high doses of prednisone will produce weight gain. The following section reviews the evidence for diet, exercise, and prevention obesity, as well as the epidemiology over the past decade.

Is the Increase in Obesity a Recent Phenomenon?

Although the beginning of this chapter documented the increase in obesity over the past decade, Helmchen and Henderson,[24] in a review of 12,312 randomly drawn Union Army Veterans examined between 1890 and 1900, compared these with 4059 National Health and Nutrition

Examination Survey participants examined between 1976 and 2000. They documented that the average annual growth rate of median BMI was lowest between 1900 and 1976 and has been rising to 0.5% per annum between 1988 and 2000. In short, their data suggest that the current epidemic started sooner than the past decade and may date back as far as 40 years. If this is true, then some of the currently cited causes may be less likely.

What Role Do Sugar-Sweetened Beverages Play in Childhood Obesity?

A commonly cited cause of obesity among children and adolescents is the regular consumption of sweetened, high-caloric beverages. Ebbeling et al[25] randomly assigned 103 adolescents, aged 13 to 16 years, who regularly consumed sugar-sweetened beverages to intervention and control groups in which all of the participants completed the study. Consumption of the sugar-sweetened beverages decreased by 82% in the intervention group. The net difference, 0.14 ± 0.21 kg/m^2, was not significant overall. In a more current study in 2012, Ebbeling et al[25] randomly assigned 224 overweight and obese adolescents who regularly consumed sugar-sweetened beverages to experimental (1.7 servings per day) and control groups (0 servings). With retention rates of 97% at 1 year and 93% at 2 years, they documented that the increase in BMI was significantly smaller in the experimental group than in the control group after 1 year but at the 2-year follow-up there was no longer any significant difference. In a less controlled setting, it will be interesting to see the effects of the measure to ban the sale of large sodas and other sugary drinks at restaurants, street carts, and movie theaters, championed by former Mayor Bloomberg in New York City. The ban seems to be a reasonable attempt to affect childhood obesity but, so far, the evidence supporting such an effort is not strong.

Does "Snacking" Play a Role?

Snacking is also frequently indicated as a cause of obesity. Field et al,[26] however, in a prospective observational study of 8203 girls and 6774 boys, 9 to 14 years in age, concluded that "although snack foods may have low nutritional value, they were not an important independent determinant of weight gain among children and adolescents."

Bertéus Forslund et al[27] pursued the question further with a prospective study involving 140 patients (36 men and 104 women), aged 18 to 60 years and BMI > 30. The patients were randomized to 2 groups: (1) 3 meals a day and 3 snacks per day or (2) just 3 meals per day for a year. They concluded that "recommending snacks or not between meals does not influence 1-year weight loss." Snacking and the ready availability of food may indeed play a role, but there is no sound evidence to support that hypothesis.

What if We Increase Physical Activity in the Schools?

The decrease in physical education (PE) programs in schools is also often cited as a cause of the recent increase in obesity. Cawley et al[28] studied this question with the nationwide data from the Youth Risk Behavior Surveillance System for 1999, 2001, and 2003 merged with data on state minimum PE requirements from the 2001 Shape of the Nation Report. They found that high school students with a binding PE requirement reported an average of 31 additional minutes per week spent physically active in PE class. Their results also indicated that additional PE time raises the number of days per week that girls report having exercised vigorously or having engaged in strength-building activity. However, they found no evidence that PE lowers BMI or the probability that a student is overweight. They concluded that raising PE credit requirements may make girls more physically active overall, but there is not yet the scientific base to declare raising PE requirements as an anti-obesity initiative for either boys or girls.

Does Increasing Fruits and Vegetables in the Diet Promote Weight Loss?

The common recommendation that an increase in fruits and vegetables would improve weight loss was tested by Whybrow et al[29] in 34 males and 28 females who were provided with 0, 300, or 600 g of fruits and vegetables over 8 weeks using a randomized parallel design. They concluded that "consumption of mandatory food and vegetable supplements for 8 weeks produced beneficial changes in diet composition but did not result in lower reported energy or fat intakes and did not result in loss of body weight."

What if We Make the Public Aware of the Caloric Content of Foods?

Aaron et al[30] explored the effects of providing nutritional information to consumers in 1995 and found that the experimental group actually increased its purchased kilocalories from 870 to 910 with a $p < .05$. Although there are a number of national and international initiatives for informing the purchasing public of the nutritional and caloric content of foods, a recent review by Storksdieck Genannt Bonsmann et al[31] of the efforts in the European Union concluded that "no real-life evidence exists linking nutrition label use with measured changes in body weight."

RESPONDING TO THE EPIDEMIC

The best approaches to the obesity epidemic are prevention and appropriate treatment. While the epidemic has raged on for decades, we still lack enough knowledge to fully understand the pathophysiology that underlies the development of obesity, nor do we comprehend the metabolic changes that follow the best treatment—bariatric surgery.

Prevention

So far, none of the preventive approaches have proven to be effective for general use. In December 2012, Look AHEAD (Action in Health and Diabetes), the most intensive long-term National Institutes of Health trial of lifestyle interventions for the prevention and treatment of obesity and type 2 diabetes, was stopped due to suboptimal results. The trial enrolled 4503 adults over the span of 4 years and was halted with the following conclusion: "In these exploratory analyses of overweight adults, an intensive lifestyle intervention was associated with a greater likelihood of partial remission of type 2 diabetes compared with diabetes support and education. However, the absolute remission rates were modest."[32] The accompanying editorial in the *Journal of the American Medical Association* was even more straightforward: "Other recent trials found similar, disappointing results for intensive medical management of type 2 diabetes."[33] The Action to Control Cardiovascular Disease in Diabetes (ACCORD), Action in Diabetes and Vascular Disease (ADVANCE), and Veterans Affairs Diabetes Trial (VADT) showed unexpectedly small effects on cardiovascular event rates and mortality in people with type 2 diabetes. In fact, the ACCORD trial reported 19% more deaths in the intensive glucose-management group than in the standard glucose-management group during the 5-year study period. All of these trials failed to reduce end-stage microvascular complications during their study periods, although they reported some mixed benefits on multiple measures of early microvascular disease. Perhaps future analyses of Look AHEAD, ACCORD, ADVANCE, and the VADT will identify subgroups of patients with type 2 diabetes that may warrant intensive lifestyle or medical intervention to reduce cardiovascular risk. However, a more potent intervention—bariatric surgery—already appears to achieve what intensive medical and lifestyle interventions cannot—reducing cardiovascular events and mortality rates among severely obese patients with type 2 diabetes.[32]

Treatment

Although the evidence is limited, treatment of the overweight and Class I obese patients can be successful. Wadden at al,[34] in an excellent review of the current approaches to obesity, concluded that "a comprehensive program of lifestyle modification produces a 7% to 10% reduction in initial weight that is associated with clinically meaningful improvements in several cardiovascular disease risk factors, including the prevention of type 2 diabetes." They also expressed hope that the new technological resources including Facebook, Twitter, smartphones, and other approaches to rapid and easy communication could provide better results.

For patients with Class II and higher levels of obesity, Arterburn and O'Connor summarize it well: "Evidence is increasing that bariatric surgery is more effective than medical or lifestyle interventions for weight loss and diabetes remission."[33] In a recent analysis of severely obese patients with diabetes, the adjusted probability of initial remission was 12- to 24-fold greater for the 1395 patients who had bariatric surgery than for the 62,322 who received usual medical care alone. In a recently reported 6-year prospective study,[35] remission of type 2 diabetes was significantly more common among patients who underwent Roux-en-Y gastric bypass (62%) than among severely obese patients with diabetes who initially sought but did not undergo bariatric surgery (6%) and those who never sought bariatric surgery (8%). In another long-term analysis,[36] remission of type 2 diabetes occurred in 68% of 4434 patients who had Roux-en-Y gastric bypass surgery, with a median duration of remission of 8 years.

Research

Even though obesity and its comorbidities are the most common and most serious diseases confronting the United States and the world, support for research in this area remains limited. The causes of the obesity epidemic are multifactorial, but many areas still have a dearth of research, especially in the effects of the microbiome; the effects of food additives, herbicides, pesticides, and fertilizers; and in the epigenetics and investigation of the underlying mechanisms for satiety and metabolic syndrome.

Summary

The epidemic of obesity and its comorbidities has become the most serious health problem of the world, more serious and more costly than yellow fever, malaria, tuberculosis, and cancer, the pressing health care challenges of the past. The combinations of diet, exercise, behavioral modification, and drugs, though effective in a few, have had little long-term success. Bariatric surgery, although remarkably effective and safe, is not a widely useful advance. We cannot operate on the whole world. Hopefully research can provide more solid answers, especially in prevention, through a far better understanding of the effects of our "progress" in the development of food additives; new genetic forms of seeds, herbicides, pesticides, and fertilizers; and pollution of our air and water in our environment. Let's hope these answers come soon.

References

1. Flegal KM, Carroll MD, Kit BK, Ogden CL. Prevalence of obesity and trends in the distribution of body mass index among US adults, 1999-2010. *JAMA*. 2012;307(5):491-497.
2. Bright-See E. Doctor, how can I lose weight? *Can Fam Physician*. 1983;29:2164-2168.
3. Jackson AS, Stanforth PR, Gagnon J. The effect of sex, age, and race on estimating percent body fat from BMI: the HERITAGE Family Study. *Int J Obes*. 2002;26:789-796.

4. Katz EG, Stevens J, Truesdale KP, Cai J, North KE, Steffen LM. Associations of body mass index with incident hypertension in American white, American black and Chinese Asian adults in early and middle adulthood: the Coronary Artery Risk Development in Young Adults (CARDIA) study, the Atherosclerosis Risk in Communities (ARIC) study and the People's Republic of China (PRC) study. *Asia Pac J Clin Nutr.* 2013;22(4):626-634.
5. Pories WJ, Dohm GL, Mansfield CJ. Beyond the BMI: the search for better guidelines for bariatric surgery. *Obesity.* 2010;18:5:865-871.
6. Uccioli L, Fleury M, De Gregorio M et al. Can the body mass index and the waist:hips ratio (WHR) affect the correlation between impedance measurement and anthropometry in the evaluation of body composition? *Minerva Endocrinol.* 1990;15(4):251-255.
7. Pischon T, Boeing H, Hoffmann K, et al. General and abdominal adiposity and risk of death in Europe. *N Engl J Med.* 2008;359:2105-2120.
8. Pories WJ. Unpublished data. 1990.
9. Moon JR, Tobkin SE, Smith AE, et al. Percent body fat estimations in college men using field and laboratory methods: a three-compartment model approach. *Dyn Med.* 2008;7:7.
10. Andreoli A, Scalzo G, Masala S, Tarantino U, Guglielmi G. Body composition assessment by dual-energy X-ray absorptiometry (DXA). *Radiol Med.* 2009;114:286-300.
11. McCarthy EA, Strauss BJ, Walker SP, Permezel M. Determination of maternal body composition in pregnancy and its relevance to perinatal outcomes. *Obstet Gynecol Surv.* 2004;59:731-742.
12. Moon JR, Eckerson JM, Tobkin SE, et al. Estimating body fat in NCAA Division I female athletes: a five-compartment model validation of laboratory ethods. *Eur J Appl Physiol.* 2009;105:119-130.
13. Lee SY, Gallagher D. Assessment methods in human body composition. *Curr Opin Clin Nutr Metab Care.* 2008;11(5):566-572.
14. Haas VK, Allen JR, Kohn MR, et al. Total body protein in healthy adolescent girls: validation of estimates derived from simpler measures with neutron activation analysis. *Am J Clin Nutr.* 2007;85:66-72.
15. Neovius M, Hemmingsson E, Freyschuss B, Uddén J. Bioelectrical impedance underestimates total and truncal fatness in abdominally obese women. *Obesity (Silver Spring).* 2006;14:1731-1738.
16. Gray DS, Bray GA, Gemayel N, Kaplan K. Effect of obesity on bioelectrical impedance. *Am J Clin Nutr.* 1989;50(2):255-260.
17. Ridker PM. Cardiology patient page. C-reactive protein: a simple test to help predict risk of heart attack and stroke. *Circulation.* 2003;108:e81-e85.
18. Vasques AC, Rosado LE, Rosado GP, et al. Different measurements of the sagittal abdominal diameter and waist perimeter in the prediction of HOMA-IR. *Arq Bras Cardiol.* 2009;93(5):511-518.
19. Pajunen P, Rissanen H, Laaksonen MA, Heliövaara M, Reunanen A, Knekt P. Sagittal abdominal diameter as a new predictor for incident diabetes. *Diabetes Care.* 2013;36(2):283-288.
20. Flegal KM, Kit BK, Orpana H, Graubard BI. Association of all-cause mortality with overweight and obesity using standard body mass index categories: a systematic review and meta-analysis. *JAMA.* 2013;309(1):71-82.
21. Heymsfield SB, Cefalu WT. Does body mass index adequately convey a patient's mortality risk? *JAMA.* 2013;309(1):87-88.
22. US Department of Health and Human Services. *Preventing chronic diseases: investing wisely in health: preventing diabetes and its complications.* http://www.cdc.gov/nccdphp/publications/factsheets/Prevention/pdf/diabetes.pdf
23. Novo Nordisk. *Ten states bear brunt of diabetes burden.* http://www.prnewswire.com/news-releases/ten-states-bear-brunt-of-diabetes-burden-118160629.html
24. Helmchen LA, Henderson RM. Changes in the distribution of body mass index of white US men, 1890-2000. *Ann Hum Biol.* 2004;31(2):174-181.
25. Ebbeling CB, Feldman HA, Chomitz VR, et al. A randomized trial of sugar-sweetened beverages and adolescent body weight. *N Engl J Med.* 2012;367(15):1407-1416.
26. Field AE, Austin SB, Gillman MW, Rosner B, Rockett HR, Colditz GA. Snack food intake does not predict weight change among children and adolescents. *Int J Obes Relat Metab Disord.* 2004;28(10):1210-1216.
27. Bertéus Forslund H, Klingström S, Hagberg H, Löndahl M, Torgerson JS, Lindroos AK. Should snacks be recommended in obesity treatment? A 1-year randomized clinical trial. *Eur J Clin Nutr.* 2008;62(11):1308-1317.
28. Cawley J, Meyerhoefer C, Newhouse D. The impact of state physical education requirements on youth physical activity and overweight. *Health Econ.* 2007;16(12):1287-1301.
29. Whybrow S, Harrison CL, Mayer C, James Stubbs R. Effects of added fruits and vegetables on dietary intakes and body weight in Scottish adults. *Br J Nutr.* 2006;95(3):496-503.
30. Aaron JI, Evans RE, Mela DJ. Paradoxical effect of a nutrition labeling scheme in a student cafeteria. *Nutrition Research.* 1995;15(9):1251-1261.
31. Storcksdieck Genannt Bonsmann S, Wills JM. Nutrition labeling to prevent obesity: reviewing the evidence from Europe. *Curr Obes Rep.* 2012;1(3):134-140.
32. Gregg EW, Chen H, Wagenknecht LE, et al for the Look AHEAD Research Group. Association of an intensive lifestyle intervention with remission of type 2 diabetes. *JAMA.* 2012;308(23):2489-2496.

33. Arterburn DE, O'Connor PJ. A look ahead at the future of diabetes prevention and treatment. *JAMA*. 2012;308(23):2517-2518.
34. Wadden TA, Webb VL, Moran CH, Bailer BA. Lifestyle modification for obesity: new developments in diet, physical activity, and behavior therapy. *Circulation*. 2012;125(9):1157-1170.
35. Arterburn D, Bogart A, Coleman KJ, et al. Comparative effectiveness of bariatric surgery vs. nonsurgical treatment of type 2 diabetes among severely obese adults. *Obes Res Clin Pract*. 2013;7(4):e258-e268.
36. Arterburn DE, Bogart A, Sherwood NE, et al. A multisite study of long-term remission and relapse of type 2 diabetes mellitus following gastric bypass. *Obes Surg*. 2013;23:93-102.

2

Adolescent Obesity and Weight Loss Surgery

Wendy Jo Svetanoff, MD;
R. Armour Forse, MD, CM, PhD, FRCS(C), FACS, FCCM, FASMBS; and
Caroline M. Apovian, MD

Obesity in the United States has taken a rapid rise over the past 3 decades and is now becoming a major epidemic; extreme obesity (body mass index [BMI] > 40 kg/m^2) has quadrupled to 2% of the adult population from 1986 to 2000.[1] With this rise, there are more people who have developed comorbidities, who are hospitalized, and who eventually expire from diseases related to obesity. One-seventh of the cancer deaths in men and one-fifth of the deaths in women were related to obesity,[2] and obesity has become the second leading cause of death in the United States.[3]

Unfortunately, this trend has also taken effect in the pediatric and adolescent populations. More adolescents are obese now than ever before. In the past 30 years, obesity in the adolescent population has tripled to 15.5% of all adolescents.[1,4-6] More than 50% of adolescents meet the criteria for metabolic syndrome, which include being diagnosed with hypertension, increased fasting glucose, hyperlipidemia, and excess body weight.[7] As the obesity rates continue to climb, we will soon see that the current generation will have a lower life expectancy than the previous ones.[6] With the recent push to reverse this trend, more research is being poured into weight loss surgery. Long term effects of obesity studies have shown that not only can adolescents develop the same comorbidities as adults who are overweight (such as type 2 diabetes),[4] but adolescents who are overweight are more likely than their counterparts to have obesity as adults (55% to 77% will become obese adults).[4,6,8] Research has even shown that high waist circumference and triglycerides in childhood (9 to 10 years old) can predict that these patients will develop metabolic syndrome by young adulthood (18 to 19 years old).[9] Children who were obese in childhood were also found to have shorter life spans than their counterparts in adulthood, starting at age 45.[5,8]

In 1988, a long-term (55-year) follow-up of patients enrolled in the Harvard Growth Study was performed. Children were categorized as "overweight" if their BMI > 75th percentile on 2 consecutive measurements between the ages of 13 to 18, while "lean" patients were those whose BMI was in the 25th to 50th percentile during the same time period. Phone or personal interviews were performed, looking at medical, reproductive, and exercise histories. Two big trends were seen. The first was that 52% of those who had been overweight as children were still overweight 55 years later.[8] Likewise, children who were overweight were more likely as adults to have a higher morbidity due to coronary heart disease, atherosclerosis, colorectal cancer, and gout in men. Women who

Forse RA, Apovian CM, eds.
Bariatric Surgery: What Every Provider Needs to Know (pp 15-21).

were overweight as children were more likely to have coronary heart disease, arthritis, and overall lower functional status.[8] To prevent this trend from continuing to rise, the aim of current research is to look at the effects of early intervention, mainly weight loss surgery, to curb adolescent obesity before long-standing complications and comorbidities arise.

Indications

In adolescents and pediatrics, weight is measured in percentile. Just over 16% of adolescents fall into the category of being overweight (>95th percentile).[4] A BMI>99th percentile in older adolescents has been shown to be equivalent for a BMI between 35 and 40 in adults,[1] a BMI of which weight loss surgery is to be considered. The most recent Best Practice Guidelines stated that "children with BMI>99th percentile become obese adults (BMI>30) with more health complications and a higher mortality rate than those who become obese in adulthood."[9] The Bogalusa Heart Study confirmed this, finding that 39% of children with a BMI>95th percentile had 2 risk factors for heart disease, while 59% of those with a BMI>99th percentile had them.[1] Due to these statistics and associated comorbidities, a BMI>99th percentile has been recommended as an appropriate BMI to consider weight loss surgery in adolescents.

Severe comorbidities can also have a patient qualify for weight loss surgery. The Best Practice Guidelines had recommended patients with a BMI>40 with one serious comorbidity (type 2 diabetes, obstructive sleep apnea, severe hypertension, and pseudotumor cerebri), BMI>50, failure of nonsurgical treatment, or adolescents with BMI>35 and life-threatening comorbidities.[4,10] However, a more recent statement by the American Society for Metabolic and Bariatric Surgery increased the eligibility criteria to include those with a BMI of 30 to 35 and type 2 diabetes.[6] Otherwise, surgery should only be an option for those patients who meet the more recent National Institutes of Health guidelines: BMI>40 or BMI>35 with comorbidities.[10]

Type 2 diabetes mellitus, severe hypertension, and pseudotumor cerebri are all indications for weight loss surgery.[4] Type 2 diabetes, especially, is an indication for weight loss surgery, as diabetes mellitus can progress more rapidly in adolescents, with 30% to 40% developing microalbuminemia within 5 years of diagnosis.[9] The presence of diabetes in childhood leads to early atherosclerosis and heart disease early in adulthood. Childhood obesity is associated with left ventricular hypertrophy in young adults (20 to 38 years).[9] Studies in adolescent obesity have also shown a parallel increase between obesity and cardiovascular disease, type 2 diabetes, sleep apnea, polycystic ovary syndrome, nonalcoholic steatohepatitis, and gynecological cancer.[11-13]

Oberbach and colleagues also looked at levels of serum uric acid in adolescents and its effect on comorbidities. By regulating the production of macrophage chemoattractant protein 1 (a protein that is involved in insulin resistance and fatty acid catabolism) and decreasing nitric oxide production, an abundance of serum uric acid has led to increasing insulin resistance, arterial hypertension, and cardiovascular disease.[14] They compared the metabolic characteristics of a small group of adolescent patients who underwent laparoscopic sleeve gastrectomy (LSG) or Roux-en-Y gastric bypass (RYGB) to normal cohorts. Preoperatively, fasting insulin levels, insulin resistance, triglycerides, and gamma-glutamyl transpeptidase were all elevated in the overweight patients compared to the control group. In both the LSG and RYGB groups, fasting insulin levels were significantly lower than their normal-weight counterparts; insulin resistance, triglycerides, and liver enzymes had also decreased to a normal level.[14] Similarly, patients with patients had significantly higher levels of serum uric acid preoperatively, which decreased after surgery. This was linked to a reduction in BMI and diastolic blood pressure, adding evidence to the theory that high levels of serum uric acid can lead to future cardiovascular disease. By implementing weight loss surgery in these morbidly obese adolescents, the metabolic abnormalities can be regulated, leading to a reduction in cardiovascular disease and other comorbidities.

Before weight loss surgery can be considered in children and adolescents, the Best Practice Guidelines committee recommends that patients have already completed skeletal and psychological maturity to minimize the risk of potential nutritional deficiencies on final maturation.[4] For most, skeletal maturity occurs around 13 years of age in women and 15 years of age in men; those who have not reached skeletal maturity (as determined by bone age on radiographs) or physical maturity (Tanner stage IV) should not be considered for weight loss surgery.[4] Psychological assessment is also needed to ensure that the patients and their families understand the lifestyle changes and rigorous follow-up that will be required after the surgery. Patients in this age group are more likely to have depression and engage in harmful or suicidal behaviors as a result of the effects of peer pressure and poor body image.[15] These issues should be addressed (especially drug abuse or suicidal tendencies) before the patient is cleared for surgery. Having a multidisciplinary team that includes a surgeon, pediatrician, dietician, and psychologist are crucial to the successful outcome in these patients.

Pregnancy is another controversial topic in the area of adolescent weight loss surgery. Mothers who are obese are more likely to have gestational diabetes, preeclampsia, cesarean sections, and anesthesia-related complications.[3] Werler et al also found that mothers who are obese were more likely to have babies born with neural tube defects.[16] The reason hypothesized was that the daily recommended intake of folate was not sufficient once a mother reached a body weight of 70 kg; they also found that the risk of neural tube defects increase with increasing maternal weight, regardless of folic acid intake.[16] Because of these risks for both the mother and the baby, attention has now been placed on performing weight loss surgery before becoming pregnant.

This proposition comes with its own set of complications, however. Mothers who become pregnant within the first 2 years of weight loss surgeries have a higher risk of having nutritional deficiencies during pregnancy due to the rapid weight loss that happens during this time period. A Danish study, looking specifically at both obstetric and neonatal outcomes in women who have undergone weight loss surgery, showed that infants born to mothers who previously had weight loss surgery had significantly lower birth weights that their normal-weighted counterparts.[17] These neonates are also more likely to be admitted to the neonatal intensive care unit at some point during the first month of life. Both of these statistics add to the concern about fetal malnourishment with mothers who have undergone weight loss surgery.[17] Two years has been deemed the cut-off point as this is when weight loss is the most and when the potential for nutrient deficiencies is the highest.

One study looking at prenatal and fetal complications when becoming pregnant soon after weight loss surgery found that those who became pregnant earlier (<2 years) had more miscarriages than those who waited. There was no difference in preeclampsia or preterm labor and no congenital defects were noted in either set of babies.[3] Other studies have shown that despite the rapid weight loss, as long as the patients are closely monitored for vitamin deficiencies, there were not any more problems for the mother or the baby if the mother became pregnant within the first 18 months after weight loss surgery. One study done by Berlac et al compared outcomes in pregnant females who had previously undergone RYGB (but were still overweight) to those who were overweight but did not have weight loss surgery and expectant mothers who were of normal weight.[17] Mothers who had already undergone RYGB were significantly less likely to have preeclampsia, emergency cesarean sections, or infant asphyxia than their overweight counterparts. However, they were still more likely to have hypertension and gestational diabetes than their normal-weight counterparts. Of concern was the result that mothers with previous RYGB were significantly more likely to come to the hospital with acute abdominal pain and ileus (most of which required exploration) compared to either the overweight or normal-weighted controls.[17] The Best Practice Guidelines recommend that patients who are pregnant, breast-feeding, or plan on becoming pregnant in the next 2 years should be excluded from weight loss surgery due to the concern of birth defects, low birth rate, and increased admissions to the neonatal intensive care unit from potential nutrient deficiencies.[4,10,17]

Weight Loss Surgeries

Many different weight loss surgeries have been implemented in the adult population, including adjustable gastric band (AGB), RYGB, LSG, vertical banded gastroplasty, biliopancreatic diversion with duodenal switch, and ileal-jejunal bypass. Vertical banded gastroplasty has gone out of favor as an adequate weight loss procedure; both biliopancreatic diversion with duodenal switch and ileal-jejunal bypass lead to extreme malabsorption that can be detrimental to the physical maturation of patients who undergo the procedure before full maturity.[4] These extreme malabsorptive procedures can likewise lead to nutritional complications during pregnancy.[9] Therefore, the 3 weight loss surgeries most often studied (and recommended by the national guidelines) include AGB, RYGB, and LSG.

For adolescents, weight loss surgeries were first implemented in the 1980s.[9] However, there has been a relative hesitancy to include weight loss surgery as part of the repertoire for weight loss management in adolescents. In the mid-2000s, only 1% of bariatric surgeries were performed on adolescents.[18] The RYGB has shown, among adults, to be the most effective weight loss procedure and has become the standard of care for future surgeries and research studies to be compared to.[5] In this procedure, a limb of jejunum is divided 30 to 50 cm to the ligament of Treitz. The fundus of the stomach will remain attached to the duodenum, allowing for drainage of bile from the biliary system.[19] This "biliary limb" is reanastomosed to the jejunum 75 to 150 cm distal to the gastrojejunal anastomosis. The length of the jejunum that is being bypassed can be altered depending on how much weight loss the patient is trying to achieve—less jejunum will be bypassed in patients with a smaller BMI or those receiving a RYGB for severe reflux.[18] Similarly, those who are severely morbidly obese (BMI > 55) will have up to 150 cm of jejunum bypassed. The Roux limb is then brought up to the level of the stomach in an antegastric and antecolic position.[18,19] The stomach is stapled upward toward the angle of His to make a 15- to 20-cc pouch and the Roux limb is anastomosed to the posterior side of the gastric pouch to complete the RYGB.

This procedure results in both a restrictive (small gastric pouch) and malabsorptive (bypass) procedure contributing to weight loss.[4,19] There is also an added component of hormonal changes that contributes to the RYGB becoming the most successful surgery for weight loss: reduced hunger and augmented satiety from decreased levels of ghrelin and increased energy expenditure.[20] It is also the best procedure for adolescents who also experience gastroesophageal reflux symptoms[11] as Roux-en-Y procedures have also become an option for patients with severe reflux disease and failed fundoplications. The biggest concerns of this procedure are the potential complications, which include anastomotic leak, biliary limb obstruction, and internal hernia. The rate of complications in adolescents, though, is similar to what is seen in adults. When comparing adolescents who underwent RYGB with adults of similar demographics, the weight loss was similar, with 95% losing > 50% excess weight and an average of 75% excess weight loss by the end of the second year postoperatively.[18,20] It has also been shown that adolescents undergoing RYGB have the same resolution of comorbidities as their adult counterparts, including decreasing the incidence of diabetes and hypertension, decreasing the proinflammatory state, and improving renal function without any increase in complications.[6,18,20] The initial practice guidelines for pediatric weight loss surgery recommended RYGB as the procedure with the best long-term outcome. It is the most studied among adolescents and has been deemed to be safe for adolescents with appropriate long-term follow-up.

AGB first became approved in 2001 with the first research publication coming in 2003.[21] With AGB, a band is placed around the upper part of the stomach with a port in the subcutaneous tissue, resulting in a small gastric pouch and the patient feeling full after only small quantities of food.[21] The band can then be adjusted depending on how much the patient can eat by adding water to the port. This has been an attractive option for adolescents as this is not a permanent procedure and the band can be removed if complications arise. Unfortunately, AGB, although resulting in more weight loss than behavorial changes, does not have the large weight loss or reduction of comorbidities that is seen with either the LSG or RYGB.[6,21] It is also associated with an 8% to 10% reoperation rate due to band slippage, gastric prolapse, and port displacement.[9,21]

LSG is the newest surgery to be performed in adolescent patients and is the fastest-growing bariatric procedure worldwide.[6] It involves resecting the greater curvature of the stomach, making the stomach into the shape of a tube.[2] The gastrocolic ligament is dissected and then the short gastric vessels are taken down approximately 6 cm from the pylorus until the angle of His is reached.[15] A bougie is then inserted to act as a guide for the gastrectomy. The gastric remnant with a sleeve gastrectomy is between 100 to 150 cc, compared to the 20 cc of a Roux-en-Y gastric pouch.[22] The postoperative diet is very similar to patients undergoing RYGB, where a liquid diet with protein supplementation is maintained for the first few weeks, followed by gradual introduction of more complex foods. The advantages of an LSG include the lack of bowel anastomosis and maintenance of the pylorus, while bringing restrictive and hormonal changes to weight loss.[7] Those who undergo sleeve gastrectomy have been found to release less ghrelin, a hormone known for stimulating appetite. Therefore, not only does the smaller stomach restrict the amount of food a patient can consume at one time, the decreased ghrelin suppresses the hunger drive, making these patients want to eat less.[2] The biggest concerns with this procedure compared to RYGB are leaks from the stomach line (which may require stent placement)[15] and increased reflux following the procedure.[15,22] Patients with any history of gastroesophageal reflux disease should be directed toward the RYGB as up to 21% of patients were noted to have reflux symptoms after LSG.[15] There is also a concern about lack of follow-up among the adolescent population due to travel for school, work, etc; the LSG provides an appealing option for these patients, as adequate weight loss has been shown without the long-term concerns (internal hernias, anastomotic strictures) that come with bowel anastomosis and intestinal rearrangement.[15] This surgery was not approved under the most recent Best Practice Guidelines due to lack of long-term research outcomes[9]; however, recent studies show that LSG may be a good option for patients (33% to 90% of excess weight loss at 2 years, with 45% to 95% complete resolution of comorbidities)[2,7] without the risk of malnutrition that is associated with RYGB. A database query of the Kids' Inpatient Database done by Zwintscher et al confirmed previous studies, showing that children were able to lose up to 90% of excess weight at 2 years after LSG and had a lower risk of nutritional deficiencies.[6] This has been corroborated in studies done around the world, including France and Kuwait.[15,22]

Long-Term Outcomes

All weight loss surgeries have been shown to be more effective than behavorial interventions at producing weight loss, even AGB[6,9]; it is also the only intervention that has resulted in sustained weight loss for adolescents.[1] As a result, the number of adolescent weight loss procedures being performed has tripled in the past 10 years and increased 5-fold since 1997.[6,8] The highest percentage (34%) of surgeries are being done in the South as 10 out of 12 states with adolescent obesity rates greater than 15% were in the South.[6] The American Society of Metabolic and Bariatric Surgery emphasized the need for earlier surgical intervention in order to prevent and/or reverse the comorbities associated with extreme obesity.[11] Studies have also shown that diabetes (if caught early), obstructive sleep apnea, nonalcoholic steatohepatitis, and increased inflammatory markers can be reversed with weight loss surgery.[9,20] In a study done by Cozacov et al, who compared LSG with RYGB at 55 months postoperative, the highest satisfaction scores after the surgery were in social relationships, self-esteem, and sexual activity, indicating the importance the image of being overweight has on an adolescent patient's psyche and feeling of self-worth.[11]

Due to the increasing trend of adolescent weight loss surgery, the Teen-Longitudinal Assessment of Bariatric Surgery study (Teen-LABS) was initiated to review not only preoperative characteristics but safety outcomes in those undergoing weight loss surgery.[8] The original study, published in January 2014, enrolled 242 patients with a mean age of 17, who underwent weight loss surgery at 1 of 5 academic institutions. Mean BMI was 50, with 76% of participants being female. Dyslipidemia, sleep apnea, and hypertension were the most common comorbidities found in these individuals, with close to 40% of participants having 4 or more comorbidities at the time of enrollment.[8] There was an 8% development of major complications (leak, bleeding, pulmonary embolism, etc) and 15% development of minor complications (urinary tract infections, dehydration, wound infection, etc). There were no deaths; however, this initial study only looked at the 30-day safety profile. Although the complications rates are similar to statistics for adult weight loss surgery, more long-term analysis will be needed to fully assess the safety of these procedures. Many studies have recommended having a multidisciplinary team in place in order to promote successful outcomes.[1,4,9] This team should include a surgeon, pediatrician, dietician, psychologist, along with pediatric subspecialists.[1] In the Teen-LABS study, all centers included a core team of a psychologist, registered dietician, physical activity specialist, and bariatric administrative program coordinator along with the surgeons and pediatricians.[13] This strong support system, as well as frequent evaluations in the postoperative period, will help keep these adolescents on track in terms of lifestyle choices, vitamin supplementation, and overall health.[13] Overall, with the presence of a good team of doctors, therapists, and nutritionists, weight loss procedures such as RYGB and LSG are viable options for adolescents who need to lose weight.[4]

Summary

Obesity is on the rise, not only in adults, but also in the pediatric population. Adolescents with obesity face many of the same health concerns as adults, including hypertension, diabetes mellitus, and polycystic ovary syndrome, but also can succumb to depression and poor images of self-worth. Obesity in the childhood and adolescent population frequently continues into adulthood, leading to a higher incidence of coronary artery disease, colorectal cancer, gynecological cancer, and a shorter life expectancy for the current generation. By pursuing weight loss surgery for adolescents with obesity, these health risks can be curbed or even reversed. RYGB has been the most studied procedure for adolescent weight loss and is the current standard of care. LSG, however, is on the rise due to similar weight loss results without the nutritional deficiencies or need for intestinal rearrangement. Long-term results are still lacking, but with a support group of surgeons, pediatricians, psychologists, and dieticians, weight loss surgery is an appropriate option for adolescents with obesity.

References

1. Xanthankos S, Inge T. Extreme pediatric obesity: weighing the health dangers. *J Pediatrics*. 2007;150:3-5.
2. Shi X, Karmali S, Sharma AM, Birch DW. A review of laparoscopic sleeve gastrectomy for morbid obesity. *Obes Surg*. 2010;20:1171-1177.
3. Dao T, Kuhn J, Ehmer D, Fisher T, McCarty T. Pregnancy outcomes after gastric-bypass surgery. *Am J Surg*. 2006;192:762-766.
4. Apovian CM, Baker C, Ludwig DS, et al. Best practice guidelines in pediatric/adolescent weight loss surgery. *Obes Res*. 2005;13:274-282.
5. Inge T. Bariatric surgery for morbidly obese adolescents: is there a rationale for early intervention? *Growth Horm IGF Res*. 2006;16(Suppl A): S15-S19.
6. Zwintscher NP, Azarow KS, Horton JD, Newton CR, Martin MJ. The increasing incidence of adolescent bariatric surgery. *J Pediatr Surg*. 2013;48(12):2401-2407.
7. Raziel A, Sakran N, Szold A, et al. Mid-term follow-up after laparoscopic sleeve gastrectomy in obese adolescents. *Isr Med Assoc J*. 2014;16:37-41.
8. Must A, Jacques PF, Dallal GE, Bajema CJ, Dietz WH. Long-term morbidity and mortality of overweight adolescents: a follow-up of the Harvard Growth Study of 1922 to 1935. *N Engl J Med*. 1992;327:1350-1355.

9. Pratt JS. Best practice updates for pediatric/adolescent weight loss surgery. *Obesity.* 2009;17:901-910.
10. Wasserman H, Inge T. Bariatric surgery in obese adolescents: opportunities and challenges. *Pediatr Ann.* 2014;43:230-236.
11. Cozacov Y, Roy M, Moon S, et al. Mid-term results of laparoscopic sleeve gastrectomy and Roux-en-Y gastric bypass in adolescent patients. *Obes Surg.* 2014;24:727-752.
12. Inge TH, Zeller MH, Jenkins TM, et al. Perioperative outcomes of adolescents undergoing bariatric surgery: the Teen-Longitudinal Assessment of Bariatric Surgery (Teen-LABS) study. *JAMA Pediatr.* 2014;168:47-53.
13. Michalsky MP, Inge TH, Teich S, et al. Adolescent bariatric surgery program characteristics: the Teen Longitudinal Assessment of Bariatric Surgery (Teen-LABS) study experience. *Semin Pediatr Surg.* 2014;23:5-10.
14. Oberbach A, Neuhaus J, Inge T, et al. Bariatric surgery in severely obese adolescents improves major comorbidities including hyperuricemia. *Metabolism.* 2014;63:242-249.
15. Nocca D, Nedelcu M, Nedelcu A, et al. Laparoscopic sleeve gastrectomy for late adolescent population. *Obes Surg.* 2014;24:861-865.
16. Werler MM, Louik C, Shapiro S, Mitchell AA. Prepregnant weight in relation to risk of neural tube defects. *JAMA.* 1996;275:1089-1092.
17. Berlac JF, Skovlund CW, Lidegaard O. Obstetrical and neonatal outcomes in women following gastric bypass: a Danish national cohort study. *Acta Obstet Gynecol Scand.* 2014;93:447-453.
18. DuCoin C, Moon RC, Mulatre M, Teixeira AF, Jawad MA. Safety and effectiveness of Roux-en-Y gastric bypass in patients between the ages of 17-19. *Obes Surg.* 2015;25:464-469.
19. Fischer JE. Laparoscopic gastric bypass. *Fischer's Mastery of Surgery.* 6th ed. Philadelpha, PA: Lippincott Williams & Williams; 2012:1121-1128.
20. Gothberg G, Gronowitz E, Flodmark C-E, et al. Laparoscopic Roux-en-Y gastric bypass in adolescents with morbid obesity: surgical aspects and clinical outcome. *Semin Pediatr Surg.* 2014;23:11-16.
21. Zitsman JL. Laparoscopic adjustable gastric banding in adolescents. *Semin Pediatr Surg.* 2014;23:17-20.
22. Al-Sabah SK, Almazeedi SM, Dashti SA, Al-Mulla AY, Ali DA, Jumaa TH. The efficacy of laparoscopic sleeve gastrectomy in treating adolescent obesity. *Obes Surg.* 2015;25:50-54.

3

Medical Treatment of Obesity

W. Scott Butsch, MD, MSc and Nadia N. Ahmad, MD, MPH

Obesity is a complex chronic disease. The etiology of this disease can be traced to macrolevel factors, such as industrialization and national food policy, as well as microlevel factors, such as the behavioral, genetic, and molecular determinants of energy balance within an individual. While the former are more appropriately addressed by public health initiatives, the latter are amenable to assessment and treatment in the clinical setting and will form the basis for our discussion of the medical management of obesity in this chapter.

We begin the chapter with 6 core Principles of Obesity Care that we believe can serve as a guide for the physician through the spectrum of care from diagnosis and assessment through treatment and follow-up. Next, in the Evaluation of the Patient With Obesity, we describe the measurement of adiposity and disease risk and introduce a nuanced approach to the patient history, physical exam, and diagnostic testing. This is followed by a series of sections on medical treatment options, including Lifestyle Interventions, such as diet, exercise, sleep, and behavioral change, and Pharmacotherapy, including on- and off-label use of single and dual agents. We have included a brief section on the Emerging Field of Weight Loss Devices to keep the physician abreast of upcoming therapeutic advances in the field. Practitioners who medically manage challenging cases of obesity may be interested in Indications for Referral to obesity medicine specialists and/or comprehensive weight management centers. In the next section, Weight Stigma, we emphasize the importance of addressing this pervasive phenomenon throughout the evaluative and therapeutic process. We conclude the chapter with Addressing Weight Issues After Bariatric Surgery, a critical area in which medical evaluation and/or treatment are needed to combat the issues of suboptimal weight loss or, more commonly, weight regain after gastrointestinal weight loss surgery. Throughout this chapter, we have sought to convey the application of a chronic disease-based model of care in which the complexity and biologic basis of obesity is recognized and translated into effective clinical strategies and therapeutic interactions that should be rewarding for both the patient and the provider.

Forse RA, Apovian CM, eds.
Bariatric Surgery: What Every Provider Needs to Know (pp 23-58).

Principles of Obesity Care

Through our training and practice, we have identified 6 core principles for providers treating obesity (Table 3-1).

Principle 1: Obesity Has a Complex Biological Basis

"Life is at bottom a competition for energy,"[1] and it is no wonder then that our energy regulatory system has evolved to be both complex and efficient at the cellular and whole organism level. It is composed of redundant and interconnected neurohumoral pathways designed to protect against energy deprivation.[2] Since the discovery of leptin in the 1990s, which heralded a new era in the scientific investigation of energy regulation, we now know that the system involves dozens of neurotransmitters and hormones including a host of adipokines, gut incretins, and, more recently, myokines.[3-6] An in-depth review of these individual players is beyond the scope of this chapter. However, a basic conceptual understanding of the system is important for appropriate medical management of obesity.

For the sake of simplicity, we can divide the system into 2 parts: central and peripheral. Central refers to the central nervous system (CNS) that receives a variety of signals from the rest of the body. The peripheral signals to the CNS include the following:

- Those from sensory organs that relay the availability of energy and specific nutrients in the environment through our senses of vision, smell, taste, and touch
- Those from the gastrointestinal tract that signal to the brain precisely what nutrients are coming on board
- Those from tissues such as muscle and bone relaying the body's energy needs
- Those from our organs of energy storage (eg, adipose tissue, liver) that relay how much and what type of energy stores are already on board

These peripheral afferent signals communicate with the brain's homeostatic and hedonic circuitry (ie, the hypothalamus and dopaminergic mesocorticolimbic pathways, respectively). This circuitry, in turn, has bidirectional communication with the frontal cortex, an area of the brain that guides our executive function and decision making. The complex interplay of neurohumoral signals in the CNS essentially determines the "adiposity set point" (ie, how much fat the body needs to store). Efferent signals then emanate from the CNS to the periphery dictating our appetitive drive (ie, food intake) and nutrient handling (ie, energy storage and expenditure) such that the "set point" is achieved and maintained.[7]

In an appropriately functioning system, any excess energy stores (eg, in the form of adipose tissue) should be "sensed" by the CNS (via afferent neurohumoral signaling pathways). The CNS, in turn, should signal decreased food intake, increased energy expenditure, and decreased energy storage via efferent pathways. Energy balance should thereby be maintained and is maintained in many individuals who effortlessly remain a healthy weight in today's obesogenic environment. The development of excess adiposity, therefore, can be conceived as the dysfunction of an energy regulatory system that is no longer sensing the excess and is regulating to an abnormally higher set point. The precise molecular basis of the pathophysiology has yet to be determined and likely varies among individuals, although leptin resistance has been proposed as one potential contributing mechanism to the accumulation of adiposity.[8]

Like most of biology, the physiology of energy regulation can be modulated by a variety of factors, including genetics, epigenetics, developmental exposures, behavior, and environmental and psychosocial influences. Of these, individual behavior has been the sole target of obesity assessment and treatment for decades. Recognizing that obesity has a biological basis does not negate the

Table 3-1

The BEHAVE Model of Obesity Treatment: Six Principles for Providers

Biological basis	The body's degree of adiposity falls under the control of the energy regulatory system, a complex network of neurohumoral pathways. This network can be modulated by genetic, developmental, environmental, and behavioral factors leading to the accumulation of excess adiposity (ie, overweight and obesity).
Education	Educating patients about the biological basis of their condition: Helps to reduce weight bias and patient blame Helps patients better understand their body's response to prior weight loss attempts Equips patients with the necessary background information to engage in the decision-making process regarding treatments
Heterogeneity	Given the complexity of the energy regulatory system and the many ways in which it may be modulated by genetic, developmental, environmental, and behavioral factors, it is not surprising that the population with overweight and obesity is physiologically, and therefore clinically, heterogeneous. Patients vary in their age of onset, weight distribution, hunger and satiety cues, cravings, metabolic rates, propensity to exercise, and response to sleep and stress as well as a host of other clinically measurable factors.
Assessment	Understanding that your patient population with obesity is clinically heterogeneous allows for a line of clinical questioning that will help you decipher subpopulations of patients. Through a more nuanced assessment, you may learn over time to tailor treatments to individual phenotypes.
Variability in response	Given physiologic heterogeneity in the patient population, there is generally a broad distribution of response to weight loss treatments, including diets, pharmacotherapy, and bariatric surgery. A single treatment does not suit all patients. However, for each treatment you are likely to find a subpopulation of high-responders.
Expectation	Upon trialing a treatment for obesity, if you expect variability in response among patients, you are less likely to blame the patient for noncompliance if the treatment is ineffective. You are also able to better manage patient expectations so that if the treatment is not resulting in substantial weight loss, the patient is prepared to move onto the next therapy, continues to follow up, and remains engaged in the therapeutic process.

etiologic role of behavior or environment. Rather, it places these factors in perspective. As in most other chronic diseases (eg, type 2 diabetes, cardiovascular disease, cancer), individual behavior and the external environment contribute to the disease state by working through the framework of an organism's physiology and disrupting its normal processes.

Principle 2: Educating Patients About the Basis of the Condition Is a Prerequisite to Effective Clinical Care

We are often products of our society, and unfortunately societal views of obesity as a characterological flaw, a failure of individual willpower, and a solely behavioral condition of excessive intake and sedentary lifestyle are what prevail in the minds of most patients. If this internalized weight bias is not countered by patient education regarding the biological basis of the condition, most patients will fail to understand the rationale for specific treatment strategies (nutritional, behavioral, pharmacologic, or surgical), will become frustrated when a particular treatment strategy does not work to expectation, and will find it difficult to remain compliant and engaged in the therapeutic process. Therefore, to only educate the patient on his or her disease risk associated with obesity is unsatisfactory. It is also of paramount importance to inform the patient in layperson's terms how his or her adiposity is determined by biological processes (in addition to the psychosocial and behavioral factors) and how these processes can potentially be modified to varying degrees by lifestyle (eg, diet, physical activity, stress, sleep), medications, or surgery.

Principle 3: Obesity Is a Heterogeneous Condition

Biological complexity naturally gives rise to phenotypic heterogeneity. To illustrate, imagine there are only 3 genes involved in energy regulation and 1 genetic variation predisposing to obesity is possible in each of those genes. Then there are 8 possible subpopulations of individuals carrying 0, 1, 2, or all 3 of those variations. Although all result in obesity as defined by excess adiposity, each subpopulation has defining phenotypic characteristics based on its particular combination of genetic variations. Now, in reality, energy regulation involves innumerable pathways and genes (not just 3) and for many of these genes specific variations favoring energy efficiency have been evolutionary selected for and likely may be found in different segments of the population. The distribution of genetic variations in the population combined with differences among individuals in environmental exposures, development, behavior, and other "modulating" factors is what results in tremendous heterogeneity in obesity presentation and treatment response.

Principle 4: Understanding of Heterogeneity Allows for a More Comprehensive and Thorough Assessment and an Individualized Treatment Plan

The most direct clinical translation of Principle 3 (disease heterogeneity) is a more sophisticated and nuanced assessment that attempts to identify clinically relevant subpopulations of patients. The nuanced patient assessment, as will be discussed, involves far more than a simple history of diet and exercise. It attempts to identify patients with different ages of onset, comorbidities, adiposity distribution, taste preferences and cravings, inclination for exercise, specific weight gain triggers such as sleep deprivation or stress, tendency for weight gain on specific medications, and so on. Although response to specific anti-obesity medications or even surgery cannot yet be accurately predicted by these clinical characteristics, certain therapies can be individually tailored based on a detailed assessment. Moreover, an assessment that appreciates the heterogeneity of the disease changes the verbal landscape of the clinical encounter leading to a less biased and more productive dialogue between patient and provider.

Principle 5: There Is Considerable Variability in Response to All Weight Loss Treatments

Due to the tremendous heterogeneity of obesity, all anti-obesity treatments have a broad range of weight loss response. This has been shown in clinical trials of diets, exercise, medications, and surgery. In the case of surgery, such as Roux-en-Y gastric bypass (RYGB), the average response is 60% to 70% excess weight loss (EWL). However, when interpreting the distribution of treatment response, there are 5% to 10% of patients who have < 30% EWL (at the low end of the distribution), while another 5% to 10% of patients have > 90% EWL (at the high end).[9] In the case of most behavioral and medication treatments, the average weight loss is modest, but there are a small percentage of patients who have a robust response (which may be as great, if not greater, than some responses to surgery).[10,11]

Principle 6: Expecting a Broad Range of Treatment Responses Manages Expectations for Both Patient and Provider and Serves to Strengthen the Therapeutic Alliance

One of the myths of obesity treatment is that some treatments (namely diets and medications) do not work. When one particular behavioral approach or one particular medication does not have a robust response in a patient, both patient and provider are likely to give up on the treatment approach altogether. This negatively impacts both patient compliance and the physician's confidence in using the same treatment again on another patient. However, if one expects variability in treatment response, where some treatments will not work and others will, then these negative treatment outcomes become less discouraging. If both provider and patient expectations are managed with every treatment trial, then it is more likely that treatments will be trialed sequentially until a robust response is achieved with the treatment that best suits the patient's phenotype. For this process to occur, the patient must be engaged in the therapeutic relationship over a long period of time. Managing expectations, therefore, becomes a critical component of the medical management of obesity.

Evaluation of the Patient With Obesity

The primary objectives of the evaluation include elucidation of the underlying mechanism(s) responsible for the excess weight, detection of any underlying illnesses presenting with weight gain, and determination of the risks the excess weight confers.

Initial steps of the assessment should estimate the amount and distribution of fat, followed by a consideration of other risk factors and underlying conditions that add to morbidity and mortality risks. As described previously, it is important to understand the heterogeneity of obesity and that individuals at the same level of obesity may have completely different metabolic profiles and thus disease risk. Individuals with obesity who lack its metabolic complications have a reduced risk of cardiovascular disease—they are referred to as metabolically healthy obese—whereas others with a normal body mass index (BMI) and a high body fat content may develop metabolic disease and have an increased cardiovascular disease risk.[12] These differences highlight the importance of considering obesity not as a single disorder, but rather as a spectrum of diseases.

Defining and Measuring Obesity by Body Mass Index

The associated health risks of overweight/obesity are primarily related to the amount and distribution of excess adipose tissue as both are independent determinants of disease risk.

BMI = weight (kg) / height (m^2) = weight (lb) x 703 / height (in)

The classification of obesity by BMI is shown in Table 3-2.

BMI is the most commonly used tool to assess the degree of total adiposity and quantify disease risk. Although the numerator in this ratio, weight, does not distinguish lean body mass and fat mass, BMI highly correlates with the percentage body fat and its associated health risks.

TABLE 3-2

DEFINITION AND CLASSIFICATION OF EXCESS WEIGHT

Class		BMI (kg/m^2)	Disease Risk[a]
Underweight		< 18.5	
Normal		18.5 to 24.9	*
Overweight		25.0 to 29.9	Increased*
Obesity	Class I	30.0 to 34.9	High*
	Class II	35.0 to 39.9	Very high
	Class III	≥40.0	Extremely high

BMI = body mass index.

[a]Relative to normal weight and waist circumference. Risk for development of type 2 diabetes, hypertension, coronary artery disease.

*Increased risk if waist circumference > 102 cm (40 in) in men, > 88 cm (35 in) in women.

Adapted from National Institutes of Health NHLBI and North American Association for the Study of Obesity. *The Practical Guide: Identification, Evaluation and Treatment of Overweight and Obesity in Adults.* Washington, DC: Author; 2000.

Limitations of BMI include an overestimation of body fat in individuals with higher than average lean body mass (eg, body builders) and an underestimation in individuals with higher than average body fatness (eg, elderly). Furthermore, BMI may differ by gender and ethnicity. For example, women have greater body fat mass compared with men at a similar BMI. Hispanic women have a greater body fat mass when compared with Black and White women, while Black men and women have greater lean body mass and less body fat mass compared with White men and women at a given BMI. Asian populations have greater visceral adiposity at a similar BMI when compared with White and Black populations; therefore, BMI cut-offs for Asian populations are at 23 for overweight and 27 for obesity (instead of 25 and 30, respectively). Although the BMI range of 20 to 24.9 is classified as "normal" body weight, individuals with normal weight but excess body fat content may be at increased risk to develop metabolic syndrome or insulin resistance.[13]

BMI remains the preferred measure for evaluating weight status because it provides the best estimate of disease risk and is easily calculated. However, the aforementioned limitations must be entertained when using BMI alone as a measurement of adiposity in a clinical setting.

Measurements of Adiposity and Its Distribution

Waist circumference is a simple and effective method to assess body fat distribution and complements BMI measurement during physical examination. As a reflection of visceral adiposity, it is independently associated with increased relative risk of cardiovascular disease and mortality;

however, it provides no additional risk in individuals with a BMI > 35 kg/m^2. The waist circumference should be obtained at the level of the iliac crest or at 1 fingerbreadth above the umbilicus; gender-specific cutoffs (> 102 cm [40 in] in men and > 88 cm [35 in] in women) vary widely by ethnicity.

The ratio of waist-to-hip circumference (ie, waist-hip ratio [WHR]) is another indicator of visceral adiposity; ratios above 0.8 (for women) and 1.0 (for men) are associated with increased cardiovascular risk and metabolic disease. The hip circumference is measured at the maximal gluteal protrusion. WHR may be beneficial when adjusting for ethnicity and in the elderly.

Skinfold thickness has been used to quantify subcutaneous adiposity. Calipers are used to measure skinfold thickness in at least 3 regions, including chest, abdomen, and thigh. However, age and racial differences, low interrater reliability, and the presence of large skinfolds limit its usefulness in patients with obesity.

The most accurate techniques to measure body composition or distribution of body fat include computed tomography, magnetic resonance imaging, dual x-ray absorptiometry, and air-displacement plethysmography. These, however, are typically reserved for research. Although bioelectric impedance analysis is more easily used in the clinical setting to measure total body fat, it remains inaccurate in individuals with obesity.[12]

History of Present Illness

The purpose of the history and physical examination is to identify underlying conditions contributing to weight gain and to assess for potential complications of excess body weight.

The history should begin with obtaining a weight history, in particular the age of onset of obesity, family history of obesity, and any identifiable circumstances (eg, smoking cessation, menopause, medications) associated with the onset of weight gain. (See Table 3-3 for review of weight gain promoting medications.) The state of physical activity and proclivity toward exercise should be identified. Dietary composition and quantity need to be ascertained to determine total caloric intake. Social and cultural routines as well as psychological and situational stressors may influence eating behaviors and therefore should be explored for both their possible contribution to weight gain and as potential barriers to lifestyle modification. Aside from the 2 most common eating disorders, anorexia nervosa and bulimia, providers should identify other eating and sleep disorders associated with weight gain (eg, binge eating disorder [BED], night eating syndrome [NES], and sleep-related eating disorder [SRED]). BED, the most common of the 3, is characterized by uncontrollably eating large amounts of food in a discrete amount of time, at least once weekly over the course of 3 months. This is accompanied by at least 3 of the following characteristics:

- Eating to uncomfortable fullness
- Eating in absence of hunger
- Eating more rapidly than normal
- Eating alone due to embarrassment
- Having guilt after the episode, without inappropriate compensatory actions (eg, purging)

NES is characterized by evening hyperphagia, frequent nocturnal awakenings associated with conscious episodes of compulsive eating, and morning anorexia. SRED is more aligned with an abnormal circadian rhythm and is characterized by unconscious episodes of compulsive food intake. Therefore, it is important to take a sleep history. Not only is sleep dysfunction implicated in weight gain, but studies have also demonstrated that lack of sufficient sleep may compromise efforts to lose weight with lifestyle modification.[14] Other potential contributors to weight gain and complications of excess weight are listed in Table 3-4.

Table 3-3
Medications Associated With Weight Gain

MEDICATION CLASS, *Drug**	ALTERNATIVE MEDICATION *
Atypical Antipsychotics	
Clozapine (Clozaril) **Olanzapine (Zyprexa)** **Quetiapine (Seroquel)** **Risperidone (Risperdal)** **Aripiprazole (Abilify)** **Haloperidol (Haldol)** Perphenazine (Trilafon) Chlorpromazine (Thorazine)	Ziprasidone (Geodon)
Anticonvulsants/Mood Stabilizers	
Lithium **Valproic acid (Valproate)** **Carbamazepine (Tegretol)** **Vigabatrin (Sabril)** **Gabapentin (Neurontin)** Phenytoin (Dilantin) Divalproex sodium (Depakote) Oxcarbazepine (Trileptal)	Topiramate (Topamax) Zonisamide (Zonegran) Lamotrigine (Lamictal)
Antidepressants	
Selective Serotonin Reuptake Inhibitors: **Paroxetine (Paxil)** **Citalopram (Celexa)** Fluoxetine (Prozac) Sertraline (Zoloft)	Fluoxetine, Sertraline (substitute for paroxetine) Bupropion (Wellbutrin)
Tricyclic Antidepressants: **Amitriptyline (Elavil)** Nortriptyline (Pamelor) Imipramine (Tofranil)	Desipramine (Norpramin)
Monoamine Oxidase Inhibitors: Phenelzine (Nardil)	Tranylcypromine (Parnate)
Other Antidepressants: **Mirtazapine (Remeron)** Trazodone (Desyrel)	Nefazodone (Serzone)

(continued)

Table 3-3 (continued)

Medications Associated With Weight Gain

MEDICATION CLASS, *Drug**	ALTERNATIVE MEDICATION *
Antidiabetic Medications	
Insulin	
Sulfonylureas:	
Glyburide (Diabeta)	Glimepiride (substitute for glyburide, glipizide)
Glipizide (Glucotrol)	GLP-1 agonists (exenatide [Byetta, Bydureon], liraglutide [Victoza])
Glimepiride (Amaryl)	Amylin agonist (pramlintide [Symlin])
	SGLT2 inhibitors (canagliflozin [Invokana])
	DPP-IV inhibitors (sitagliptin [Januvia])
Thiazolidinediones:	
Pioglitazone (Actos)	
Rosiglitazone (Avandia)	
Other Classes	
Antihypertensive Medications:	
ß-blockers (propranolol [Inderal])	Carvedilol (Coreg), ACEI, ARBs
Metoprolol (Lopressor, Toprol), atenolol (Tenormin)	Doxazosin (Cardura)
α-blockers (clonidine [Catapres], prazosin [Minipress], terazosin [Hytrin])	
Corticosteroids:	
Prednisone, hydrocortisone, dexamethasone	Immunosuppressants, TNF-α blockers, NSAIDs (when clinically appropriate)
Antihistamines:	
Diphenhydramine (Benadryl)	Loratadine (Claritin)
Hormonal Contraceptives:	
Depot medroxyprogesterone acetate (Depo-Provera)	Barrier methods

*Drugs are listed in order from greatest to least weight gain. Bold drugs have the greatest degree of weight gain. Alternative medications are weight neutral or cause less weight gain.

ACEI = angiotensin-converting-enzyme inhibitors, ARBs = angiotensin II receptor blockers, DPP-IV = dipeptidyl peptidase-4, NSAIDs = nonsteroidal anti-inflammatory drugs, SGLT2 = sodium-glucose co-transporter 2.

Table 3-4

History and Physical Exam in the Patient With Obesity

FINDINGS ON HISTORY AND THEIR SIGNIFICANCE	PHYSICAL EXAM AND/OR RECOMMENDATIONS FOR MANAGEMENT
Weight History	
• If early onset or strong family history, consider genetic etiology • If rapid gain, consider exposure to medications, cessation of a restrictive diet, or onset of an endocrine disorder (eg, Cushing's syndrome). If gradual gain, consider more of a behavioral etiology.	• Genetic testing (eg, MC4R, leptin mutations [if highly suspicious]) • Review medications • Targeted endocrine exam and management of endocrine disorders (see endocrine section in Review of Systems)
Medications	
• May be potential contributor(s) to weight gain	• Review medications for weight-promoting drugs • Consider substitution or discontinuation when applicable
Sleep Patterns	
• If positive for snoring, witnessed apnea, choking/gasping for breath at night, morning headaches, and/or daytime sleepiness, consider obstructive sleep apnea • Altered sleep patterns, insomnia, or sleep deprivation may reflect altered circadian rhythm, a potential source of altered eating habits and weight gain • Use of sleep medications may promote weight gain • History of shift work may be a source of altered sleep or eating behaviors	• On exam look for oropharyngeal crowding, large neck circumference (> 16 cm, women; > 17 cm, men) • Refer for polysomnography • Consider referral to sleep medicine specialist and/or psychologist to help with sleep hygiene • Decrease or discontinue medications for sleep • Counsel on sleep and diet patterns in shift workers
Stress	
• Personal and work-related stressors are potential contributors to weight gain; may cause hormonal changes and altered sleep and eating behaviors • Weight discrimination can be a source of stress	• Refer to psychologist for cognitive behavioral therapy • Consider alternative therapies for stress (eg, mind-body approaches [yoga, meditation, relaxation techniques])

(continued)

Table 3-4 (continued)

History and Physical Exam in the Patient With Obesity

FINDINGS ON HISTORY AND THEIR SIGNIFICANCE	PHYSICAL EXAM AND/OR RECOMMENDATIONS FOR MANAGEMENT
Social History	
• Tobacco cessation is a potential contributor to weight gain	• Counsel on tobacco cessation; reassure weight gain will be addressed • Consider bupropion in patients wanting to quit smoking (if clinically appropriate)
• Alcohol use is a potential contributor to weight gain; may cause altered sleep and eating behaviors	• Counsel on decreasing/avoiding alcohol
Diet and Exercise History	
• Responsiveness to any past diets may indicate future therapeutic potential • Increased caloric intake at night, eating in the middle of the night/while asleep, excessive food intake at one sitting (eg, NES, BED, SRED) • History of eating disorders (eg, bulimia, anorexia nervosa)	• Consider implementing change in diet composition if previously successful (eg, low carb or low fat) • Encourage self-directed tools (web-based [eg, myfitnesspal.com]) • Referral to dietician for medical nutrition therapy and nutrition education and/or psychologist to confirm/treat eating disorders
• Barriers to exercise	• Water-based exercise therapies may be helpful in patients with musculoskeletal pain or physical limitations • Identify resources for exercise (use of devices [eg, FitBit, Fuelband], exercise trainer, online apps [eg, Couch to 5K])
Review of Systems	
• Skin: Increased susceptibility to candidal infections, cellulitis (due to venous insufficiency), hidradenitis suppurativa, psoriasis, lymphedema • Lipomas may be benign, but alert to lipodystrophies, lipomatoses, MEN1	• On exam: Redness and irritation with satellite lesions under the breasts and abdominal fold(s) and in the inguinal area suggest candidal infections, lipoatrophy suggests lipodystrophy; acanthosis nigricans suggests insulin resistance • Painful subcutaneous nodules should be investigated • Absorbant powders, better fitting clothes may decrease irritation • Topical antifungals (eg, creams, powders) • Compression stockings for lymphedema

(continued)

Table 3-4 (continued)

History and Physical Exam in the Patient With Obesity

FINDINGS ON HISTORY AND THEIR SIGNIFICANCE	PHYSICAL EXAM AND/OR RECOMMENDATIONS FOR MANAGEMENT
Cardiac: At risk for atrial fibrillation, hemorrhagic stroke, congestive heart failure, adipositas cordis* (heart failure specific to obesity)	• On exam: Lower extremity edema, venous stasis changes in skin
Pulmonary: Increased risk for asthma, deep vein thrombosis, and/or pulmonary embolism	• On exam: Lower extremity edema, wheezing, distant breath sounds • Screen for deep venous thrombosis (ultrasound)
Gastrointestinal: At risk for gallstones (post prandial abdominal pain) and nonalcoholic fatty liver disease (abdominal fullness)	• Screen for nonalcoholic fatty liver disease, choleliathiasis (ultrasound, hepatic transaminases) if clinically suspicious
Endocrine: • Symptoms of diabetes: Polyuria, polydipsia, polyphagia • Symptoms of hypothyroidism: Constipation, fatigue, dry skin, coarse hair • Symptoms of Cushing's syndrome: Weight gain, irregular menstrual cycles, anxiety, high blood pressure, moon facies • Symptoms of polycystic ovary syndrome: Hirsutism, irregular menstrual cycles, anovulation, acne • Post partum weight retention • Menopause, association with insulin resistance and reduced energy expenditure in some	• On exam: Acanthosis nigricans suggests insulin resistance; hirsutism, acne suggest polycystic ovary syndrome (females); moon facies, pigmented abdominal striae, truncal obesity, dorsal cervical fat pad, supraclavicular fat pad suggest Cushing's syndrome; ask patient to look up (stretch neck) for better access to the thyroid • Consider serum fasting insulin to screen for polycystic ovary syndrome • Screen diabetes (HbA1c), hypothyroidism (serum thyroid-stimulating hormone) • Work-up (24-hour urine cortisol, 1 mg dexamethasone suppression test, computed tomography of the sella turcica) and/or referral to endocrinologist for Cushing's syndrome
Musculoskeletal: At risk for arthritis, degenerative joint disease	• On exam: Proper positioning is helpful to best examine
Neurological: Symptoms of pseudotumor cerebri, headaches, visual difficulty, tinnitus	• On exam: Papilledema, visual field loss, sixth nerve palsy • Referral to ophthalmology

(continued)

Table 3-4 (continued)

History and Physical Exam in the Patient With Obesity

FINDINGS ON HISTORY AND THEIR SIGNIFICANCE	PHYSICAL EXAM AND/OR RECOMMENDATIONS FOR MANAGEMENT
Cancer screening • Associated increased risk of cancers of the esophagus, colon, rectum, breast (postmenopausal), endometrium (the lining of the uterus), kidney, pancreas, thyroid, gallbladder, and possibly more types • Disparities in cancer screening in patients with obesity	• On exam: Examine females in lateral decubitus position to best examine breasts, hirsutism, acne • Aggressive screening for cancer (Pap smear, digital rectal examination, prostate-specific antigen, mammography, colonoscopy)

* Poirier P, Giles TD, Bray GA, et al. Obesity and cardiovascular disease: pathophysiology, evaluation and effect of weight loss: an update of the 1997 American Heart Association scientific statement on obesity and heart disease from the obesity committee of the council on nutrition, physical activity, and metabolism. *Circulation.* 2006;113:898-918.

BED = binge eating disorder, HbA1c = hemoglobin A1c, MC4R = melanocortin receptor 4, MEN1 = multiple endocrine neoplasia type 1, NES = night eating syndrome, SRED = sleep-related eating disorder.

Physical Examination

The physical examination of a patient with obesity may be challenging for multiple reasons, ranging from the amount and distribution of adiposity to the physical environment of the examination room. Therefore, it is essential to overcome potential environmental barriers (eg, by providing gowns that can fit larger patients and using large blood pressure cuffs when appropriate) in order to perform the detailed examination required to generate an accurate differential diagnosis.[15] Proper physical examination includes the search for both etiologic causes and possible complications of obesity (see Table 3-4), with specific attention to signs and symptoms of metabolic syndrome, obstructive sleep apnea, and polycystic ovary syndrome. A careful examination of the skin and lower extremities, in particular, potential unreachable areas like the feet, is suggested as these areas may be less frequently addressed. Diagnosis of an endocrine disorder, such as Cushing's syndrome, may be difficult as signs and symptoms of hypercortisolemia (eg, striae and central adiposity) may overlap with some obesity phenotypes with hyperinsulinemia.

Laboratory Testing

Laboratory testing should complement the physical examination in elucidating the diagnosis of an underlying medical etiology and the detection of the metabolic consequences of obesity (see Table 3-4). Hypothyroidism is rarely a direct cause of obesity in an individual, but thyroid function should still be checked. Screening for metabolic syndrome is also essential, and therefore, waist circumference, fasting glucose, and lipid profile should be routinely measured. Serum insulin levels provide a more direct measurement of hyperinsulinism, but assays are not well standardized.

Measurements of gastrointestinal hormones involved in weight regulation (ie, glucagon-like peptide-1 [GLP-1], ghrelin, and peptide YY [PYY]), as well as serum leptin levels, are not currently used in the clinical setting but may be useful in the future. Similarly, measures of energy expenditure, thermogenesis, and most genetic testing are relegated to the research laboratory. However, if a patient has clinical features of a syndromic form of obesity (eg, Prader-Willi syndrome) or a monogenic cause (eg, MC4R or leptin deficiency), specific genetic assays would be appropriate.

Treatment Approach

Recent guidelines[16] direct providers to offer a comprehensive lifestyle program to individuals who are overweight with a weight-related comorbidity or have obesity and are interested in losing weight. Principal components of a comprehensive lifestyle program include a reduction in caloric intake, a regular exercise routine, and behavioral strategies to facilitate long-term lifestyle change. Goals of treatment should aim for a 5% to 10% weight loss in the first 6 months. In those individuals who do not respond to intensive lifestyle therapy, strategy should include a stepwise approach to weight loss, with adjunctive therapies. Pharmacotherapy (for BMI $\geq$ 27 with at least one obesity-related medical condition or BMI $\geq$ 30) and gastrointestinal weight loss surgery (for BMI $\geq$ 35 with one or more obesity-related medical conditions or BMI $\geq$ 40) are used as adjunctive therapy to a lifestyle program. Although these guidelines are based on BMI, the aggressiveness of therapy can be determined by the extent and severity of the weight-related comorbidities, psychosocial and functional limitations, and overall quality of life.

It is difficult to determine who will be successful in the treatment of obesity. Although assessment of patient readiness is one of the first steps in predicting the effectiveness of behavioral interventions, a recent review concluded there are insufficient data to support the benefits of self-reported readiness in terms of predicting patient adherence and weight loss.[17]

In those individuals who are not ready to make a lifestyle change, providers should educate the patient on cardiovascular disease risks related to excess weight and schedule periodic visits to assess readiness. Regardless of the patient's interest or readiness to engage in a weight loss intervention, attempts should be made to increase awareness of the health risks of excess weight. Studies have shown that merely informing the patient of his or her abnormal weight/BMI may be helpful in not only raising patient awareness but promoting weight loss attempts.[18] Finding an effective weight loss intervention for patients can be challenging, and clinicians need to be as committed as their patients to the search. In the end, "success" need not be measured only by the numbers on the scale. Rather, reductions in blood pressure and cholesterol or improvements in the quality of life (eg, ability to sit comfortably in a chair) may act as the best measures of success for a particular patient.

Lifestyle Interventions

Lifestyle modification, consisting of changes in patterns of dietary intake, exercise, sleep, and other behaviors, is considered the cornerstone of obesity management. The 2 longest randomized lifestyle trials, the Diabetes Prevention Program[19] and the Look AHEAD,[20] have both provided insight into the health benefits of modest weight loss and highlighted the difficulty in achieving sustained weight loss through lifestyle interventions. Nonetheless, the reality for clinicians is that there are no data to help effectively match a specific diet or lifestyle intervention to an individual's biology in order to produce durable weight loss. Substantial variation in weight loss response to lifestyle modification further complicates treatment goals.

Historically, patients and providers have focused on "dieting" as the first step in weight reduction. This narrowed approach, based on the assumption that a temporary change in diet will lead to long-term weight loss, typically provides 500 to 1000 fewer calories to achieve a weight loss of 0.5 to 1.0 kg/week. However, this approach fails to address the metabolic adaptation[21] and hormonal compensation[22] that occur with diet-induced weight loss. As a result, not surprisingly, a majority of patients reach an early plateau and/or regain weight after "dieting." Thus starts the cycle of repeated diet attempts accompanied by perpetual frustration and self-blame.

With an understanding of the complex biological pathways of obesity and the heterogeneity of treatment response (previously discussed in Principles of Obesity Care), providers should develop an individualized obesity treatment plan focused on achieving a more gradual, permanent lifestyle change. As weight loss may be limited with lifestyle change alone, focus should be directed toward the many additional health benefits of lifestyle changes. Special attention should be given to specific lifestyle factors in addition to diet that may contribute to an individual's increased body weight (eg, sleep deprivation and/or fragmentation, increased internal and external stressors, a lack of regular exercise). A more targeted approach may center only on one area at a time (eg, first on stress reduction then on sleep hygiene) if the history suggests that these are potentially strong contributors to the patient's increased body weight. We find this simple sequential treatment strategy allows the clinician to more easily measure progress while also addressing nonweight outcomes (eg, hours of sleep), prolongs patient engagement by providing several potential treatment options (beyond diet and exercise), and creates a healthy environment where both the provider and patient appreciate the complexity of obesity and avoid the repetitive recommendation of "eat less and exercise more." Depending on the area of lifestyle modification addressed, referrals to a dietician, psychologist, exercise trainer, social worker, and/or sleep medicine specialist may be necessary.

Diet

Extensive research of diets has failed to identify an optimal diet for weight loss. Although changes in diet composition (ie, low fat, low carbohydrate, high protein, low glycemic, and Mediterranean diets) have been shown to modestly reduce weight and risk of cardiovascular disease and diabetes,[23-25] the weight loss effect is attributed entirely to the degree of caloric restriction and adherence rather than the composition.[26,27] Therefore, most long-term diet interventions follow a similar course, one of maximum effect at 6 months, followed by a period of sustained weight and weight regain.[28] Commercial and self-help programs have a similar outcome, but are less studied.[29] It is suggested that the lack of adherence and the return to past eating behaviors (unfortunately often described in the literature as recidivism—see section on Weight Stigma) account for the ineffectiveness of diet interventions. However, the aforementioned hormonal compensation (eg, increased ghrelin, reduced leptin, PYY, amylin, and cholecystokinin) that occurs with weight loss may not only explain individual variation in adherence, but supports the hypothesis that weight regain has a strong physiological basis and may not be as simple as once thought.

Very low calorie diets (VLCDs) are medically supervised diets (500 to 800 calories/day) with a high protein (1.5 g/kg) content to preserve lean body mass. VLCDs are safe and considered for use in adults with a BMI > 30 who require rapid significant weight loss (eg, prior to an elective surgery). Contraindications include pregnancy, type 1 diabetes, pancreatitis, severe renal or hepatic impairment, active cancer, and severe psychological disturbance. Most VLCDs are generally offered in liquid form as part of a commercial program and achieve 15% to 25% body weight loss in the 3- to 6-month initial phase, with a sustained weight loss of 8% to 9% after 1 year. Gradual weight regain begins after solid foods of a higher caloric content are reintroduced, reaching up to 50% of lost weight after 1 to 2 years. High dropout rates and poor long-term maintenance are discouraging aspects of this form of treatment.[27,30]

Exercise

Exercise plays an important role in every weight loss intervention. Although exercise alone achieves only modest weight loss, it is most effective when combined with a reduction in caloric intake.[31] There are 2 forms of exercise: aerobic and resistance. Aerobic exercise (eg, walking briskly, running, swimming, biking) increases fitness, which strongly correlates with cardiovascular and all-cause mortality[32]; whereas resistance exercise is usually in the form of weight lifting or use of resistance bands and increases muscle mass. In combination, these forms of exercise are effective in weight loss, in particular in reducing fat mass. It is important to emphasize to patients that exercise has a stronger role in weight maintenance than weight loss. Exercise helps to preserve lean body mass and maintain increased energy expenditure in the weight-reduced state. In fact, physical activity has been shown to be one of the best predictors of successful weight maintenance.[33]

A specific exercise prescription, including both aerobic and resistance exercise, should be prescribed. Implementation of an exercise program can occur at any time, but to ensure compliance, it should be physically realistic, medically safe, and able to fit into the patient's daily routine. Recommendations for prevention of weight gain are at least 150 minutes per week or 30 to 60 minutes 5 days per week of moderately intense physical activity, or 20 to 60 minutes per week of vigorous activity.[34] However, researchers estimate more than 200 minutes per week of moderately intense physical activity is needed for weight loss, and more than 250 minutes is needed for weight maintenance.[35]

As seen with caloric reduction, there is broad variation in response to exercise and adaptation occurs to limit the amount of energy expended.[36] Compensatory changes in diet and behavior related to neuroendocrine hormones such as GLP-1 and ghrelin are plausible explanations.[37] Variability of response to exercise may also be explained by changes in nonexercise activity thermogenesis (NEAT). NEAT can be represented by unintentional activities (eg, fidgeting) or informal physical activities (eg, parking farther away, taking the stairs), and also is highly variable.[38] As a result, exercise recommendations are best adjusted according to individual responses and preferences. Patients should be encouraged to use pedometers (aiming to achieve more than 8000 to 10,000 steps per day) or other tracking devices to promote physical activity.

Behavioral Modification

Behavioral modification is an integral part of the treatment of overweight/obesity. The goal of behavioral therapy is to develop practical alternative behaviors that are likely to lead to long-term decreased caloric intake and increased physical activity.[39] Strong evidence exists to support the application of a combination of behavioral theory and cognitive behavior theory to facilitate modification of habits. Individuals with eating disorders (eg, BED, NES, SRED) or emotionally triggered eating behaviors may benefit from behavioral modification.

Targeted sleep behavioral therapy is particularly beneficial in those patients with poor sleep hygiene and interrupted sleep due to circadian-rhythm dysfunction. Behavioral therapy can also be used for continuous positive airway pressure (CPAP) desensitization to promote adherence to treatment for patients with sleep-disordered breathing (eg, obstructive sleep apnea).

Behavioral strategies, such as self-monitoring, goal setting, stimulus control, and motivational interviewing, are important as they often target patient barriers to adherence. Goal setting provides patients with a sense of accountability and should include easily measured outcomes. Self-monitoring, which consists of keeping records of eating behaviors and weighing oneself weekly, has been effective in long-term weight control. Patients should be instructed to keep detailed records of all eating behaviors, including specific portion sizes, time and place of eating, stimuli preceding eating, and a description of surroundings. Stimulus control consists of the behavioral change around food choices and food preparation, in addition to visual cues. Distracting activities, such as watching television or reading while eating, are discouraged. Eating behavior is made to be associated with highly specific stimuli. Meal-replacement and partial meal-replacement programs and structured meal plans have been studied and found to be effective as forms of stimulus control.

Motivational interviewing is designed to elicit behavior change by assisting patients in exploring and resolving ambivalence to change. Open-ended questions, reflective listening, affirmations, and summarization are used to help patients explore and resolve ambivalence and barriers to change.

Behavioral treatment is provided on a weekly basis initially and becomes less frequent with time and progress. Group sessions are more effective than individual, enhanced by both social support and healthy competition.[40] The effectiveness of behavioral modification is similar to diet and

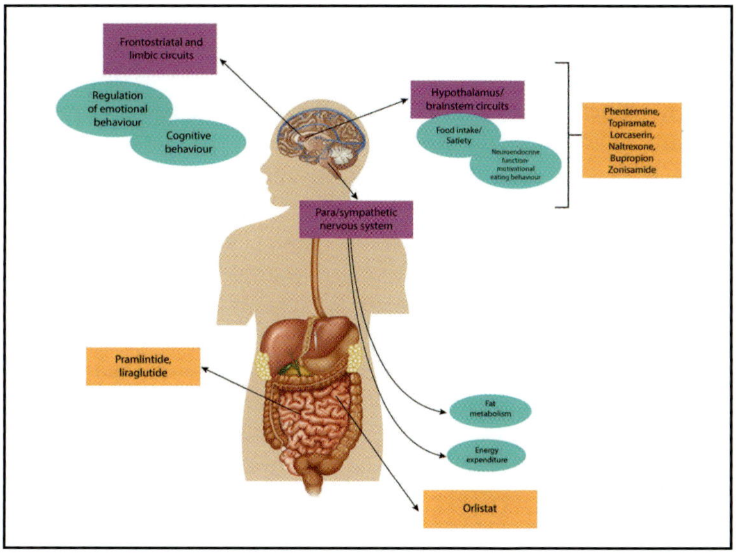

Figure 3-1. Anti-obesity medications target different aspects of the energy regulatory system. (Adapted from Ioannides-Demos LL, Piccenna L, McNeil JJ. Pharmacotherapies for obesity: past, current, and future therapies. *J Obes*. 2011;2011:179674.)

exercise interventions, reaching a modest maximum weight loss at 6 months followed by weight regain once treatment is terminated. Remote counseling (eg, using email, telephone, and web-based interface programs) is comparable to the traditional face-to-face counseling.[41] There are numerous online self-directed programs that can assist patients in monitoring caloric intake, energy expenditure, and sleep duration. Combination therapy involving the addition of a weight loss medication to a comprehensive behavioral modification program has been shown to augment weight loss.[42]

Pharmacotherapy

Biological Basis

As discussed in Principle 1, both sides of the energy balance equation (energy input and energy expenditure) are regulated by identifiable physiologic processes. As these biological pathways that determine energy homeostasis have been uncovered, many molecular targets have emerged for the pharmacologic treatment of obesity. Not surprisingly, the majority of these targets are located in the CNS, the key integrator of peripheral input and regulator of energy expenditure and storage (Figure 3-1). The first physiologic pathways to be targeted by medications were the adrenergic, serotonergic, and dopaminergic neurotransmitter systems.[43] Central increases in these 3 neurotransmitters are known to decrease food intake either through decreasing hunger or increasing satiety (homeostatic pathways) or blunting nonhunger-related drives to eat such as cravings or the "appeal" and "reward" of food (hedonic pathways). Stimulation of the adrenergic system also increases energy expenditure.[43] As described below, some agents have been specifically developed to increase one or more of these neurotransmitters for the purpose of weight loss (eg, phentermine, lorcaserin). Additionally, centrally acting agents approved for other uses (ie, depression or epilepsy) have been found to lower appetitive drive likely through their actions on the same neurotransmitter systems (eg, bupropion). Some of these latter agents are used "off-label" for weight loss by obesity medicine specialists. Other central processes involved in weight regulation are the opioid and cannabinoid receptors.[43] Blocking these receptors by drugs like naltrexone (off-label) or rimonabant (discontinued), respectively, has been shown to promote weight loss. Additionally, γ-aminobutyric acid (GABA) and glutamate have been found to contribute to energy regulation and at least one drug (topiramate) is thought to evoke its weight loss effects through the glutamatergic system.[44] In addition to the neural pathways of energy homeostasis, research has illuminated the hormonal regulation of energy balance, giving rise to investigational drugs such as leptin and amylin analogues.[45] The appetite suppressive effects of GLP-1 analogues approved for the treatment of type 2 diabetes and obesity are now also well known.[46]

As will be discussed, monotherapy with any of the above agents has 2 main limitations: toxicity and low to modest efficacy, both of which are rooted in characteristics of the energy regulatory system. The system is intricate and complex and involves innumerable players, so no 1 or 2 pathways or pharmacologic targets dictate the system. This limits the effect size of single agents; to achieve a clinically significant effect in the drug development phase, weight loss agents are then necessarily pushed to higher doses (ie, they have a narrow therapeutic window and therefore increased rate of side effects). Furthermore, the system is highly redundant and energy efficient, so that manipulating a single neurohumoral pathway often results in counterregulation and an early weight loss plateau. Targeting multiple pathways via combination therapy has the advantage of requiring lower doses of the individual drugs (lowering the rate of side effects) and suppressing counterregulation (increasing the weight loss effect).

Indications

Pharmacotherapy for obesity is considered in adults with a BMI $\geq$ 27 plus one or more obesity-related medical conditions or a BMI $\geq$ 30 who have had an inadequate response to lifestyle and behavior modification.

Efficacy and Effectiveness

Pharmacological agents for obesity, when prescribed with lifestyle interventions in clinical trials, have shown additional weight loss benefit on the scale of 3% to 6% over 1 to 2 years with monotherapy and nearly 10% with combination therapy.[42,47-49] In most cases, the maximal effect appears to occur within the first year of therapy with partial regain of lost weight thereafter. However, the individual response to each medication varies widely; a small percentage (2% to 5%) of patients may achieve significantly more than average weight loss, while the majority (30% to 60%) experience no weight loss.[49,50]

Effectiveness of each agent is based on the ability to achieve 3% to 5% weight loss after 3 months. A proposed guideline suggests using the 4 x 3 rule (ie, losing 4 lb per month for the first 3 months = 12 lb over 3 months).[50] If this short-term goal is not met, discontinuation of the medication should be entertained. Continuation of the agent is recommended in those individuals who respond within the first 3 months. Long-term use is necessary to sustain the weight loss effect as cessation of an effective drug is almost always met with weight regain.

Adverse Effects

Adverse effects from weight loss medications may occur. Therefore, the decision to use weight loss medications should be made for those individuals in whom the benefit exceeds the risk. If side effects are experienced, it is reasonable to reduce the dose of the medication prior to discontinuation. Close monitoring is necessary and may involve vital signs and serology depending on the agent.

Agents

Based on our past understanding of obesity, drug therapy was directed either at appetite suppression or impairment of nutrient absorption with the goal of reducing caloric intake and thus body weight. However, advances in understanding mechanisms of appetite control, energy expenditure, and nutrient sensing promise a host of new, more effective agents (Table 3-5).

Table 3-5
Agents Used for Obesity Treatment

DRUG (BRAND NAME)	EXAMPLE OF USUAL DOSES, STARTING DOSE (DOSAGE RANGE)	SIDE EFFECTS (SE)/ CONTRAINDICATIONS (CI)*	COMMENTS
Diethylpropion (Tenuate)	75 mg QD (75 mg QD ER caps)	SE: Elevated BP/HR, dry mouth, constipation, insomnia, headache CI: CAD, CVA, cardiac arrhythmia, seizures, uncontrolled HTN	• FDA approved for short-term use • Monitor BP, HR • Available in immediate release form but not studied • DEA Schedule IV drug
Liraglutide (Saxenda)	0.6 mg QD (0.6 to 3.0 mg QD)	SE: Nausea, vomiting, hypoglycemia, pancreatitis, C-cell hyperplasia of thyroid CI: Medullary thyroid carcinoma, MEN type II	• FDA approved for long-term use • Injectable medication • Take before meals • Pregnancy Category X
Lorcaserin (Belviq)	10 mg QD (10 to 20 mg QD)	SE: Nasopharyngitis, HA CI: Preexisting depression	• FDA approved for long-term use • Caution in CHF, priapism • Monitor for depression • Pregnancy Category X
Orlistat (Xenical, Alli)	120 mg QD (120 mg QD to TID) Alli (60 mg QD to TID)	SE: Flatulence, diarrhea, bloating/ cramping, liver failure CI: Chronic malabsorption	• FDA approved for long-term use • Advise daily multivitamin • Take with meals • Monitor fat-soluble vitamins • Alli is an OTC form of orlistat

(continued)

Table 3-5 (continued)
Agents Used for Obesity Treatment

DRUG (BRAND NAME)	EXAMPLE OF USUAL DOSES, STARTING DOSE (DOSAGE RANGE)	SIDE EFFECTS (SE)/ CONTRAINDICATIONS (CI)*	COMMENTS
Phentermine (Adipex-P, Ionamin)	15 mg QD (15 to 30 mg QD) ½ tablet of 37.5 mg (37.5 mg tablet QD)	SE: Elevated BP/HR, dry mouth, constipation, insomnia, headache CI: CAD, CVA, cardiac arrhythmia, seizures, uncontrolled HTN	• FDA approved for short-term use • Monitor BP, HR • Inexpensive • Most widely prescribed drug • DEA Schedule IV drug
Phentermine + topiramate (Qsymia)	3.75/23 mg QD (3.75/23 to 15/92 mg QD)	SE: Similar to phentermine and topiramate CI: Similar to phentermine and topiramate	• FDA approved for long-term use • Increased risk of oropalatal clefts • Pregnancy Category X
Naltrexone + bupropion (Contrave)	8/90 mg QD (8/90 to 2 8/90 mg tablets BID)	SE: Constipation, HA, nausea, vomiting, dizziness, insomnia CI: Seizures, bulimia, long-term opioids use	• FDA approved for long-term use • Avoid coadministration with high fat meals • Pregnancy Category X
Off-Label Use for Treatment of Obesity			
Bupropion (Wellbutrin)	150 mg QD (150 to 450 mg QD)	SE: Insomnia, anxiety, HA, diarrhea, dry mouth CI: Seizures, bulimia, cardiac arrythmia	• Monitor HR, BP • Avoid in bipolar disorders • Synergistic combination with naltrexone
Exenatide (Byetta, Bydureon)	5 µg BID (5 to 10 µg BID) Bydureon (2 mg every 7 days)	SE: Nausea, hypoglycemia, pancreatitis CI: Medullary thyroid carcinoma, MEN type II	• Injectable medication • Take before meals • Bydureon is an ER exenatide

(continued)

Table 3-5 (continued)
Agents Used for Obesity Treatment

DRUG (BRAND NAME)	EXAMPLE OF USUAL DOSES, STARTING DOSE (DOSAGE RANGE)	SIDE EFFECTS (SE)/ CONTRAINDICATIONS (CI)*	COMMENTS
Metformin (Glucophage, Glumetza)	500 mg QD (500 to 2000 mg QD)	SE: Nausea, diarrhea, vitamin B_{12} deficiency, lactic acidosis. CI: Renal insufficiency (Cr > 1.4 ng/mL).	• Useful in antipyschotic-induced weight gain • Useful in PCOS • Increased risk of lactic acidosis in combination with topiramate
Pramlintide (Symlin)	60 µg TID (60 to 120 µg TID)	SE: Hypoglycemia, nausea, vomiting, HA CI: Gastroparesis	• Useful in persons with diabetes on insulin • Take before meals
Topiramate (Topamax)	25 mg QD (25 to 150 mg QD)	SE: Paresthesias, taste aversion, somnolence, memory impairment, acute angle glaucoma CI: Kidney stones, glaucoma	• Useful in antipyschotic-induced weight gain • Useful in binge eating • Abrupt withdrawal is not recommended • Increased risk of lactic acidosis in combination with metformin • Pregnancy Category D
Zonisamide (Zonegran)	100 mg QD (100 to 400 mg QD)	SE: Altered taste, HA, impaired memory, gastrointestinal and musculoskeletal problems CI: Sulfa allergy, kidney stones, glaucoma	• Monitor serum Cr • Used in combination with bupropion • Abrupt withdrawal is not recommended

*This is an incomplete list of all the side effects and contraindications of the medications.

BID = 2 times a day, BP = blood pressure, CAD = coronary artery disease, CHF = congestive heart failure, Cr = creatinine, CVA = cerebrovascular accident, HA = headache, HR = heart rate, HTN = hypertension, OTC = over-the-counter, PCOS = polycystic ovary syndrome, QD = daily, TID = 3 times a day.

Although the number of US Food and Drug Administration (FDA)-approved weight loss medications is small, there are several medications approved for other medical conditions that are used off-label for weight loss.

Agents for obesity treatment are chosen based on efficacy, safety, and so-called "double benefit." For example, bupropion may be chosen in patients with obesity who are depressed or need to stop smoking and topiramate may be considered in those who have migraine headaches.

Phentermine and Other Sympathomimetic Agents

Phentermine (Ionamin, Adipex-P) is the most widely prescribed weight loss medication and is one of several sympathomimetics, including diethylpropion (Tenuate), phendimetrazine (Bontril), and benzphetamine (Didrex), that is FDA approved for short-term use. They are grouped together because they act to increase the levels of norepinephrine in the CNS. Early clinical trials of these drugs were generally short as it was thought that obesity was a result of poor behaviors and could be cured with time. As a result, few studies of sympathomimetics have extended beyond 6 months. A meta-analysis of phentermine trials ranging from 2 to 24 weeks showed an average of 3.6 kg (confidence interval [CI], 0.6 to 6.0 kg) of additional weight loss over placebo.[51] One of the longest trials compared intermittent and continuous use of phentermine vs placebo for 36 weeks. Although both regimens of phentermine produced weight loss over placebo, there was no significant difference in weight loss between continuous and intermittent dosing.[52] In a recent 1-year trial, diethylpropion produced modest sustained weight loss over placebo, with maximum effect at 6 months.[53] These medications are only approved for short-term use (interpreted as up to 12 weeks of treatment), but clinical experts often continue treatment in those who have an early therapeutic response.

The adverse effect profile of sympathomimetic drugs includes dry mouth, insomnia, nervousness, palpitations, hypertension, and constipation. Due to potential elevations in blood pressure and heart rate, these agents are contraindicated in persons with hyperthyroidism, coronary heart disease, and tachyarrhythmias. Although phentermine was used in combination with fenfluramine (a nonspecific serotonergic agent associated with valvular heart disease), it alone has not been independently associated with heart valve issues (see discussion below on lorcaserin). Phentermine and diethylpropion are classified by the US Drug Enforcement Agency as Schedule IV drugs, indicating their potential for abuse, although this potential appears to be low. Benzphetamine and phendimetrazine are Schedule III drugs and are considered to have a substantially higher potential for abuse than the Schedule IV drugs. Careful prescribing and monitoring are essential.[54]

Lorcaserin

In 2012, a selective serotonin 2c (5-HT2c) receptor agonist, lorcaserin (Belviq), became the first drug approved by the FDA for long-term weight loss in over a decade. This agent has a high affinity for the 5-HT2c receptor that is found predominantly in the CNS and is not expressed in heart valves. In 1997, the nonspecific serotonergic weight loss agents fenfluramine and dexfenfluramine were withdrawn from the market due to valvular heart disease.[55] Subsequent analysis of 5-HT receptors and several drugs that are known or suspected to cause heart valve disease including fenfluramine implicated the 5-HT2b receptor subtype as the likely target involved in the pathogenesis of medication-induced valvulopathy. Thus, research shifted to studying the 5-HT2c receptor, and hence the creation of lorcaserin. Three placebo-controlled clinical trials of lorcaserin[56-58] have not reported an increased risk of valvulopathy or other adverse cardiovascular events. These trials did show a 3.5% to 4.0% placebo-subtracted weight loss with lorcaserin. The BLOOM-DM trial also showed a 0.5% drop in the hemoglobin A1c (HbA1c) in persons with type 2 diabetes.

The adverse effect profile of lorcaserin includes nasopharyngitis, dizziness, and upper respiratory infections. Although there were concerns over an increase in mammary tumors in animals on lorcaserin, this was associated with toxic doses of lorcaserin in early phase trials and not found in human participants. Caution should be used in patients with congestive heart failure and depression, in particular those taking selective serotonin reuptake inhibitors, as there may be a small but significant risk of serotonin syndrome. High cost may be a barrier to the selection of this agent.

Orlistat

Orlistat (Xenical, Alli) is a potent and selective inhibitor of pancreatic and gastric lipases, inhibiting absorption of approximately 30% of ingested fat. A meta-analysis of 1-year orlistat trials reported a mean of 2.89 kg (CI, 2.27 to 3.51 kg) of additional weight loss over placebo.[51] A 4-year double-blinded, randomized placebo-controlled trial with orlistat demonstrated a modest 2.8% placebo-subtracted weight reduction along with some improvements in lipid profile, HbA1c, and insulin levels.[59]

Orlistat is not absorbed, and therefore its adverse effects are mostly related to its pharmacological action. Adverse gastrointestinal effects, including abdominal cramps, flatulence, and oily stools, are common initially, but subside as patients learn to use the drug. Although a high-fat diet may serve as a potential indication for the use of orlistat, there is no evidence that it is more effective in patients with high-fat diets. Its high cost and the potential malabsorption of both healthy fats (monounsaturated and polyunsaturated fats) and fat-soluble vitamins may lower the priority of its selection. Although vitamin deficiencies are uncommon, patients should be instructed to take a daily multivitamin 2 hours before or after orlistat.

Liraglutide

The 3.0-mg dose of liraglutide (Saxenda) was approved in December 2014 for chronic weight management and is a higher dose of liraglutide (Victoza), already approved for second-line treatment of type 2 diabetes. Liraglutide is a GLP-1 agonist that shares 97% homology to native GLP-1 extending the circulating half-life of GLP-1 from 1 to 2 minutes to 13 hours.[60] GLP-1 is a hormone secreted by the L-cells in the intestine in response to food intake that decreases glucose levels through stimulation of insulin secretion and inhibition of glucagon secretion and gluconeogenesis. It also delays gastric emptying and increases satiety, through stimulations of pro-opiomelanocortin (POMC) neurons in the arcuate nucleus, which may be responsible for the reduction in calories. However, its mechanism of weight loss is not clear.

Two past randomized studies have demonstrated a 6% placebo-subtracted weight loss with 3.0 mg liraglutide,[46,61] which is comparable to other approved anti-obesity medications. This was confirmed by a recent study in nondiabetics that showed a 5.4% placebo-subtracted weight loss and significant improvements in cardiometabolic factors (eg, blood pressure, waist circumference, and fasting insulin).[62]

Common side effects are gastrointestinal complaints, specifically nausea, which subside with time. There are concerns regarding postmarketing findings of pancreatitis and pancreatic cancer that require further research to determine causality.

Other Obesity Agents

Several drugs approved for other indications have been shown in clinical trials to produce weight loss and add to the list of available agents to consider in obesity treatment. Selection of one of these medications for use in obesity may depend on its potential "double benefit" in addition to its efficacy. These agents include anticonvulsants (topiramate and zonisamide), antidepressants (bupropion), antidiabetic medications (metformin, exenatide, and pramlintide), and an opioid receptor antagonist (naltrexone). Some of these will be discussed here.

Topiramate

Topiramate (Topamax) is a weak carbonic anhydrase inhibitor approved for epilepsy, migraine prophylaxis, and mood stabilization. In addition, topiramate has been studied in the treatment of alcoholism,[63] binge-eating,[64] and medication-induced weight gain.[65] Its effects on weight loss and food intake were first noted as a side effect in the clinical trials for the treatment of epilepsy. The precise mechanism of action behind weight loss is not clear, but may be related to a reduction in compulsive or addictive food craving via antagonism of α-amino-3-hydroxy-5-methyl-4-isoxazolepropionic acid (AMPA) receptors and kainate receptors, decreased lipogenesis and modification of food taste via inhibition of carbonic anhydrase isoenzymes, and increased energy expenditure via activation of GABA receptors.[66] A meta-analysis of topiramate randomized controlled trials reported a 5.34 kg (CI, 4.56 to 6.12 kg) additional weight loss over placebo.[67] Efficacy was associated with duration of the trial and dose of topiramate. Common adverse effects including paresthesias, taste perversion, and cognitive impairment are also dose dependent (more frequent with doses above 96 mg/day), but some of these effects may resolve with time. Gradual titration of topiramate is recommended from a starting dose of 25 mg/day to an effective dose not exceeding 150 mg/day, and careful monitoring should be considered.

Zonisamide

Zonisamide (Zonegran), an anti-epileptic drug with serotonergic and dopaminergic effects, has not been extensively investigated in the treatment of obesity. Like topiramate, zonisamide's weight loss effects were first noted as a side effect in clinical trials for epilepsy. In 2003, a double-blinded randomized controlled trial demonstrated 6.6% weight loss in the zonisamide group. However, there were several limitations including small study size, short duration, and poor placebo response.[68] A recent 1-year trial reported a 3.3-kg placebo-subtracted weight loss with 400 mg/day of zonisamide; however, the 200 mg/day dose was not superior to placebo.

Although zonisamide demonstrated moderate efficacy of a magnitude similar to orlistat and lorcaserin, adverse events occurred at a higher frequency relative to placebo.[69] Common adverse effects include somnolence, headache, fatigue, nausea/vomiting, and language and speech problems. A small but significant increase in creatinine has been reported.

Bupropion

Bupropion (Wellbutrin, Zyban) is a norepinephrine and dopamine reuptake inhibitor that is approved for the treatment of depression and smoking cessation. The modest weight loss seen in patients receiving bupropion therapy has been attributed to its stimulatory effect on POMC-producing neurons in the arcuate nucleus of the hypothalamus.[70] A meta-analysis of 3 studies in participants with depression or depressive symptoms treated with bupropion showed a mean additional weight loss of 2.77 kg (CI, 1.1 to 4.5 kg) in the bupropion group over placebo.[51] However, inclusion of both 6-month and 1-year duration studies, varying doses, and inconsistent control groups decreased the sensitivity of the analysis. One of these studies[71] in uncomplicated patients showed maintenance of weight after 1 year on 300 or 400 mg/day of bupropion. Nondepressed patients may respond to bupropion with weight loss to a greater extent than depressed patients.

Bupropion has also been studied in combination with zonisamide. One small phase II study concluded the combination (bupropion 200 mg/d and zonisamide 400 mg/d) was more effective (7.5% vs 1.2% body weight loss) and had less drop-out rates (22% vs 44%) than zonisamide monotherapy.[72]

Dry mouth, insomnia, headaches, nausea, and anxiety are reported as the most common side effects.

Metformin

Metformin (Glucophage) is a biguanide that is approved for the treatment of diabetes mellitus. It acts by increasing insulin sensitivity, reducing hepatic glucose production, and reducing intestinal absorption of carbohydrates. In the evaluation of metformin's weight loss effects, additional mechanisms of action related to the induction of an anorectic and lipolytic effect as well as a decrease in leptin levels have been noted. Studies primarily evaluating the weight loss effects of metformin compared with placebo have been small and short in duration.[73] However, metformin has been shown to produce a modest but durable weight loss (mean 2.5 kg or 2% body weight loss) in patients with prediabetes after 10 years, with enhanced weight loss effects dependent on adherence to the medication.[74] Furthermore, other studies demonstrate that metformin can attenuate weight gain in patients with diabetes on insulin or sulfonylureas[75] and in patients on antipsychotic medications.[76,77] Metformin is well tolerated with gastrointestinal complaints (abdominal pain, dysgeusia, diarrhea) cited as the most common adverse effects. Lactic acidosis is a serious, but rare, side effect that may occur in those with renal impairment. Metformin has been used in nondiabetics without the induction of hypoglycemia.

Pramlintide

Pramlintide (Symlin) is a synthetic analogue of amylin, a hormone that is co-secreted from pancreatic ß-cells with insulin in response to nutrient stimuli. It is approved for the treatment of diabetes mellitus and has been found to produce weight loss compared to placebo. A meta-analysis showed statistically significant weight loss over placebo in patients with type 2 diabetes and obesity (-2.27 kg, CI -2.88, -1.66 kg) and nondiabetics with obesity (-2.27 kg, CI -2.88, -1.66 kg).[78] The most common adverse effect is nausea, and there is no significant increased risk of hypoglycemia.

Combination Therapies

A better understanding of the complex system of redundant physiological pathways of energy regulation and an only modest weight loss benefit from single-agent clinical trials has led to focused efforts on combination therapies. The aim of combination therapy is to enhance effectiveness while limiting toxicity through dose reduction. Several combinations have been evaluated in clinical trials, 2 have been approved.

Phentermine/Topiramate

The combination of phentermine and topiramate-extended release (Qsymia) was approved in 2012 and has produced the greatest weight loss effect of any obesity agent. Clinical trials demonstrate a greater than 10% weight loss at 1 year with sustained weight loss after 2 years.[48,79] Contraindications and adverse effects are similar to the summation of the individual agents as described above. Women of childbearing age should be cautioned of the increased risk of orofacial clefts in the fetus with the use of this medication. This medication is prescribed with a starting 3.75 mg phentermine/23-mg topiramate dose for 2 weeks before titrating up to a 7.5-mg/46-mg dose.

Bupropion/Naltrexone

The combination of naltrexone HCl plus bupropion HCl (Contrave) was approved by the FDA for weight loss in September 2014. The weight loss effect of the drug is based on the combined mechanisms of action of bupropion and naltrexone on the hypothalamic melanocortin system and the mesolimbic dopamine reward system. The mechanism of action of bupropion is described in a separate paragraph. Naltrexone is a centrally acting opioid receptor antagonist and is approved for alcohol and opioid dependence. By blocking the auto-inhibitory opioid-mediated negative feedback that suppresses POMC firing (a compensatory effect stimulated by bupropion) naltrexone enhances the effects of bupropion, and their combined effect is additive compared to monotherapy of the individual drugs.[80]

Four 56-week randomized placebo-controlled trials—Contrave Obesity Research (COR)-I,[81] COR-II,[82] COR–Behavior Modification (COR-BMOD),[83] and COR–Diabetes (COR-D)[84]—were conducted to evaluate the efficacy of naltrexone/bupropion. In patients without diabetes, the placebo-subtracted weight loss ranged from 4.2% in the COR-BMOD to 4.8% in the COR-I trial using the highest dose (32 mg/360 mg) of naltrexone/bupropion SR. In patients with diabetes, the placebo-subtracted weight loss results of 3.2% were less effective; however, there was a greater decrease in HbA1c in the naltrexone/bupropion group 0.6% compared to the placebo arm 0.1%.[85]

The most common adverse effect experienced in those on naltrexone/bupropion was nausea, followed by constipation, headache, vomiting, and dizziness. Due to the bupropion component, there is a black box warning on the package insert for the potential increased risk for suicidality and potential increased risk for neuropsychiatric symptoms in individuals taking bupropion for smoking cessation.

Emerging Field of Weight Loss Devices

Over the past decade, the field of obesity therapeutics has expanded considerably in the device development arena, with a focus on the gastrointestinal tract. After the failure of several early devices, many have been approved for clinical trials in the United States and 3 have recently been approved for use in 2015 (Table 3-6). Two of the FDA-approved devices are gastric balloons that are placed endoscopically and filled with saline. They promote satiety and weight loss by occupying space in the stomach. In the United States, the Orbera single balloon and ReShape dual balloon systems are approved for use for 6 months in conjunction with a supervised diet and exercise program in individuals with a BMI between 30 and 40 who have failed prior lifestyle therapy. In their respective pivotal clinical trials comparing the balloon plus diet and exercise to diet and exercise alone at 6 months, Orbera led to 10.5% weight loss vs 4.7% in the control group, and ReShape demonstrated 25% excess weight loss compared to 11.3% in the control group. Potential side effects with gastric balloons include nausea, vomiting, abdominal pain, gastric ulcers, indigestion, and balloon migration with obstruction. Gastric balloons are contraindicated in pregnancy and in individuals with previous gastrointestinal or bariatric surgery, inflammatory intestinal or bowel disease, large hiatal hernia, symptoms consistent with delayed gastric emptying, or active *Helicobacter pylori* infection. Balloons should also be avoided in patients on anticoagulants, aspirin, or anti-inflammatory agents.

The third device approved for use in the United States is a rechargeable electrical stimulator (Maestro, EnteroMedics). This device intermittently blocks afferent vagal signals from the gastrointestinal tract to the brain. The afferent vagus is involved in regulating hunger and satiety but the precise mechanism of weight loss with the device is unknown. The device is approved for use in individuals with a BMI > 40, or BMI between 35 and 39.9 with at least one obesity-related comorbidity, who have failed a supervised weight loss attempt in the past 5 years. Clinical trial results demonstrated 8.5% greater excess weight loss at 12 months with gastric electrical stimulation compared to control. Potential side effects include pain at neuroregulator site, nausea, vomiting, abdominal pain, heartburn, problems swallowing, belching, and chest pain. The device is contraindicated in the setting of cirrhosis, portal hypertension, esophageal varices, or clinically significant hiatal hernia. It is also contraindicated in patients needing magnetic resonance imaging or those with another permanently implanted electrically powered medical device or prosthesis.

In addition to the devices that focus on increasing satiety via manipulation of the stomach, there are 2 devices in clinical trials (the endoluminal sleeve and gastric aspiration) that are aimed at intestinal nutrient absorption and signaling. The practitioner treating obesity should anticipate the addition of more weight loss devices to the therapeutic options that will be available for patients in the future. For appropriate medical management, clinicians will need to be well versed in the efficacy and side effect profile of each device to be able to appropriately channel patients to the best therapy, monitor their prognosis, and optimize on the full potential of device therapy using multimodal combinatorial approaches.

Table 3-6

Weight Loss Devices

CATEGORY	EXAMPLES	COMPANY	MECHANISM	STATUS
Endoluminal sleeve	EndoBarrier	GI Dynamics	Reduces contact between nutrients and proximal intestinal lumen, likely altering gastrointestinal pathways involved in energy regulation	In US clinical trials Approved in Europe and Australia
Gastric aspiration	AspireAssist	Aspire Bariatrics	Reduces intestinal nutrient absorption (and possibly nutrient signaling) by removal of about 30% of stomach contents after every meal via a G-tube device	In US clinical trials Approved in Europe and Middle East
Gastroplasty	Transoral gastroplasty (TOGA)	Satiety	Decreases stomach size by the creation of a small gastric pouch along the lesser curvature using endoscopic stapling devices	Failed clinical trial
Gastric pacemakers	Maestro	EnteroMedics	Vagal blocking to reduce gastric emptying and increase satiety	Approved in US
		IntraPace		Approved in Europe
Gastric balloons	Orbera balloon	Apollo Endosurgery	Fills a large portion of the stomach and may thereby increase satiety	Approved in US
	ReShape dual balloon	ReShape Medical		Approved in US
	Adjustable balloon	Spatz FGIA		In US clinical trials Approved in Europe, parts of Asia, Africa, and South America
Gastric compression	Prevail System	Vibrynt	Device shaped like a stomach that is implanted next to the real stomach to compress it	Approved for trial
Gastric capsule	Expandable gel capsule	Gelesis	After swallowing, capsule expands in the stomach filling a large portion of the stomach and possibly increasing satiety	In US clinical trials

Indications for Referral

Behavioral modification and lifestyle interventions for obesity are only effective in a small percentage of patients seeking weight loss. When to refer a patient to a dietician or a multidisciplinary weight loss clinic (consisting of one or more of the following providers: dietician, psychologist, exercise trainer, obesity medicine specialist, bariatric surgeon) is not clear, but should be considered in patients with medically complex obesity who are resistant to lifestyle modification or when more intensive weight loss treatments (eg, VLCDs, pharmacotherapy, or weight loss surgery) are required. Other patient populations who may benefit from a referral to an obesity medicine specialist include patients seeking weight loss before surgery (general, orthopedic, transplantation), women requiring weight loss before pregnancy or in vitro fertilization, patients with psychotropic drug-induced weight gain, and those who have a BMI > 60.

Although current guidelines state weight loss surgery should be considered in patients with Class III obesity (BMI > 40) or Class II obesity (BMI 35 to 39.9) with a medical comorbidity (eg, diabetes, hypertension, dyslipidemia), those patients with Class II obesity with an overall poor quality of life due to physical disabilities should also be considered. If weight loss surgery is considered, a referral directed toward a practice with a multidisciplinary team is suggested.

Weight Stigma

Physicians managing patients with obesity should be aware of the prevalence of weight bias, the impact of weight bias on their patients, and proactive measures they can take to address bias in the health care setting. Weight bias, or weight stigma, is negative judgments of an overweight or obese individual that may result in unfair treatment, prejudice, and/or discrimination. The judgments are often based on false stereotypes of overweight or obese individuals being incompetent, lazy, or lacking in self-discipline. Weight stigma is pervasive in society for several reasons, including our cultural values of thinness, our perception of health as a solely personal responsibility, which leads to blaming the patient for being overweight or obese, and widespread negative portrayals of obesity in the media.[86] Not to mention, it is still an "acceptable" form of discrimination with no legal consequence in contrast to age, gender, and racial discrimination.[87]

There are many forms of weight bias in the community, some leading to significant disparities in education, employment, and socioeconomic status for individuals with obesity.[88] Substantial research also shows that weight bias is prevalent in the health care setting with one study reporting that more than two-thirds of patients have experienced weight bias from their doctor. Weight bias is also prevalent among medical students, nurses, dieticians, and psychologists. Importantly, patients seeking surgical treatment for obesity have reported weight bias from both medical and nonmedical staff at bariatric clinics. Research has also shown that physicians specializing in the field of obesity exhibit anti-fat bias. Among the most common biases held by physicians is that patients with obesity do not lose weight due to characterological flaws and they are noncompliant and therefore sicker. However, there are many other subtle and overt forms of bias as highlighted in Table 3-7.[88]

The physician has an ethical responsibility to understand and address weight bias because such bias has been shown to have a profound impact on a patient's life and well-being. Weight bias has been shown to lead to underutilization of health care by individuals with obesity.[88] Women with obesity in particular have been found to get less preventative medical care, including cervical, breast, and colorectal cancer screening, even though the incidence of these conditions is higher with obesity.[88] Patients will often not return to the same physician or will avoid medical visits in general if they have faced stigma in the medical setting. Weight bias also has a strong psychological impact and has been independently correlated to depression, anxiety, poor body image, low

Table 3-7

Manifestations of Weight Bias in the Medical Setting

TYPES OF WEIGHT BIAS IN HEALTH CARE	EXAMPLES
Attitudes	• Obese patients are lazy, lacking in self-discipline, and noncompliant
Language	• Obese, morbid, fat, recidivism
Behavior	• Negative comments or facial gestures while weighing patients; weighing patients in a nonprivate setting
Built environment • Office environment • Medical equipment	• Small waiting room chairs, small doorways and hallways • Lack of appropriately sized patient gowns, examination tables, blood pressure cuffs, speculums, scales, stretchers, wheelchairs, and radiologic equipment

self-esteem, and suicidal ideation and action. The social consequences of bias include barriers in education and employment, avoidance of social settings, and stigma in interpersonal relationships with peers, family, and romantic partners. Weight stigma also has a physical impact and impairs weight loss since patients who experience bias tend to engage in unhealthy eating patterns, avoid physical activity, and drop out of weight loss programs.[88]

As a practitioner treating obesity, the first step in addressing weight bias is to become self-aware of one's own prejudices and attitudes regarding weight.[89] Next, understanding the biological basis of obesity and the complex multifactorial etiology of the disease allows one to overcome the assumption that the lack of weight loss is due to a characterological flaw (such as laziness, lack of willpower, or nonadherence). This, in turn, leads to more effective and empathetic communication in which the role of many contributing factors and strategies to address those factors are explored. When discussing weight with a patient, using patient-first language is important and one should avoid stigmatizing terms such as *fat, obese,* and *morbid*.[90] Moreover, patients should be weighed in private with consent, and judgmental gestures, expressions, and comments must be avoided.[91] Creating an office environment that addresses the needs of patients with obesity is critical. This includes appropriate weigh scales, examination tables, toilets, chairs, and blood pressure cuffs. It also includes educating and training all staff (medical and nonmedical).[91] Finally, given the disparities in preventative care, the physician should address breast, cervical, and colorectal cancer screening in patients with obesity. Addressing weight bias in these ways is likely to contribute to the success of the doctor-patient relationship, the outcome of weight loss therapy, and the patient's self-perception and overall well-being.

Addressing Weight Issues After Bariatric Surgery

Suboptimal Response

Gastrointestinal weight loss surgery is currently the most effective treatment for moderate to severe obesity. However, similar to other weight loss treatments like behavioral and pharmacologic interventions, there is a broad range of weight loss response to surgery (see Principle 5). There is a subpopulation of patients who have a suboptimal response to surgical intervention. Tackling obesity in this population after the current best and most invasive treatment fails can be challenging for the medical provider.

Although the composite of several factors, such as patient compliance with postoperative appointments, decreased physical activity, higher initial BMI, diabetes, and lower educational level, has been found to predict weight loss response to RYGB, each factor on its own accounts for a surprisingly small proportion of the variation in surgical response.[92] Since RYGB exerts its effects through neurohumoral mechanisms, biology and therefore genetics play a strong role in the response to surgery.[9] Thus, the appropriate approach to patients who have a suboptimal response to weight loss surgery is usually not surgical revision, such as a longer bypass or a smaller gastric pouch. The former is associated with significant morbidity and mortality due to protein malnutrition,[93-95] while the latter has not proven to be beneficial.[96,97] Nor should treatment in this population be limited to monotherapy with behavioral/lifestyle interventions since often the reason surgery was pursued is that such interventions alone were not adequate. To address the neurohumoral dysregulation in energy balance that is not adequately reversed by a surgical intervention, trials of pharmacotherapy coupled with a healthy lifestyle are indicated.

There are currently no published data guiding providers toward one pharmacotherapeutic agent over another for poor surgical responders. However, in our experience, off-label use of topiramate in this population has shown weight loss benefit with some patients having markedly increased feelings of satiety even on small doses (25 to 75 mg). Such subjective responses appeared to mimic the immediate post-surgical symptoms of fullness and nausea that were absent in these patients, indicating that RYGB and topiramate may have additive or synergistic effects that need to be further explored.

Weight Regain

In addition to the small group of patients that has a suboptimal response to surgery, there is a much larger group of patients that experiences weight regain after surgery. Due to inconsistent definitions of excessive weight regain in the literature it is difficult to quantify the true prevalence of this issue. Weight regain often has a multifactorial etiology and requires targeted history, examination, and diagnostic testing to determine its most likely causes. The factors leading to weight regain can be divided into the following categories as described in Table 3-8: behavioral, psychological, anatomic, iatrogenic, and biological. Anatomic causes vary by the type of surgery. In the case of laparoscopic adjustable gastric band, weight regain may occur due to the patient's failure to follow up for proper band adjustment, enlargement of the gastric pouch, or proximal slippage of the band.[98-103] The latter 2 may be treated by band deflation and follow-up, although proximal slippage can also require surgical repositioning or removal.[98-103] For vertical sleeve gastrectomy, the size of the gastric sleeve is thought to be related to weight regain and as the sleeve may expand over time it has been suggested that one should evaluate for sleeve dilation with an upper endoscopy or upper gastrointestinal series.[98,104,105] For RYGB, it is often thought that dilation of the pouch may lead to weight regain, yet surgical intervention to correct the pouch size does not often lead to weight loss.[96-98,106] Enlargement of the stoma is an anatomic factor that has been most independently associated with weight regain and yet surgical correction of the stoma size does not often lead to weight loss either.[98,106-108] Gastrogastric fistulas can form between the remnant stomach and pouch essentially causing a reversal of the bypass as some food would pass through the fistula into the remnant stomach and down the bypassed intestinal limb. Gastrogastric fistulas should be considered if there is a history of ulcers and symptoms of sudden return of hunger and decreased satiety. There is some weight loss with surgical correction of gastrogastric fistulas. However, surprisingly, surgical correction does not lead to 100% loss of the regained weight.[98,109-111]

Table 3-8

Addressing Obesity After Weight Loss Surgery

CATEGORIES OF REGAIN OR SUBOPTIMAL WEIGHT LOSS	EXAMPLES	TREATMENT
Behavioral	Decreased physical activity, poor diet, disrupted or inadequate sleep, increased stress	Behavioral lifestyle intervention focused on physical activity, diet, sleep, or stress as indicated
Psychological	Depression, bipolar disorder, binge eating disorder	Treat underlying condition; avoid or change weight gain-promoting psychotropic medication whenever possible; consider adding weight loss promoting psychotropic medication if indicated (eg, bupropion, topiramate)
Anatomic	Staple line disruption, gastrogastric fistula	Referral to surgeon for consideration of surgical repair; in the case of gastrogastric fistulas, repair often does not reverse all weight regain, and weight loss medications may be considered as adjunctive treatment
Iatrogenic	Medications (eg, risperidone)	Discontinue or switch medication whenever possible; if not possible, consider adding a weight loss medication to counter the effects of the weight-promoting drug
Biological	Poor initial response to surgery	After weight stabilization, consider adding weight loss medication to achieve additive or synergistic effect with surgery

Behavioral factors leading to weight regain may include dietary indiscretion, such as poor food choices and grazing behaviors, physical inactivity, and sleep disruption.[98] Dietary indiscretion with maladaptive eating may in turn be due to psychological stressors or biologic issues such as reactive hypoglycemia.[98,112-117] Since physical activity is critical to weight maintenance, a decrease or halting of activity over time is a common contributor to regain.[92,118] Insufficient and/or fragmented sleep contributes to weight gain in the general population and should be screened for as it may lead to regain in surgical patients as well.[119]

A strong linear correlation has been found between the number of psychiatric diagnoses and weight regain.[120,121] The mechanisms underlying this correlation have not been teased out but may include maladaptive eating as aforementioned, the impact of psychological stress on energy regulation, or weight-promoting psychotropic medication.[98] In general, weight gain-promoting medications are the main iatrogenic cause of weight regain after surgery. Changes in medications should always be screened for in a patient with regain.

Finally, as with suboptimal weight loss, weight regain may be neurohumorally mediated. Increased fasting and post-prandial ghrelin levels have been correlated with a return of hunger in post-surgical patients.[98] Just as the initial neurohumoral effects of surgery determine the initial weight loss response, variations in long-term neurohumoral changes may be involved in the phenomenon of weight regain.[98]

References

1. Pollan M. *Cooked.* London, England: The Penguin Press; 2013.
2. Friedman JM. Obesity: causes and control of excess body fat. *Nature.* 2009;459:340-342.
3. Trayhurn P. The biology of obesity. *Proceedings of the Nutrition Society.* 2005;1:31-38.
4. Wozniak SE, Gee LL, Wachtel MS, Frezza EE. Adipose tissue: the new endocrine organ? A review article. *Dig Dis Sci.* 2009;54:1847-1856.
5. Suzuki K, Simpson KA, Minnion JS, Shillito JC, Bloom SR. The role of gut hormones and the hypothalamus in appetite regulation. *Endocr J.* 2010;57:359-372.
6. Pedersen BK, Febbraio, MA. Muscles, exercise and obesity: skeletal muscle as a secretory organ. *Nature Reviews Endocrinology.* 2012;8:457-465.
7. Saper CB, Chou TC, Elmquist JK. The need to feed: homeostatic and hedonic control of eating. *Neuron.* 2002;36:199-211.
8. Myers MG, Cowley MA, Münzberg H. Mechanisms of leptin action and leptin resistance. *Annu Rev Physiol.* 2008;70:537-556.
9. Hatoum IJ, Greenawalt DM, Cotsapas C, Reitman ML, Daly MJ, Kaplan LM. Heritability of the weight loss response to gastric bypass surgery. *J Clin Endocrinol Metab.* 2011;96:E1630-E1633.
10. Smith SR, Prosser WA, Donahue DJ, et al, APD356-004 Study Group. Lorcaserin (APD356), a selective 5-HT2C agonist, reduces body weight in obese men and women. *Obesity.* 2009;17:494-503.
11. Gardner CD. Tailoring dietary approaches for weight loss. *Int J Obes.* 2012;2:S11-S15.
12. Cornier M-A, Depres J-P, Davis N, et al. Assessing adiposity: a scientific statement from the American Heart Association. *Circulation.* 2011;124:1996.
13. De Lorenzo A, Del Gobbo V, Premrov MG, et al. Normal-weight obese syndrome: early inflammation? *Am J Clin Nutr.* 2007;85:40-45.
14. Nedeltcheva AV, Kilkus JM, Imperial J, et al. Insufficient sleep undermines dietary efforts to reduce adiposity. *Ann Intern Med.* 2010;153:435-441.
15. Silk AW, McTigue KM. Reexamining the physical examination for obese patients. *JAMA.* 2011;305:193-194.
16. Jensen MD, Ryan DH, Apovian CM, et al. 2013 AHA/ACC/TOS guideline for the management of overweight and obesity in adults: a report of the American College of Cardiology/American Heart Association Task Force on practice guidelines and the Obesity Society. *J Am Coll Cardiol.* 2013: doi:10.1016/j.jacc.2013.11.004.
17. Casazza K, Fontaine KR, Astrup A, et al. Myths, presumptions and facts about obesity. *N Engl J Med.* 2013;368:446-454.
18. Post RE, Mainous AG, Gregorie SH, et al. The influence of physician acknowledgement of paitents' weight status on patient persceptions of overweight and obesity in the United States. *Arch Int Med.* 2011;171:316-321.
19. Knowler WC, Fowler SE, Hamman RF, et al, Diabetes Prevention Program Research Group. 10-year follow-up of diabetes incidence and weight loss in the Diabetes Prevention Program Outcomes Study. *Lancet.* 2009;374:1677-1686.
20. Look AHEAD Research Group. Eight-year weight losses with an intensive lifestyle intervention: the Look AHEAD study. *Obesity.* 2014;22:5-13.
21. Leibel RL, Rosenbaum M, Hirsch J. Changes in energy expenditure resulting from altered body weight. *N Engl J Med.* 1995;332:621-628.
22. Sumithran P, Prendergast LA, Delbridge E, et al. Long-term persistence of hormonal adaptations to weight loss. *N Engl J Med.* 2011;365:1597-604.
23. Westerterp-Plantenga MS, Lemmons SG, Westerterp KR. Dietary protein: its role in satiety, energetics, weight loss and health. *Br J Nutr.* 2012;108:S105-S112.
24. Bray GA, Smith SR, de Jonge L, et al. Effect of dietary protein content on weight gain, energy expenditure, and body composition during overeating. *JAMA.* 2012;307:47-55.
25. Estruch R, Ros E, Salas-Salvado J, et al. Primary prevention of cardiovascular disease with Mediterranean diet. *N Engl J Med.* 2013;368:1279-1290.

26. Dansinger ML, Gleason JA, Griffith JL, et al. Comparison of the Atkins, Ornish, Weight Watchers, and Zone diets for weight loss and heart disease risk reduction: a randomized trial. *JAMA.* 2005;293:43-53.
27. Sacks FM, Bray GA, Carey VJ, et al. Comparison of weight-loss diets with different compositions of fat, protein, and carbohydrates. *N Engl J Med.* 2009;360:859-873.
28. Franz MJ, Van Wormer JJ, Crain AL, et al. Weight-loss outcomes: a systematic review and meta-analysis of weight-loss clinical trials with a minimum 1-year follow-up. *J Am Diet Assoc.* 2007;107:1755-1767.
29. Tsai AG, Wadden TA. Systematic review: an evaluation of major commercial weight loss programs in the United States. *Ann Intern Med.* 2005;142:56-66.
30. National Task Force on the Prevention and Treatment of Obesity. Very-low-calorie diets. *JAMA.* 1993;270:967-974.
31. Swift DL, Johannsen NM, Lavie CJ. The role of exercise and physical activity in weight loss. *Progress in Cardiovascular Diseases.* 2014;56:441-447.
32. Lee D, Sui X, Artero EG, et al. Long-term effects of changes in cardiorespiratory fitness and body mass index on all-cause and cardiovascular disease mortality in men: the Aerobics Center Longitudinal Study. *Circulation.* 2011;124:2483-2490.
33. McKary RA, Feskanish D, Hu F, et al. Physical activity in relation to long-term weight maintenance after intentional weight loss in premenopausal women. *Obesity.* 2010;18:167-174.
34. Garber CE, Blissmer B, Deschenes MR. Quantity and quality of exercise for developing and maintaining cardiorespiratory, musculoskeletal, and neuromotor fitness in apparently healthy adults: guidance for prescribing exercise. *Med Sci Sports Exerc.* 2011;43:1334-1359.
35. Jakicic JM, Marcus BH, Gallagher KI, et al. Effect of exercise duration and intensity on weight loss in overweight, sedentary women: a randomized trial. *JAMA.* 2003;290:1323-1330.
36. Church TS, Earnest CP, Skinner JS, Blair SN. Effects of different doses of physical activity on cardiorespiratory fitness among sedentary, overweight or obese postmenopausal women with elevated blood pressure: a randomized controlled trial. *JAMA.* 2007;297(19):2081-2091.
37. Melanson EL, Keadle JE, Donnelly B, et al. Resistance to exercise-induced weight loss: compensatory behavioral adaptations. *Med Sci Sports Exerc.* 2013;45:1600-1609.
38. Levine JA. Non-exercise activity thermogenesis (NEAT): environment and biology. *Am J Physiol Endocrinol Metab.* 2004;286:E675-E685.
39. Butryn ML, Webb V, Wadden TA. Behavioral treatment for obesity. *Psychiatr Clin North Am.* 2011;34(4):841-859.
40. Butryn ML, Phelan S, Hill JO, et al. Consistent self-monitoring of weight: a key component of successful weight loss maintenance. *Obesity.* 2007;15:3091-3096.
41. Appel JA, Clark JM, Yeh J-C, et al. Comparative effectiveness of weight loss interventions in clinical practice. *N Engl J Med.* 2011;365:1959-1968.
42. Wadden TA, Berkowitz RI, Womble LG, et al. Randomized trial of lifestyle modification and pharmacotherapy for obesity. *N Engl J Med.* 2005;353:2111-2120.
43. Rodgers RJ, Tschop MH, Wilding JPH. Anti-obesity drugs: past, present and future. *Dis Model Mech.* 2012;5:621-626.
44. Antel J, Hebebrand J. Weight-reducing side effects of the antiepileptic agents topiramate and zonisamide. *Handb Exp Pharmacol.* 2012;209:433-466.
45. Ravussin E, Smith SR, Mitchell JA, et al. Enhanced weight loss with pramlintide/metreleptin: an integrated neurohormonal approach to obesity pharmacotherapy. *Obesity.* 2009;17:1736-1743.
46. Astrup A, Carraro R, Finer N, et al. Safety, tolerability and sustained weight loss over 2 years with the once-daily human GLP-1 analog, liraglutide. *Int J Obes.* 2012;36:843-854.
47. Bray GA. Lifestyle and pharmacological approaches to weight loss: efficacy and safety. *J Clin Endocrinol Metab.* 2008;93:S81-S88.
48. Garvey WT, Ryan DH, Look M, et al. Two-year sustained weight loss and metabolic benefits with controlled-release phentermine/topiramate in obese and overweight adults (SEQUEL): a randomized, placebo-controlled, phase 3 extension study. *Am J Clin Nutr.* 2012;95:297-308.
49. Yanovski SZ, Yanovski JA. Long-term drug treatment for obesity: a systematic and clinical review. *JAMA.* 2014;311(1):74-86.
50. Kaplan LM. Pharmacologic therapies for obesity. *Gastroenterol Clin N Am.* 2010;39:69-79.
51. Li Z. Meta-analysis: pharmacologic treatment of obesity. *Ann Intern Med.* 2005;142:532-546.
52. Munro JF, MacCuish AC, Wilson EM, Duncan LJP. Comparison of continuous and intermittent anorectic therapy in obesity. *BMJ.* 1968;1:352-354.
53. Cercato C, Roizenblatt VA, Leanc CC, et al. A randomized double-blind placebo-controlled study of the long-term efficacy and safety of diethylpropion in the treatment of obese subjects. *Int J Obes.* 2009;33:857-865.
54. Bray GA. Medications for weight reduction. *Med Clin N Am.* 2011;95:989-1008.
55. Rothman RB, Baumann MH, Savage JE, et al. Evidence for possible involvemenet of 5-HT(2B) receptors in the cardiac valvulopathy associated with fenfluramine and other serotonergic medications. *Circulation.* 2000;102:2836-2841.

56. Smith SR, Weissman NJ, Anderson CM, et al. Behavioral Modification and Lorcaserin for Overweight and Obesity Management (BLOOM) Study Group. Multicenter, placebo-controlled trial of lorcaserin for weight management. *N Engl J Med.* 2010;363:245-256.
57. Fidler MC, Sanchez M, Raether B, et al. A one-year randomized trial of lorcaserin for weight loss in obese and overweight adults: the Blossom Trial. *J Clin Endocrinol Metab.* 2011;96:3067-3077.
58. O'Neil PM, Smith SR, Weissman NJ, et al. Randomized placebo-controlled clinical trial of lorcaserin for weight loss in type 2 diabetes mellitus: the Bloom-DM study. *Obesity.* 2012;20:1426-1436.
59. Torgerson JS, Hauptman J, Boldrin MN, Sjöström L. Xenical in the prevention of diabetes in obese subjects (XENDOS) study: a randomized study of orlistat as an adjunct to lifestyle changes for the prevention of type 2 diabetes in obese patients. *Diabetes Care.* 2004;27:155-161.
60. Bray GA. Medical treatment of obesity: the past, present and the future. *Best Pract and Res Clin Gastr.* 2014;28:665-684.
61. Wadden TA, Hollander P, Klien S, et al. Weight maintenance and additional weight loss with liraglutide after low-calorie-diet-induced weight loss: the SCALE Maintenance randomized study. *Int J Obes.* 2103;37:1443-1451.
62. Pi-Sunyer X, Astrup A, Fujioka K, et al. A randomized, controlled trial of 3.0 mg liraglutide in weight management. *N Engl J Med.* 2015;373:11-22.
63. Johnson BA, Rosenthal N, Capece JA, et al. Topiramate for treating alcohol dependence: a randomized controlled trial. *JAMA.* 2007;298(14):1641-1651.
64. McElroy SL, Arnold LM, Shapira NA. Topiramate in the treatment of binge eating disorder associated with obesity: a randomized controlled trial. *Am J Psychiatry.* 2003;160:255-261.
65. Mahmood S, Booker I, Haung J, Coleman CI. Effect of topiramate on weight gain in patients receiving atypical antipsychotic agents. *J Clin Psychopharmacol.* 2013;33:90-94.
66. Verrotti A, Scaparrotta A, Agostinelli S, Di Pillo S, Chiarelli F, Grosso S. Topiramate-induced weight loss: a review. *Epilepsy Res.* 2011;95:189-199.
67. Kramer CK, Leitao CB, Pinto LC, et al. Efficacy and safety of topiramate on weight loss: a meta-analysis of randomized controlled trials. *Obes Rev.* 2011;12:e338-e347.
68. Gadde KM, Franciscy DM, Wagner HR II, Krishnan KR. Zonisamide for weight loss in obese adults: a randomized controlled trial. *JAMA.* 2003;289:1820-1825.
69. Gadde KM, Kopping MF, Wagner HR II, et al. Zonisamide for weight reduction in obese adults: a 1-year randomized controlled trial. *Arch Intern Med.* 2012;172:1557-1564.
70. Goldstein MG. Bupropion sustained release and smoking cessation. *J Clin Psychiatry.* 1998;59:66-72.
71. Anderson JW, Greenway FL, Fujioka K, et al. Bupropion SR enhances weight loss: a 48-week double-blind placebo-controlled trial. *Obes Res.* 2002;10:633-641.
72. Gadde KM, Yonish GM, Foust MS, Wagner HR. Combination therapy of zonisamide and bupropion for weight reduction in obese women: a preliminary, randomized, open-label study. *J Clin Psychiatry.* 2007;68(8):1226-1229.
73. Golay A. Metformin and body weight. *Int J Obes.* 2008;32:61-72.
74. The DPP Research Group. Long-term safety, tolerability, and weight loss associated with metformin in the Diabetes Prevention Program Outcomes Study. *Diabetes Care.* 2012;35:731-737.
75. Desilets AR, Dhakal-Karki S, Dunican KC. Role of metformin for weight management in patients without type 2 diabetes. *Ann Pharmacother.* 2008;42:817-826.
76. Ellinger LK, Ipema HJ, Stachnik JM. Efficacy of metformin and topiramate in prevention and treatment of second-generation antipsychotic–induced weight gain. *Ann Pharmacother.* 2010;44:668-679.
77. Maayan L, Vakhrusheva J, Correll CU. Effectiveness of medications used to attenuate antipsychotic-related weight gain and metabolic abnormalities: a systematic review and meta-analysis. *Neuropsychopharmacol.* 2010;35(7):1520-1530.
78. Singh-Franco D, Perez A, Harrington C. The effect of pramlintide acetate on glycemic control and weight in patients with type 2 diabetes mellitus and in obese patients without diabetes: a systematic review and meta-analysis. *Diab Obes Metab.* 2011;13(2):169-180.
79. Gadde KM, Allison DB, Ryan DH, et al. Effects of low-dose, controlled-release, phentermine plus topiramate combination on weight and associated co-morbidities in overweight and obese adults (CONQUER): a randomised, placebo-controlled, phase 3 trial. *Lancet.* 2011;377:1341-1352.
80. Greenway FL, Whitehouse MJ, Guttaduria M, et al. Rational design of a combination medication for the treatment of obesity. *Obesity.* 2009;17:30-39.
81. Greenway FL, Fujioka K, Plodkowski RA, et al; COR-I Study Group. Effect of naltrexone plus bupropion on weight loss in overweight and obese adults (COR-I): a multicentre, randomized double-blind, placebo-controlled, phase 3 trial. *Lancet.* 2010;376:595-605.
82. Apovian CM, Aronne L, Rubino D, et al; COR-II Study Group. A randomized, phase 3 trial of naltrexone SR/bupropion SR on weight and obesity-related risk factors (COR-II). *Obesity.* 2013;21(5):935-943.
83. Wadden TA, Foreyt JP, Foster GD, et al. Weight loss with naltrexone SR/bupropion SR combination therapy as an adjunct to behavior modification: the COR-BMOD trial. *Obesity.* 2011;19:110-120.

84. Hollander P, Gupta AK, Plodkowski R, et al. Effects of naltrexone sustained-release/bupropion sustained-release combination therapy on body weight and glycemic parameters in overweight and obese patients with type 2 diabetes. *Diabetes Care.* 2013;36:4022-4029.
85. Ruede-Clausen CF, Padwal RS, and Sharma AM. New pharmacological approaches for obesity management. Nat Rev Endocrinol. 2013;9:467-78.
86. Puhl RM, Brownell KD. Psychosocial origins of obesity stigma: toward changing a powerful and pervasive bias. *Obes Rev.* 2003;4:213-227.
87. Pomeranz JL, Puhl RM. New developments in the law for obesity discrimination protection. *Obesity.* 2013;21:469-471.
88. Puhl RM, Heuer CA. The stigma of obesity: a review and update. *Obesity.* 2009;17:941-964.
89. Rudd Center for Food Policy and Obesity. Increasing self-awareness of weight bias. http://www.uconnruddcenter.org/resources/bias_toolkit/module1.html
90. Kyle TK, Puhl RM. Putting people first in obesity. *Obesity.* 2014;1. doi: 10.1002/oby.20727
91. Rudd Center for Food Policy and Obesity. Office environment strategies to reduce weight loss. http://www.uconnruddcenter.org/resources/bias_toolkit/module4.html
92. Hatoum IJ, Stein HK, Merrifield BF, Kaplan LM. Capacity for physical activity predicts weight loss after Roux-en-Y gastric bypass. *Obesity.* 2009;17:92-99.
93. Fobi M, Lee H, Igwe D, et al. Revision of failed gastric bypass to distal Roux-en-Y gastric bypass: a review of 65 cases. *Obes Surg.* 2001;11:190-195.
94. Sugerman H, Kellum J, DeMaria E. Conversion of proximal to distal gastric bypass for failed gastric bypass for superobesity. *J Gastrointest Surg.* 1997;1:517-525.
95. Muller M, Rader S, Wildi S, et al. Matched pair analysis of proximal vs. distal laparoscopic gastric bypass with 4 years follow-up. *Surg Endosc.* 2007;21:S369.
96. Schwartz R, Strodel W, Simpson W, Griffen W. Gastric bypass revision: lessons learned from 920 cases. *Surgery.* 1988;104:806-812.
97. Muller M, Wildi S, Scholz T, et al. Laparoscopic pouch resizing and redo of gastro-jejunal anastomosis for pouch dilatation following gastric bypass. *Obes Surg.* 2005;15:1089-1095.
98. Karmali S, Brar B, Shi X, Sharma AM, de Gara C, Birch DW. Weight recidivism post-bariatric surgery: a systematic review. *Obes Surg.* 2013;23:1922-1933.
99. Kuzmak LI, Burak E. Pouch enlargement: myth or reality? Impressions from serial upper gastrointestinal series in silicone gastric banding patients. *Obes Surg.* 1993;3:57-62.
100. DeMaria EJ, Sugerman HJ, Meador JG, et al. High failure rate after laparoscopic adjustable silicone gastric banding for treatment of morbid obesity. *Ann Surg.* 2001;233:809-818.
101. Eid I, Birch DW, Sharma AM, et al. Complications associated with adjustable gastric banding for morbid obesity: a surgeon's guide. *Can J Surg.* 2011;54:61-66.
102. Lanthaler M, Strasser S, Aigner F, et al. Weight loss and quality of life after gastric band removal or deflation. *Obes Surg.* 2009;19:1401-1408.
103. Stroh S, Hohmann U, Schramm H, et al. Fourteen year long term follow-up after gastric banding. *J Obes.* 2011;2011:1-6.
104. Weiner RA, Weiner S, Pomhoff I, et al. Laparoscopic sleeve gastrectomy—influence of sleeve size and resected gastric volume. *Obes Surg.* 2007;17:1297-1305.
105. Braghetto I, Cortes C, Herquiñigo D, et al. Evaluation of the radiological gastric capacity and evolution of the BMI 2–3 years after sleeve gastrectomy. *Obes Surg.* 2009;19:1262-1269.
106. Heneghan HM, Yimcharoen P, Brethauer SA, et al. Influence of pouch and stoma size on weight loss after gastric bypass. *Surg Obes Relat Dis.* 2012;8:408-415.
107. Catalano MF, Rudic G, Anderson AJ, et al. Weight gain after bariatric surgery as a result of a large gastric stoma: endotherapy with sodium morrhuate may prevent the need for surgical revision. *Gastrointest Endosc.* 2007;66:240-245.
108. Thompson CC, Slattery J, Bundga ME, et al. Peroral endoscopic reduction of dilated gastrojejunal anastomosis after Roux en Y gastric bypass: a possible new option for patients with weight regain. *Surg Endosc.* 2006;20:1744-1748.
109. Cucchi SG, Pories WJ, MacDonald KG. Gastrogastric fistulas. A complication of divided gastric bypass surgery. *Ann Surg.* 1995;221:387-391.
110. Filho AJ, William K, Nassif LS, et al. Gastrogastric fistula: a possible complication of Roux-en-Y gastric bypass. *JSLS.* 2006;10:326-331.
111. Capella JF, Capella RF. Gastro-gastric fistulas and marginal ulcers in gastric bypass procedures for weight reduction. *Obes Surg.* 1999;9:22-27.
112. Kalarchian MA, Marcus MD, Wilson GT, et al. Binge eating among gastric bypass patients at long-term follow-up. *Obes Surg.* 2002;12:270-275.
113. Odom J, Zalesin KC, Washington TL, et al. Behavioral predictors of weight regain after bariatric surgery. *Obes Surg.* 2010;20:349-356.

114. Colles SL, Dixon JB, O'Brien PE. Grazing and loss of control related to eating: two high-risk factors following bariatric surgery. *Obesity.* 2008;16:615-622.
115. Freire RH, Borges MC, Alvarez-Leite JI, et al. Food quality, physical activity, and nutritional follow-up as determinant of weight regain after Roux-en-Y gastric bypass. *Nutrition.* 2012;28(1):53-58.
116. Kofman MD, Lent MR, Swencionis C. Maladaptive eating patterns, quality of life, and weight outcomes following gastric bypass: results of an Internet survey. *Obesity.* 2010;18(10):1938-1943.
117. Roslin M, Damani T, Oren J, et al. Abnormal glucose tolerance testing following gastric bypass demonstrates reactive hypoglycemia. *Surg Endosc.* 2011;25(6):1926-1932.
118. King WC, Belle SH, Eid GM, et al. Physical activity levels of patients undergoing bariatric surgery in the longitudinal assessment of bariatric surgery study. *Surg Obes Relat Dis.* 2008;4:721-728.
119. Beccuti G, Pannain S. Sleep and obesity. *Curr Opin Clin Nutr Metab Care.* 2011;14:402-412.
120. Rutledge T, Groesz LM, Savu M. Psychiatric factors and weight loss patterns following gastric bypass surgery in a veteran population. *Obes Surg.* 2011;21(1):29-35.
121. Kinzl JF. Psychosocial predictors of weight loss after bariatric surgery. *Obes Surg.* 2006;16:1198-1204.

II

Surgical Issues and Procedures

4

Why Surgery?

Bruce M. Wolfe, MD, FACS, FASMBS

The basis for bariatric surgery to accomplish weight loss can be simplified into a straightforward statement: bariatric surgery induces substantial and durable weight loss among severely obese patients who have failed other interventions to accomplish such weight loss. Severe obesity is a disease that is associated with multiple comorbid conditions, psychosocial impairment, and premature mortality. Medical treatment for severe obesity may achieve transient success but usually fails to achieve lasting weight loss; however, bariatric surgery is effective in producing both short- and long-term weight loss.[1] The safety of bariatric surgery has improved dramatically over the past 20 years. If the treatment of severe obesity was as straightforward as the above construct suggests, the number of potential bariatric surgical candidates who actually undergo surgery in any given year would greatly exceed the present 1% to 2%. This percentage has remained remarkably unchanged over many years despite the progress made to improve the safety and define the outcomes of bariatric surgery. The explanation for this low utilization of bariatric surgery has been incompletely studied. Involved factors include fear of complication, hesitancy to undergo substantial rearrangement of one's anatomy, lack of financial coverage to pay for surgery and postoperative care, and a lack of knowledge or understanding of the risks of severe obesity and the benefits of bariatric surgery on the part of patients, their families, and primary care providers. Thus, a closer examination of the current status of each of these considerations is appropriate.

Obesity as a Disease

The designation of obesity as a disease by the Obesity Society and subsequently the American Medical Association continues to be met with resistance.[1] It follows that if obesity is a disease, effective treatment is indicated. Widespread anti-obesity bias continues to be prevalent, holding that obesity is secondary to inappropriate lifestyle choices such that allocation of health care resources to treatment is inappropriate.[2] As understanding of the mechanisms involved in the dysregulation of energy homeostasis progresses, the inappropriateness of such a biased opinion is evident.

Forse RA, Apovian CM, eds.
Bariatric Surgery: What Every Provider Needs to Know (pp 61-66).

Obesity Comorbidities

By definition, an obesity-related comorbidity is a condition that is caused by or contributed to/worsened by obesity. In addition, improvement if not induction of remission occurs following effective weight loss.

Type 2 Diabetes

Type 2 diabetes is a complex condition composed of insulin resistance and beta-cell dysfunction manifested by insufficient insulin secretion to overcome insulin resistance and hyperglycemia. The components of insulin resistance and causes of beta-cell dysfunction are multifactorial and vary among individuals with type 2 diabetes. For instance, approximately 20% of persons with type 2 diabetes are lean. Several of the hypothesized causes of beta-cell deterioration are associated with obesity, and the obesity epidemic closely parallels the epidemic of type 2 diabetes. Finally, remission of type 2 diabetes is induced in the majority of patients who undergo effective weight loss by bariatric surgery.[3] A diagnosis of type 2 diabetes is present in 25% to 33% of bariatric surgery patients.[4]

Hypertension

Greater than 50% of bariatric surgery patients experience hypertension.[4] Improvement, if not remission, of hypertension is expected following effective weight loss. However, hypertension appears to be one of the least responsive obesity-related comorbidities to long-term effective weight loss.[5]

Dyslipidemia

The abnormalities of lipid metabolism associated with severe obesity are hypertriglyceridemia and low circulating high-density lipoprotein. Most affected patients experience substantial improvement if not complete remission of these abnormalities following bariatric surgery. Hypercholesterolemia may respond to effective weight loss, although this response has a greater variability.[6]

Obstructive Sleep Apnea

The association of obstructive sleep apnea with severe obesity has been more recently established. The lack of routine polysomnography to identify unrecognized obstructive sleep apnea has limited definition of the true prevalence of the association of obstructive sleep apnea and severe obesity.[7] Similarly, incomplete utilization of post-bariatric surgery sleep studies has limited the ability to accurately define the response rate to bariatric surgery. Symptomatic improvement or patient perception may overestimate the incidence of complete remission of obstructive sleep apnea and the need for treatment following bariatric surgery.

Musculoskeletal/Functional Impairment

The prevalence of degenerative joint disease is often attributed to obesity. Increased joint pain leading to impaired function exceeds the population of patients with clearly identified joint degeneration.[4] Effective weight loss leads to variable asymptotic and functional improvement, particularly among those who are newly eligible for joint replacement after being denied due to the presence of the severe obesity.

Cancer

The incidence of multiple cancers has been demonstrated to be increased by the presence of obesity in multiple epidemiologic studies.[8] This relationship holds for most common cancers that are associated with mortality, with lung cancer being the primary exception. Cancers associated with estrogen compounds, such as ovary, breast, and endometrial, are particularly common among women with obesity. Gastrointestinal cancers, including liver as well as kidney, are increased in both males and females. A remarkable reduction in the incidence of cancers and cancer mortality has been demonstrated following bariatric surgery.[9,10] This effect is most dramatically demonstrated regarding breast cancer.[11]

Psychosocial Impairment

Multiple aspects of psychosocial impairment have been extensively studied and shown to be affected by severe obesity. These include but are not limited to depression, anxiety, multiple components of quality of life, employment and economic status, and others. All of these impairments are improved on average following bariatric surgery, although variable responses of each have been reported. Increased concern regarding possible suicide as well as a slight but definite increase in alcohol abuse has been reported.[12,13]

Premature Mortality

The relationship of overweight and progressively severe obesity to longevity or premature mortality has been reported by various epidemiologic studies involving the US population, international populations, and specific populations, such as the Asian population or those who are greater than 50 years of age.[14] These studies have consistently shown a progressively increased relative risk of mortality as body mass index (BMI) rises above 30 kg/m^2, the accepted definition of obesity. Reported data for BMI > 40 have been limited. It is reasonable to assume the relative risk continues to steeply rise as BMI rises. A randomized clinical trial comparing long-term survival among patients eligible for bariatric surgery, comparing bariatric surgery to usual care, has not been feasible. Three trials with matched comparator groups of surgery vs usual care have shown substantial improvement in mortality risk.[12,15,16] The most carefully matched trial is the Swedish Obese Subjects study, which showed improved survival at 12 years following bariatric surgery, consistent with the interval of time required for a change to be demonstrated in the risk profile for cardiovascular events and death. Thus, trials that report no mortality benefit to bariatric surgery of less than 12 years' duration must be interpreted with caution.

Most recently a somewhat reduced relative risk of overweight and obesity has been reported, particularly among those with a BMI of 25 to 30 and 30 to 35.[17] There are 3 potential explanations for these recently reported data:

1. The data are international, deriving cases from a variety of environments and available interventions for complications of obesity.
2. The identification and treatment of obesity-related comorbid conditions. The medical management of diabetes to tighter glucose control, identification and treatment of hypertension with multiple drugs, the widespread use of statins for dyslipidemia, and the increased identification and treatment of obstructive sleep apnea with continuous positive airway pressure (CPAP) all have the potential to reduce obesity-related mortality as mediated by these comorbid conditions. Thus, updated research to take into account the prevalence and effective treatment of these comorbid conditions, each of which independently is known to increase mortality risk, is needed.
3. An apparent survival benefit for a number of conditions, such as congestive heart failure, as well as improved outcomes following certain surgical procedures, such as vascular

reconstruction, has been reported for populations with BMI ≤ 35. There has been no such report for individuals with BMI ≥ 35. The mechanism (or mechanisms) by which what has been considered overweight or Class I obesity provides a protective effect of some degree remains to be defined. Furthermore, there is controversy in the field as to whether the obesity paradox is real and will be sustained by further research.

Weight Loss

There is agreement that bariatric surgical procedures consistently produce superior short- and long-term weight loss over as many as 20 years over any medical intervention, including intense behavior modification with or without medications. Most recently this observation has been confirmed among participants with BMI 30 to 40 in several randomized clinical trials that have proved feasible.[18,19] Weight loss following virtually every surgical procedure tends to show some regain of lost weight between years 1.5 and 4.[15] Thereafter weight appears to be stable, with a maintained weight loss in the range of 15% to 30% of initial body weight.

The weight loss has been found to be highly variable among a seemingly homogeneous population, as defined by BMI, undergoing a relatively standardized procedure such as gastric bypass.[20] Correlation analyses published to date have failed to fully explain this remarkable degree of variable weight loss. Several predictors of some of the variability have been identified to include the presence of preoperative diabetes. Comorbidity responses and induction of remission of these comorbidities appears to be roughly correlated with the extent of the weight loss, although research of this question is incomplete.

Complications of Bariatric Surgery

The previously reported benefits of bariatric surgery (weight loss and the results of gastrointestinal tract alteration) must be weighed against the risk of complications. In the past, complications of bariatric surgery have been a substantial problem with procedures such as the jejunoileal bypass, the first bariatric surgical procedure to be done on a widespread basis to achieve major weight loss. Perioperative and metabolic complications and mortality were reduced by a shift to gastric bypass and later vertical banding gastroplasty and adjustable gastric banding. Continued mortality was problematic, however, as demonstrated by Flum and Dellinger, who reported the mortality rate following gastric bypass to be 2%.[21] More recently, perioperative mortality has been reported to be 0.3%, with serious complications occurring in approximately 4% of patients.[22] Large registries of population-based studies most recently have indicated perioperative mortality has been reduced to 0.1% or less. Complications continue to occur in a small but definite percentage. The capacity of bariatric surgical programs to identify and correct complications has greatly improved in recent years.

Longer term complications have been well defined on an anecdotal basis, but the true incidence is not well defined. These include problematic regain of weight with recurrence of previously remitted comorbid conditions and gastrointestinal complications such as small bowel obstruction and peptic ulcer disease.

Micronutrient deficiencies have been reported, particularly by referral centers that collect cases from multiple surgical centers, making determination of the true incidence of these complications unknown.[23] The most common nutrient deficiency is iron deficiency (anemia), which can generally be corrected with supplemental iron, although parenteral iron is required in some cases. Concern regarding calcium malabsorption has been raised by vitamin D deficiency and increased parathormone secretion and occasional fractures. Nephrolithiasis is another potential complication in later years due to increased oxalate absorption leading to calcium oxalate stones. The prevalence of nephrolithiasis among the severely obese is elevated, such that the impact of gastric bypass on long-term nephrolithiasis remains to be determined.

In general, these nutrient complications can be corrected when promptly identified and replacement therapy delivered. Due to the possibility that these complications may occur 10 years or more following surgery, systems for surveillance, early detection, and treatment of these deficiencies are necessary to avoid severe complications such as neuropathies.

Summary

Bariatric surgery induces substantial and durable weight loss among severely obese patients who have failed other interventions to accomplish such weight loss. The health benefits have been studied and documented repeatedly. Short- and long-term complications have been greatly diminished, but cannot be completely eliminated. Long-term follow-up for micronutrient deficiencies is indicated.

References

1. Allison DB, Downey M, Atkinson RL, et al. Obesity as a disease: a white paper on evidence and arguments commissioned by the Council of the Obesity Society. *Obesity.* 2008;16:1161-1177.
2. Wolfe BM. Presidential address—obesity discrimination: what can we do? *Surg Obes Relat Dis.* 2012;8:495-500.
3. Pories WJ, Swanson MS, MacDonald KG, et al. Who would have thought it? An operation proves to be the most effective therapy for adult-onset diabetes mellitus. *Ann Surg.* 1995;222:339-350.
4. Belle SH, Berk PD, Chapman WH, et al. Baseline characteristics of participants in the Longitudinal Assessment of Bariatric Surgery-2 (LABS-2) study. *Surg Obes Relat Dis.* 2013;9:926-935.
5. Sjostrom L, Lindroos AK, Peltonen M, et al, Swedish Obese Subjects Study Scientific Group. Lifestyle, diabetes, and cardiovascular risk factors 10 years after bariatric surgery. *N Engl J Med.* 2004;351:2683-2693.
6. Jensen MD, Ryan DH, Apovian CM, et al. 2013 AHA/ACC/TOS guideline for the management of overweight and obesity in adults: a report of the American College of Cardiology/American Heart Association Task Force on practice guidelines and the Obesity Society. *J Am Coll Cardiol.* 2014;63(25 Pt B):2985-3023.
7. Khan A, King WC, Patterson EJ, et al. Assessment of obstructive sleep apnea in adults undergoing bariatric surgery in the Longitudinal Assessment of Bariatric Surgery-2 (LABS-2) study. *J Clin Sleep Med.* 2013;9:21-29.
8. Calle EE, Rodriguez C, Walker-Thurmond K, Thun MJ. Overweight, obesity, and mortality from cancer in a prospectively studied cohort of U.S. adults. *N Engl J Med.* 2003;348:1625-1638.
9. Christou NV, Lieberman M, Sampalis F, Sampalis JS. Bariatric surgery reduces cancer risk in morbidly obese patients. *Surg Obes Relat Dis.* 2008;4:691-695.
10. Adams TD, Stroup AM, Gress RE, et al. Cancer incidence and mortality after gastric bypass surgery. *Obesity.* 2009;17:796-802.
11. Sjöström L, Gummesson A, Sjöström CD, et al, Swedish Obese Subjects Study. Effects of bariatric surgery on cancer incidence in obese patients in Sweden (Swedish Obese Subjects study): a prospective, controlled intervention trial. *Lancet Oncol.* 2009;10:653-662.
12. Adams TD, Gress RE, Smith SC, et al. Long-term mortality after gastric bypass surgery. *N Engl J Med.* 2007;357:753-761.
13. King WC, Chen JY, Mitchell JE, et al. Prevalence of alcohol use disorders before and after bariatric surgery. *JAMA.* 2012;307:2516-2525.
14. Calle EE, Thun MJ, Petrelli JM, Rodriguez C, Heath CW Jr. Body-mass index and mortality in a prospective cohort of U.S. adults. *N Engl J Med.* 1999;341:1097-1105.
15. Sjöström L, Narbro K, Sjöström CD, et al, Swedish Obese Subjects Study. Effects of bariatric surgery on mortality in Swedish obese subjects. *N Engl J Med.* 2007;357:741-752.
16. Christou NV, Sampalis JS, Liberman M, et al. Surgery decreases long-term mortality, morbidity, and health care use in morbidly obese patients. *Ann Surg.* 2004:240:416-423.
17. Flegal KM, Kit BK, Orpana H, Graubard BI. Association of all-cause mortality with overweight and obesity using standard body mass index categories: a systematic review and meta-analysis. *JAMA.* 2013;309:71-82.
18. Schauer PR, Bhatt DL, Kirwan JP, et al; STAMPEDE Investigators. Bariatric surgery versus intensive medical therapy for diabetes—3-year outcomes. *N Engl J Med.* 2014;370:2002-2013.

19. Ikramuddin S, Korner J, Lee WJ, et al. Roux-en-Y gastric bypass vs intensive medical management for the control of type 2 diabetes, hypertension, and hyperlipidemia: the Diabetes Surgery Study randomized clinical trial. *JAMA.* 2013;309:2240-2249.
20. Courcoulas AP, Christian NJ, Belle SH, et al, Longitudinal Assessment of Bariatric Surgery (LABS) Consortium. Weight change and health outcomes at 3 years after bariatric surgery among individuals with severe obesity. *JAMA.* 2013;310:2416-2425.
21. Flum DR, Dellinger EP. Impact of gastric bypass operation on survival: a population-based analysis. *J Am Coll Surg.* 2004;199:543-551.
22. The Longitudinal Assessment of Bariatric Surgery (LABS) Consortium. Perioperative safety in the Longitudinal Assessment of Bariatric Surgery. *N Engl J Med.* 2009;361:445-454.
23. Gletsu-Miller N, Wright BN. Mineral malnutrition following bariatric surgery. *Adv Nutr.* 2013;4:506-517.

5

Choice of Bariatric Surgery

Sayeed Ikramuddin, MD; Elizabeth Colsen, MD; and Daniel B. Leslie, MD

Over the past 10 years, the population of the United States has gotten progressively more obese. The Centers for Disease Control and Prevention estimates that more than one-third of US adults (35.7%) and approximately 17% (or 12.5 million) of children and adolescents aged 2 to 19 years are obese.[1] As the population becomes more obese, the prevalence of certain obesity-related illness increases. This includes, but is not limited to, diabetes mellitus, obstructive sleep apnea, and hypertension. These comorbid illnesses pose a significant problem to the health care field. So much that the American Medical Association recently declared obesity as a disease.[2] With this new declaration comes an increased push to treat morbid obesity and its related complications.

Many techniques have been utilized for weight management throughout the past 20 years including fad diets, medications, and more recently weight loss surgery. Many patients have had success with medically supervised dietary restriction plans. However, the durability of medically based weight loss interventions is less when compared to surgical interventions. Because of the long-term successful weight loss with surgical intervention, bariatric surgery has become an increasingly popular technique for weight loss. There are 4 operations commonly performed: laparoscopic adjustable gastric band (AGB), laparoscopic vertical sleeve gastrectomy (VSG), laparoscopic Roux-en-Y gastric bypass (RYGB), and the laparoscopic/open duodenal switch biliopancreatic diversion procedure (BPD-DS).

This chapter will cover a brief history of the evolution of modern bariatric surgery. It will also discuss the indications, approach, and results for each of the 4 surgical options.

History

Bariatric surgery is the product of decades of development starting with the observation that patients who had surgical procedures like the Billroth II operation (Owen Wangensteen, University of Minnesota) and jejunoileal bypass had the side effect of significant weight loss.[3] The Billroth II gastric resection (for duodenal ulcer disease) was described as a subtotal gastrectomy with a short loop retrocolic gastrojejunostomy. The subtotal gastrectomy limited the amount of food that the

Forse RA, Apovian CM, eds.
Bariatric Surgery: What Every Provider Needs to Know (pp 67-78).

patient was able to eat, thus restricting his or her intake. The jejunoileal bypass operation was described as joining the proximal small intestine to the distal ileum, bypassing a large segment of small bowel.[3] This bypass limited digestion of food and thus absorption of nutrients and calories, which stimulated weight loss.[3] These operations created restriction and malabsorption, which has become the basis for modern-day bariatric surgical procedures.

The development of the restrictive procedures began in 1971 by Mason in association with Printen.[3,4] These procedures included variations of stapling off a small portion of the stomach to create restriction. Later modifications added a stapled gastric tube (sleeve) plus a silastic ring (vertical banded gastroplasty). These procedures led the way for the introduction of an inflatable silastic band connected to a subcutaneous port in 1986 by Kuzmak.[5] A similar adjustable silastic band is used today, but implanted using the laparoscopic technique. Additionally, the vertical banded gastroplasty as a restrictive surgical option has yielded way to the current sleeve gastrectomy.

The first gastric bypass was performed in 1977 by Dr. Edward Mason (University of Iowa). This procedure involved dividing the stomach horizontally into a small upper pouch (10%) and larger lower remnant stomach (90%). A loop gastrojejunostomy was connected to the proximal gastric pouch.[3] This operation provided significant restriction due to the small gastric pouch, and the patients achieved successful weight loss. Over the next decade, the gastric bypass was modified to the Roux-en-Y configuration, which is the current configuration of the operation.

The malabsorptive procedures originated with the jejunoileal bypass in 1953.[4] In 1979, Scopinaro et al began performing the biliopancreatic diversion operation in Italy.[6] This operation provided weight loss, but was ultimately discontinued due to complications associated with malabsorption, liver failure, kidney stone formation, arthralgias, and bacterial overgrowth. The biliopancreatic diversion was replaced by the BPD-DS in 1993 by Marceau et al[7] and later revised by Hess and Hess.[8] Their modification included a division of the duodenum, creation of a longitudinal gastric tube with closure of the distal duodenal stump, and an end-to-end anastomosis of the enteric limb to the post-pyloric duodenum with a long Roux (food) and a short common (digestive) channel. The short common or digestive channel provides significant malabsorption, thus creating weight loss. This operation is currently being performed with the open, laparoscopic, and robotic techniques.

Options

Currently, there are 4 different surgical weight loss options: laparoscopic AGB, laparoscopic VSG, laparoscopic RYGB, and the laparoscopic or open BPD-DS. The indication for each of the weight loss operations varies based on a patient's preexisting comorbidities and his or her goals for weight loss.

To qualify for bariatric surgery, a person's body mass index (BMI) must generally be ≥ 40 kg/m^2 without or ≥ 35 with comorbid conditions. These comorbid conditions include hypertension, hyperlipidemia, obstructive sleep apnea, and type 2 diabetes mellitus. Specific qualifications for bariatric surgery are determined by the major insurance providers. While the patient's BMI is the entry point into the system, many additional factors should be considered when choosing the type of bariatric surgical procedure.

Indeed, procedure selection is at best an inexact science. There are a number of other considerations that may impact the choice of surgery including improvement of comorbid illness, sustained weight loss, avoidance of nutritional and technical complications, maintenance of psychological stability, and smoking status. Each weight loss operation affects these factors differently. Specific associations will be discussed in the context of each of the individual operative procedures. However, all operations seek to have successful weight loss.

There are numerous definitions of successful weight loss following bariatric surgery. One common term used is *percent excess weight loss* (EWL). This is calculated by looking at the excess weight a patient needs to drop. For example, if a patient is 100 lb overweight and drops 50 lb, then he or she has 50% EWL. Excellent, good, and poor weight loss can be defined as EWL of greater than 50%, 30% to 50%, and less than 30%, respectively. Another definition is the attainment of a BMI < 30 if the patient's beginning BMI is 40 to 50 and 35 if starting BMI is > 50. Regardless of definition, in those patients with a starting BMI > 50, the likelihood that they will have EWL > 50 is only 45%.[9] It bears emphasis that each of these operations should be used only as a tool for the treatment of obesity. The patient must comply with the dietary and exercise requirements for the rest of his or her life.

Current Operative Procedures

Laparoscopic Adjustable Gastric Band

Indications

The laparoscopic AGB is a purely restrictive procedure that can provide the patient approximately 30% to 40% EWL. This would be 30 to 40 lb in someone who is 100 lb overweight. It does not alter the anatomy of the gastrointestinal tract and is performed minimally invasively. Hence, it is one of the safest and fastest bariatric operations performed.[10,11] It does not, however, have quite as robust an effect on comorbid conditions like diabetes mellitus as the other bariatric surgical procedures.[11]

Approach

The current approach to placing the Lap-Band (Apollo Endosurgery) or Realize Band (Ethicon Endo-Surgery) is the pars flaccida technique. This technique has been demonstrated to have lower postoperative complications, specifically posterior slippage.[12] Briefly, patients are placed supine on the operating table, and steep reverse Trendelenburg position is utilized. We use a 5-trocar technique that includes a 15-mm port in the left mid-abdomen for band placement. It is important to identify and close any hiatal hernia defect seen. The band is placed parallel to the gastroesophageal junction in this technique. The band is snapped together and 3 gastrogastric sutures can be used to secure the band in place. The tubing for the band is exteriorized to the subcutaneous pocket where the port is secured to the fascia. Port adjustments can start after 6 weeks, though in some bands fluid can be placed at the time of surgery.

Risk

There are 3 main complications following band placement: slippage, erosion, and concentric dilation of the stomach. The most common is slippage of the band in 1% to 20% of cases.[13] Slippage can involve either the anterior part of the stomach herniating through the band or the posterior stomach. The risk of posterior slippage is low using the pars flaccida approach. Slippage is often preceded by difficulty swallowing or acute abdominal pain. A flat plate and upper gastrointestinal study will demonstrate the band to be at an inappropriate angle, and possibly stomach herniated asymmetrically through the band. Acute obstruction that is not relieved by removing fluid from the band necessitates emergent surgery with reduction of the stomach and removal of the band as delay may cause strangulation of the slipped gastric tissue. Erosion of the band into the stomach occurs 1% of the time.[14] This has previously been due to the band's buckle eroding through the stomach.[14] With some bands this might be reduced by turning the buckle of the band away from the greater curvature of the stomach at the time of implantation. Concentric dilation of both the stomach pouch and/or esophageal dilation are other challenging problems. If the size of the pouch exceeds the size of the band on fluoroscopic examination, then the fluid must be removed from the band or the band removed completely if resolution does not occur.

Vertical Sleeve Gastrectomy

Indications

The VSG is a procedure in which the stomach is stapled to create a small tube and the excess stomach removed. This operation has become increasingly popular in the past 10 years. It has been shown to have weight loss comparable but slightly less than the RYGB. However, the RYGB has been shown to be more effective in meta-analysis for weight loss and controlling type 2 diabetes mellitus.[15] This factor must be taken into consideration when choosing the VSG vs the RYGB for the patient with diabetes. Overall, the VSG has had great success in the short term with weight loss and resolution of comorbid conditions; however, there is a paucity of long-term data.[16,17]

Approach

The VSG has been in evolution for the past several years. Debate exists as to whether the procedure should be antrum preserving and the optimal bougie size used to calibrate the gastric tube. Five laparoscopic ports are used, with one of the working ports as a 15-mm port (to remove the partial gastrectomy specimen). To begin the operation, the short gastric and epiploic vessels are dissected with the harmonic scalpel. This is started at a point 6 cm proximal to the pylorus (opposite the nerves of Latarjet). The dissection is completed once the left crus is identified. Also, any hiatal hernia defects are repaired if identified. The gastric sleeve is constructed over a 40 Fr. bougie with 3.5-mm staples,[18] though this must be individualized based on the perceived thickness of the stomach. Oversewing and buttressing of the staple line have not been conclusively studied.

Risk

The leak rate following VSG is very low, and in most centers less than 1%.[19,20] In one study, more than 529 consecutive cases were performed without a single leak.[19] Leakage from patients following the sleeve gastrectomy is a far more challenging clinical problem than that of the other bariatric operations. There are, however, many common issues following the VSG, including nausea, vomiting, and reflux symptoms. These are often successfully treated with medical management and resolve over time. Patients rarely have significant vitamin deficiencies as the gastrointestinal tract remains intact, but we currently place these patients on a multivitamin postoperatively. Gastroesophageal reflux disease (GERD) can complicate the postoperative course in these patients more so than other procedures[15]; accordingly, it is prudent to fix any obvious hiatal hernias if feasible at the time of surgery. It is unclear but the presence of significant esophageal pathology due to GERD might be an indication for an alternative procedure if suitable.

Laparoscopic Roux-en-Y Gastric Bypass

Indications

The RYGB has rapidly become the most popular weight loss surgery performed worldwide. This is due, in part, to the lasting effects on weight loss, the significant effects on comorbid conditions, and the overall low complication rate of the operation. Patients should expect to have at least a 60% to 70% EWL.[21] It combines restriction with a small component of malabsorption. The metabolic effects of the operation are the focus of intense study, particularly as the procedure is thought to increase satiety and insulin secretion via separate hormonal mechanisms. The recent observations that RYGB may change the levels of bile acids and favorably change the gut microbiome to a lean profile are intriguing.

The RYGB's effects on comorbid conditions is an area of increasing interest as studies have shown a lasting effect on control of diabetes mellitus.[22,23] This is an important factor when considering which operation to perform. Figure 5-1 is a current algorithm used at our center to help guide procedure choice. The presence of diabetes and the patient's starting BMI are important factors to consider when choosing which operation the patient will have.

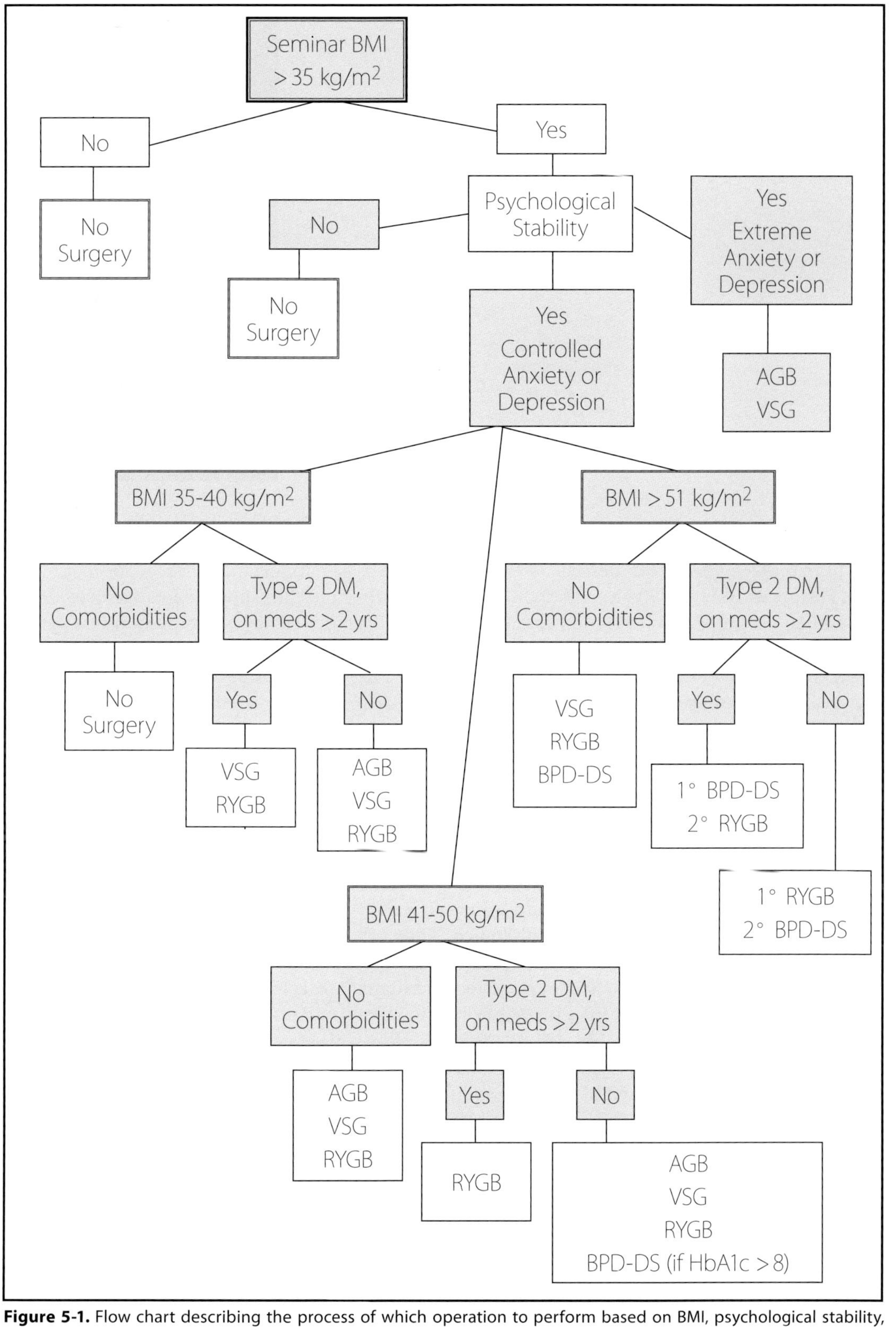

Figure 5-1. Flow chart describing the process of which operation to perform based on BMI, psychological stability, and comorbidities. AGB=adjustable gastric band, BMI=body mass index, BPD-DS=biliopancreatic diversion with duodenal switch, DM=diabetes mellitus, HbA1c=hemoglobin A1c, RYGB=Roux-en-Y gastric bypass, VSG=vertical sleeve gastrectomy.

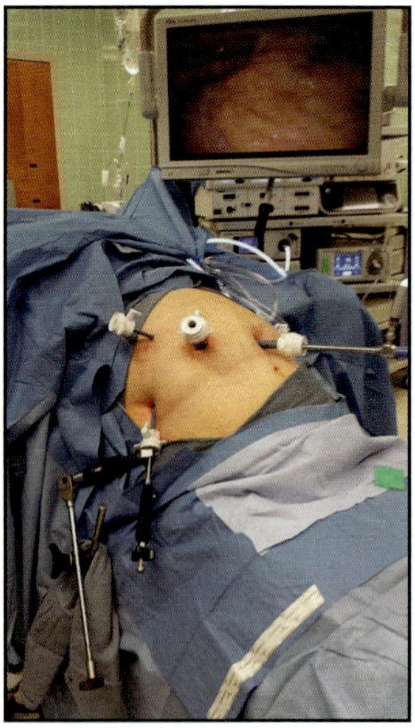

Figure 5-2. Port placement for RYGB.

Another important factor to consider is that in an RYGB, the remnant stomach, duodenum, and proximal jejunum are bypassed. These digestive areas are important for absorption of nutrients. Postoperatively, RYGB patients should take a variety of vitamin supplements and have levels checked on a regular basis to avoid becoming deficient. Iron deficiency is common in this patient population pre- and postoperatively; occasionally parenteral iron might be used to correct low levels. Vitamin D deficiency is ubiquitous before and after surgery. B_{12} deficiency is seen much less given the ease of supplementation. Prolonged emesis can be associated with B_1 deficiency that should be corrected. Patients must also strive to maintain a high protein intake of 60 g a day to maintain their nutritional status.

Approach

The laparoscopic RYGB is performed with the patient in supine position. It is important to have a foot board and safety strap in place as the steep reverse Trendelenburg position is utilized throughout the procedure. The abdomen is insufflated with carbon dioxide via a left upper quadrant 15-cm Veress needle (Ethicon Endo-Surgery). A 5-mm port is placed through this incision and a camera inserted to inspect the abdomen. Four other ports are placed over the abdomen including a 12-mm working and camera port along with a 5-mm liver retractor port and 5-mm working port (Figure 5-2). The liver is retracted and hiatus inspected for a hiatal hernia, which is repaired if found. Attention is then turned to creation of a small 20- to 30-mL vertically oriented gastric pouch with 3.5-mm staple size. We then perform an antecolic antegastric gastrojejunostomy. The ligament of Treitz is identified and 100 cm of jejunum is measured and a Penrose drain looped around the small bowel at this location. This loop of jejunum is brought up to the pouch in an antecolic antegastric fashion so that the Roux limb is oriented toward the patient's right and the biliopancreatic limb is oriented toward the left.[24] The gastrojejunostomy is created using an Endo Stitch (Covidien) with a posterior running seromuscular suture of 3-0 braided nylon. The gastrotomy and enterotomy are then made with a harmonic scalpel, and the gastrojejunostomy created using a linear staple with 3.5-mm load no larger than 2 cm in diameter. The remainder of the anastomosis is created in 2 layers with the Endo Stitch device over a 30 Fr. endoscope introduced through the patient's mouth. The jejunum is divided to the left of the anastomosis with a white staple load. Once created, the anastomosis is tested for leak by placing a bowel clamp 5 cm distal to the anastomosis and insufflating air into the anastomosis while it is submerged, looking for signs of bubbling. Once no leak is ensured, a 150-cm Roux limb is measured out from the gastrojejunostomy. The biliopancreatic limb is sutured to the Roux limb on the antimesenteric border at the 150-cm point. A functional side-to-side anastomosis is formed by making enterotomies in both limbs with a harmonic scalpel and a 6-cm white cartridge utilized for the jejunojejunostomy. The common enterotomy is closed using a white load of the stapler device. The jejunojejunostomy mesenteric defect is closed using an Endo Stitch device in a running fashion, and the Petersen defect closed with a purse string suture in a similar fashion. The trocars are removed and skin closed with staples.

Risk/Complications

The RYGB is a very safe operation, but there are many potential complications that can occur following the detachment, rearrangement, and anastomosis of the gastrointestinal tract. Several of the complications require operative intervention. The most dreaded of these is leak. Luckily, it is uncommon occurring less than 1% (0.5%) of the time.[13] However, it can make the patient very ill, so all of our patients have a swallow study on postoperative day 1 before starting a clear liquid diet. Symptoms of a leak include tachycardia, increasing abdominal pain, and hemodynamic instability. If a leak is detected, early exploration with washout and repair will avoid further complications.

Stricture formation is more common than leak and occurs 7% of the time.[25,26] The classical presentation is 3 to 4 weeks after initial operation; however, late strictures can also occur. During the weeks following surgery, diet is gradually advanced from clear liquids to thicker food. Patients who develop a stricture will complain of dysphagia, the feeling of food getting stuck, and simply not being able to advance to more solid foods. The diagnosis should be made with an upper endoscopy. Our current approach for early strictures is balloon dilation with or without the aid of fluoroscopy. Late strictures can also be managed with balloon dilation. Rarely will strictures require surgical revision of the anastomosis.

Acute gastric remnant dilation is a surgical emergency as the remnant stomach and jejunojejunostomy can be at risk for perforation. The patient will present with possible abdominal distention, abdominal pain, hiccups, and left shoulder pain and could be in extremis if already perforated. Diagnosis is often confirmed by plain upright abdominal x-ray; however, a fluid-filled remnant may not be evident on x-ray and a computed tomography (CT) scan may be necessary. Once diagnosed, it is critical to decompress the remnant as soon as possible. If possible, interventional radiology can percutaneously drain the remnant stomach. If percutaneous methods are unavailable, surgical decompression via laparotomy with gastrostomy tube should be performed. During laparotomy, the surgeon should evaluate the gastrojejunostomy, the jejunojejunostomy, and the mesenteric defects for pathology.

Another potential surgical emergency is the development of an internal hernia, which occurs 1% to 3% of the time.[27] As mentioned previously, the RYGB creates mesenteric defects. The first is at the jejunojejunostomy site, and the second is the Petersen defect, which is between the transverse mesocolon and the Roux limb (in an antecolic antegastric anastomosis). Although these mesenteric defects are closed during the initial operation, the mesentery is adipose laden, and as the patient loses weight, so does the mesentery. This shrinkage can render the previous closure loose, and create a hernia defect though which bowel can traverse. Patients will often complain of colicky periumbilical pain associated with nausea and potentially vomiting following meals. The pain usually remits between episodes. The surgeon needs to have a high index of suspicion for an internal hernia because the upper gastrointestinal and CT scan may be normal. One needs to remember that the bowel has a variable position and a static imaging study may not catch the herniating intestine. Hence, it is safest to explore these patients in the operating room. It should be mentioned that these operations may be performed laparoscopically. However, they are often challenging cases due to edematous bowel that is often difficult to reduce; thus, conversion to an open procedure would not be unusual.

The complications of dumping syndrome, hypoglycemia, and marginal ulcers are common, and are treated by diet and lifestyle modification. Dumping syndrome is characterized by sweating, flushing, weakness, tachycardia, nausea, cramping, and loose stools following a meal. The symptoms can be seen in up to 70% of RYGB patients, but less than 5% will have severe symptoms.[28] The dumping syndrome is caused by hyperosmotic food entering the jejunum quickly following a meal because the pylorus is gone. This results in fluid shifting into the bowel resulting in release of vasoactive substances that cause the above symptoms. Patients can be treated with dietary modifications including small, frequent meals with a low glycemic index and high protein. Another part of the dumping syndrome is reactive hypoglycemia. Patients have an exaggerated and prolonged insulin secretion in response to a high carbohydrate meal. The carbohydrate is digested and the insulin levels remain high creating hypoglycemia.[28,29] Treatment is dietary modification with avoidance of high carbohydrate foods. The final complication is marginal ulceration at the gastrojejunostomy. It is often associated with nonsteroidal medication use, smoking, and stress.[30] Patients will complain of epigastric pain that is sharp. Diagnosis is made with upper endoscopy. Treatment includes removal of the exacerbating factors (quitting smoking), proton pump inhibitors, and coating agents like sucralfate. Some patients may require admission to the hospital for intravenous proton pump inhibitors, intravenous fluids, and nothing-by-mouth status. Ulcers should be monitored with frequent endoscopy to document resolution. They can be insidious in nature, and if not treated, can progress to perforation or chronic pain.

Laparoscopic Biliopancreatic Diversion With Duodenal Switch

Indications

The BPD-DS operation is a malabsorptive procedure that has a component of restriction with the gastric sleeve. It has been shown to have consistent and significantly greater weight loss when compared to other bariatric procedures.[31] Patients can expect to lose 70% to 80% of their excess body weight. Appropriately, it has selective acceptance among patients and physicians, which is likely due to the nutritional challenges following BPD-DS. Additionally, because of the malabsorption, patients have to maintain a very strict diet including 90 to 120 g of protein a day along with taking several vitamin supplements. The operation is, however, very effective at achieving weight loss, control of diabetes mellitus, and other comorbid conditions.

Approach

The BPD-DS can be performed as an open, laparoscopic, and laparoscopic with robot-assisted operation. For the laparoscopic and robot-assisted operation, the reverse Trendelenburg positioning is critical to the upper abdominal dissection, so the patient must have a foot board and safety strap in place. The procedure is performed through 6 abdominal trocars. Similar to the other procedures, access to the abdomen is gained via a left upper quadrant Veress needle technique with a 12-mm port placed at this site. A 15-mm port is placed just to the left and cephalad of the umbilicus. A 5-mm port is used in the left lateral flank. The right-sided ports include a 12- and 5-mm working port along with a 5-mm liver retractor port.

The harmonic scalpel is used to take down the short gastric and epiploic vessels along the greater curvature of the stomach, starting 6 cm proximal to the pylorus, and progressing to the angle of His. The gastric sleeve is created using 3.5-mm staple loads over a 48 Fr. bougie. The duodenal dissection is performed 2 cm distal to the pylorus, and a posterior tunnel is created and a Penrose drain is used as a handle to facilitate the passage of a 3.5-mm stapler to divide at this point. The duodenal stump on the pyloric side is completely mobilized for the later anastomosis.

The bowel is now measured from the ileocecal valve to 100 cm proximal with clips placed on the mesentery to mark the location of the common channel anastomosis. The small bowel is then run 150 to 200 cm more proximally with a Penrose drain looped around the bowel. The loop is brought up to the posterior aspect of the proximal duodenal remnant and the Endo Stitch device used to create a posterior row of running 2-0 nonabsorbable suture to secure the small bowel to the duodenum. Then the small bowel is divided just to the left of the duodenoileostomy with a 3.5-mm stapler dividing the alimentary limb from the biliopancreatic limb. The mesentery is divided using two 2.0-mm staple loads. The distal biliopancreatic limb is moved toward the common channel markers and stay sutures placed using the Endo Stitch device. A stapled side-to-side anastomosis is created. The ileoileostomy mesenteric defect is closed.

Attention is then focused on completing the duodenoileostomy anastomosis. First, enterotomy defects are created above the staple line in the duodenum and the ileum with the harmonic device. A 16 Fr. nasogastric tube is advanced into the enterotomies to stent the anastomosis. The actual anastomosis is created with the da Vinci Robot (Intuitive Surgical), using an inner and outer running 3-0 absorbable suture. The anastomosis is tested with methylene blue via the previously placed nasogastric tube. A nasogastric tube is left in place until postoperative day 1, and then the patient's diet is advanced with discharge by day 3 or 4.

Risk/Complications

The malabsorptive component of the BPD-DS operation also provides its greatest nutritional challenges, the most common of which is diarrhea. The common complications usually resolve with conservative measures, diet modification, and medications as needed. The most important treatment is diet modification to include limited carbohydrate calories and high protein intake up to 120 g a day. Malabsorption also causes vitamin and mineral absorption issues. Thus, BPD-DS patients have to focus on fat-soluble vitamins for the rest of their lives. Vitamin and protein levels need to be monitored on a regular basis to confirm that the patient is not becoming deficient (Table 5-1). Typically, deficiencies are able to be corrected with increased oral vitamin intake or less commonly vitamin infusions. Protein malnutrition sometimes necessitates parenteral nutrition, but initial treatment includes oral pancreatic enzymes. Sometimes the symptoms are severe enough to merit admission to the hospital and thus care plans need to be devised to reduce readmission. Indeed readmission rates have been shown to be the higher in the BPD-DS patients when compared to RYGB.[31-33]

The surgical complications of BPD-DS are similar to that of the RYGB. Leak can occur at the gastric sleeve, duodenoileostomy, or ileoileostomy. In a recent study from Quebec of 1000 consecutive BPD-DS procedures performed both laparoscopically and open, the 2 groups had a 3.5% vs 4% ($p = .1$) leak or intra-abdominal abscess rate. The study included all patients with an abscess in the leak group as they were unable to identify if a leak had contributed to the abscess.[32] The authors changed their laparoscopic technique to hand sewing of the duodenoileostomy anastomosis, and have since had no leaks.[32] Several other studies have shown the leak rates to be consistent with that of the RYGB.[31,33]

Other surgical complications can occur like internal hernia; however, they are rare.[31-33] Marginal ulceration can also occur after a BPD-DS procedure, but again, it is infrequent and usually resolves with proton pump inhibitor therapy.[31-33]

Results

Weight Loss Results

The best long-term data for weight loss post bariatric surgery are from the Swedish Obese Subjects study.[34] The study followed patients who had surgical management for their obesity as well as exceedingly well-matched surgical controls. The surgical groups included nonadjustable banding, vertical banded gastroplasty (70%), and the RYGB. All surgical groups had improved weight loss compared to the control group. At 2 years, the gastric bypass had lost 32% of weight compared to the 20% weight loss in the adjustable banding group. At 10 years, the weight loss had stabilized at 25% and 14% in the RYGB and band groups, respectively.

Table 5-1
Time Schedule and Laboratory Testing for Each Operation

TIME INTERVAL LABORATORY STUDIES	ADJUSTABLE GASTRIC BAND	VERTICAL SLEEVE GASTRECTOMY	ROUX-EN-Y GASTRIC BYPASS	BILIOPANCREATIC DIVERSION WITH DUODENAL SWITCH
First year after surgery	@ 3 to 6 months	@ 3 to 6 months	@ 3 to 6 months	@ 3 months
Thereafter	Annually	Annually	Annually	q 6 months

LABORATORY STUDY	AGB	VSG	RYGB	BPD-DS
Complete blood count	X	X	X	X
Platelets	X	X	X	X
Electrolytes	X	X	X	X
Glucose	X	X	X	X
Hemoglobin A1c	X	X	X	X
Iron studies, ferritin		X	X	X
Vitamin B_{12}		X	X	X
Vitamin B_6				
Folic acid			X	X
Liver panel	X	X	X	X
Lipid panel	X	X	X	X
25-Hydroyvitamin D	X	X	X	X
Parathyroid hormone	X	X	X	X
Thiamine		X	X	X
Albumin		X	X	X
Prealbumin		X	X	X
Fat-soluble vitamins				
D				X
E				X
A				X
K				X
Trace elements				
Zinc			X	X
Selenium			X	X

AGB = adjustable gastric band, BPD-DS = biliopancreatic diversion with duodenal switch, RYGB = Roux-en-Y gastric bypass, VSG = vertical sleeve gastrectomy.

Resolution of Comorbid Conditions

Diabetes Mellitus Type 2

Diabetes mellitus is strongly linked to obesity. It has been well reported that it can be significantly improved by weight loss surgery. Increasingly, studies have looked at the effects of bariatric surgery on hemoglobin A1c (HbA1c) and diabetes treatment targets. A meta-analysis by Buchwald and colleagues found that laparoscopic adjustable band patients had HbA1c decrease on average 1.3% (95% confidence interval [CI], 0.9 to 1.6) compared to a decrease of 4.0% (95% CI, 0.7 to 5.0) for the RYGB patients.[23] Another meta-analysis by Buchwald compared the AGB, RYGB, and BPD-DS in respect to their effect on type 2 diabetes mellitus. This analysis showed that patients who lost the most weight (specifically the BPD-DS patients) had the best control of diabetes, with 95.1% of patients having complete resolution of their disease. It also showed 56.7% and 80.3% resolution in the AGB and RYGB patients, respectively.[23] Even though the BPD-DS operation typically has the best results with respect to weight loss and control of diabetes mellitus, it also has the highest complication rate, which prohibits it from being the preferred operation on patients with diabetes.

An even more recent study published in the *Journal of the American Medical Association* randomized 120 patients to intensive lifestyle and medical management alone or lifestyle and medical management plus the RYGB.[22] The composite endpoint was a HbA1c $<$7.0%, low-density lipoprotein cholesterol $<$100 mg/dL, and systolic blood pressure $<$130 mm Hg. In the RYGB group, 28 patients (49%; 95% CI, 36% to 64%) achieved the endpoint vs 11 (19%; 95% CI, 10% to 32%) in the lifestyle and medical management alone group. It further showed that patients who had the RYGB were on 3 fewer medications (mean 1.7 vs 4.8; 95% CI for the difference, 2.3 to 3.6) and lost 26.1% vs 7.9% (difference, 17.5%; 95% CI, 14.2% to 20.7%) of their initial body weight when compared to the intensive lifestyle and medical management group.

Summary

This chapter explains a brief history of bariatric surgery, the 4 current surgical procedures, their possible complications, and the likely results. Bariatric surgery is a potent weight loss tool. Indeed, it is only a "tool" for the patient to use on his or her weight loss journey. In order to achieve successful weight loss, patients require a complex network of health care providers both pre- and postoperatively. They must undergo a thorough preoperative evaluation that includes dietary, psychological, and medical assessments. Each of the 4 procedures has its own risks and benefits as outlined in the chapter. Careful procedural selection based on both the patient's goals and his or her comorbid conditions is paramount to maximizing weight loss and minimizing postoperative issues. With the increasing numbers of bariatric operations being performed, the need for providers who understand the complex nutritional and metabolic needs of this multifaceted group of patients is also on the rise. Providers with an understanding of the risks, benefits, and possible complications of these bariatric operations will truly be able to help their patients to realize the full potential of the tool that we have given them.

References

1. Ogden CL, Carroll MD, Kit BK, Flegal KM. Prevalence of obesity in the United States. *NCHS Data Brief.* Jan 2012;82.
2. Moyer CS. Delegates declare obesity a disease. *American Medical News.* 2013;56(13):1-2.
3. Baker MT. The history and evolution of bariatric surgical procedures. *Surg Clin North Am.* 2011;91(6):1181-1201.
4. Buchwald H, Buchwald JN. Evolution of operative procedures for the management of morbid obesity 1950-2000. *Obes Surg.* 2002;12(5):705-717.

5. Kuzmak LI, Yap IS, McGuire L, Dixon JS, Young MP. Surgery for morbid obesity. *AORN J.* 1990;51(5):1307-1324.
6. Scopinaro N, Gianetta E, Civialleri D. Biliopancreatic bypass for obesity: II. Initial experiences in man. *Br J Surg.* 1979;66:618-620.
7. Marceau P, Biron S, Bourque RA, Potvin M, Hould FS, Simard S. Biliopancreatic diversion with a new type of gastrectomy. *Obes Surg.* 1993;3(1):29-35.
8. Hess DS, Hess DW. Biliopancreatic diversion with a duodenal switch. *Obes Surg.* 1998;8(3):267-282.
9. Reinhold RB. Critical analysis of long term weight loss following gastric bypass. *Surg Gyencol Obstet.* 1982;3:385-394.
10. Favretti F, Segato G, Ashton D, et al. Laparoscopic adjustable gastric banding in 1791 consecutive obese patients: 12-yr results. *Obes Surg.* 2007;17(2):168-175.
11. Weiner R, Blanco-Engert R, Weiner S, Matokowitz R, Schaefer L, Pomhoff I. Outcome after laparoscopic adjustable gastric banding-8 year's experience. *Obes Surg.* 2003;13(3):427-434.
12. Angrisani L, Furbetta F, Doldi SB, et al. Lap Band adjustable gastric banding system: the Italian experience with 1863 patients operated on 6 years. *Surg Endosc.* 2003;17(3):409-412.
13. Kriwanek S, Schermann M, Ali Abdullah S, Roka R. Band slippage a potentially life threatening complication after laparoscopic adjustable gastric banding. *Obes Surg.* 2006;15(1):133-136.
14. Egberts K, Brown WA, O'Brein PE. Systematic review of erosion after laparoscopic adjustable gastric banding. *Obes Surg.* 2011;21(8):1272-1279.
15. Hipens J, Dapri G, Caiere GB. A prospective randomized study between laparoscopic gastric banding and laparoscopic isolated sleeve gastrectomy: results after 1 and 3 years. *Obes Surg.* 2006;16(11):1450-1456.
16. Vidal P, Ramon JM, Goday A, et al. Laparoscopic gastric bypass versus laparoscopic sleeve gastrectomy as a definitive surgical procedure for morbid obesity. Midterm results. *Obes Surg.* 2013;23(3):292-299.
17. Keidar A, Herschkop KJ, Marko L, et al. Roux-en-Y gastric bypass vs. sleeve gastrectomy for obese patients with type 2 diabetes: a randomized trial. *Diabetologia.* 2013 Jun 13. PMID 23765156.
18. Yuval JB, Mintz Y, Cohen MJ, Rivkind AI, Elazary R. The effects of bougie caliber on leaks and excess weight loss following laparoscopic sleeve gastrectomy. Is there an ideal bougie size. *Obes Surg.* 2013;23(10):1685-1691.
19. Bellanger DE, Greenway FL. Laparoscopic sleeve gastrectomy, 529 cases without a leak: short term results and technical considerations. *Obes Surg.* 2011;21(2):146-150.
20. Weiner RA, El-Sayes IA, Theodoridou S, Weiner SR, Scheffel O. Early post-operative complications: incidence, management, and impact on length of hospital stay. A retrospective comparison between laparoscopic gastric bypass and sleeve gastrectomy. *Obes Surg.* 2013;23(12):2004-2012.
21. Carlin AM, Zeni TM, English WJ, et al. The comparative effectiveness of sleeve gastrectomy, gastric bypass, and adjustable gastric banding procedures for the treatment of morbid obesity. *Ann Surg.* 2013;257(5):791-797.
22. Ikramuddin S, Korner J, Lee WJ, et al. Roux-en-Y gastric bypass vs. intensive medical management for the control of type 2 diabetes, hypertension, and hyperlipidemia: the diabetes surgery study randomized clinical trial. *JAMA.* 2013;309(21):2240-2249.
23. Buchwald H, Estok R, Fahrbach K, et al. Weight and type 2 diabetes after bariatric surgery: systematic review and meta-analysis. *Am J Med.* 2009;122(3):248-256.
24. Ikramuddin S, Kendrick ML, Kellogg TA, Sarr MG. Open and laparoscopic Roux-en-Y gastric bypass: our technique. *J Gastrointest Surg.* 2007;11(2):217-228.
25. Carrodeguas L, Szomstein S, Zundel N, Lo Menzo E, Rosenthal R. Gastrojejunal anastomotic strictures following laparoscopic Roux-en-Y gastric bypass surgery: analysis of 1291 patients. *Surg Obes Relat Dis.* 2006;2(2):92-97.
26. Takata MC, Ciovica R, Cello JP, Posselt AM, Rogers SJ, Campos GM. Predictors, treatment and outcomes of gastrojejunostomy stricture after gastric bypass for morbid obesity. *Obes Surg.* 2007;17(7):878-884.
27. Higa KD, Ho T, Boone KB. Internal hernias after laparoscopic Roux-en-Y gastric bypass: incidence, treatment and prevention. *Obes Surg.* 2003;13(3):350-354.
28. Ritz P, Hanaire J. Post-bypass hypoglycemia: a review of current findings. *Diabetes Metab.* 2011;37(4):274-281.
29. Cui Y, Elahi D, Andersen DK. Advances in the etiology and management of hyperinsulinemic hypoglycemia after Roux-en-Y gastric bypass. *J Gastrointest Surg.* 2011;15(10):1879-1888.
30. Azagury DE, Abu Dayyey BK, Greenwalt IT, Thompson CC. Marginal ulceration after Roux-en-Y gastric bypass surgery: characteristics, risk factors, treatment, and outcomes. *Endoscopy.* 2011;43(11):950-954.
31. Dorman RB, Rasmus NF, al-Haddad BJ, et al. Benefits and complications of the duodenal switch/biliopancreatic diversion compared to the Roux-en-Y gastric bypass. *Surgery.* 2012;152(4):758-765.
32. Biertho L, Lebel S, Marceau S, et al. Perioperative complications in a consecutive series of 1000 duodenal switches. *Surg Obes Relat Dis.* 2013;9(1):63-68.
33. Hedberg J, Sundbom M. Superior weight loss and lower HbA1c 3 years after duodenal switch compared with Roux-en-Y gastric bypass a randomized controlled trial. *Surg Obes Relat Dis.* 2012;8(3):338-343.
34. Sjostrom L, Narbro K, Sjostrom CD, et al. Effects of bariatric surgery on mortality in Swedish obese subjects. *N Engl J Med.* 2007;357(8):741-752.

6

Gastric Banding

Christine Ren Fielding, MD

Background

Gastric banding surgery has historically been defined as a "restrictive" operation because of the original manner in which it was placed. Starting in the 1960s, surgeons placed a rigid band of material (ie, silicone, mesh) circumferentially around the upper stomach several inches below the gastroesophageal junction. Although many patients lost weight, the quality of life was filled with vomiting and food intolerance, which subsequently led to patient maladaptive eating of soft high-calorie items such as ice cream. This occurred because although the patient was unable to eat solid food, he or she had his or her normal appetite and suboptimal satiety. The drive to eat was not changed. The evolution of banding as a "punitive" operation into a "satiety-inducing" tool came in the 1990s when the adjustable gastric band was introduced in Europe, Australia, and South America. Presently in the United States, there are 2 companies that make the device: the Lap-Band system by Apollo Endosurgery and the Realize system by Ethicon Endo-Surgery. All bands are designed to be implanted laparoscopically and only in unusual or difficult situations need a formal laparotomy (or open procedure). Thus, the nomenclature of laparoscopic adjustable gastric banding (LAGB) is routinely used.

The Device and How It Works

For all intents and purposes, both adjustable bands work in the same manner with very minor differences. The band is composed of a silicone rind with an attached inner balloon, much like a blood pressure cuff, which is wrapped around the very upper part of the stomach immediately below the gastroesophageal junction (Figure 6-1). The band is attached via hollow tubing to an access port located just below the skin, attached to the anterior rectus sheath of the abdomen (Figure 6-2). The band can be "tightened" or "loosened" by injecting saline into the access port, which travels into the balloon portion of the band, and subsequently compresses the stomach

Forse RA, Apovian CM, eds.
Bariatric Surgery: What Every Provider Needs to Know (pp 79-88).

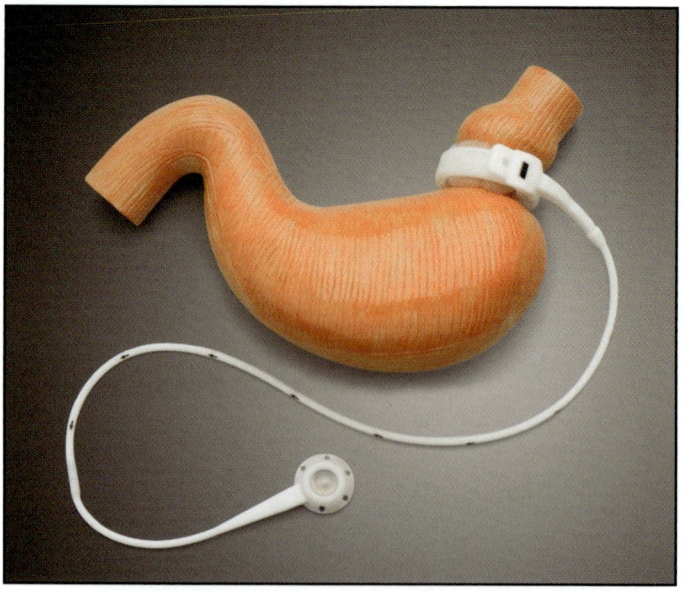

Figure 6-1. Depiction of gastric band placement around the stomach. (Used with permission of Allergan.)

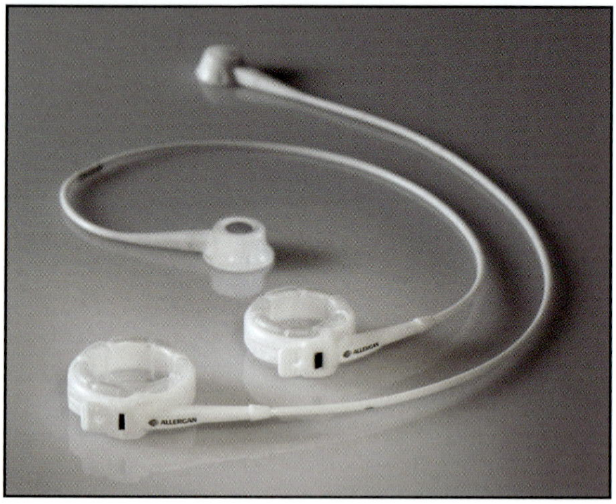

Figure 6-2. Adjustable gastric band. (Used with permission of Allergan.)

circumferentially (Figure 6-3). The band is therefore not a "static" device, but an "adjustable" interactive device that can be manipulated in its extent of compression of the stomach. It has been hypothesized that the mechanical effects of the band impact the vagal afferent signals arising from the mechanoreceptors in the upper stomach, which result in increased satiety and decreased appetite.[1] As a result, the level of satiety a patient feels can be titrated by tightening or adjusting the band, which is performed in the outpatient setting, typically the office. Dixon et al found that patients whose bands were optimally adjusted had a greater sense of satiety after a smaller meal and were found to be less hungry prior to a meal,[2] as compared to when their bands were completely loosened. Therefore, the physical compression of the stomach, or possibly the vagus nerve indirectly, allows for the patient to eat less food and subsequently lose weight.

The technical act of performing a band adjustment is straightforward but is perceived as daunting. The subcutaneous access port is similar to the Mediport used in chemotherapy, but location is in the abdominal wall rather than the upper chest. For this reason, a thick layer of subcutaneous fat may make palpation and location of the port more challenging. Strategies for port location lie in patient positioning to stabilize the rectus muscle. A common technique is to have the patient

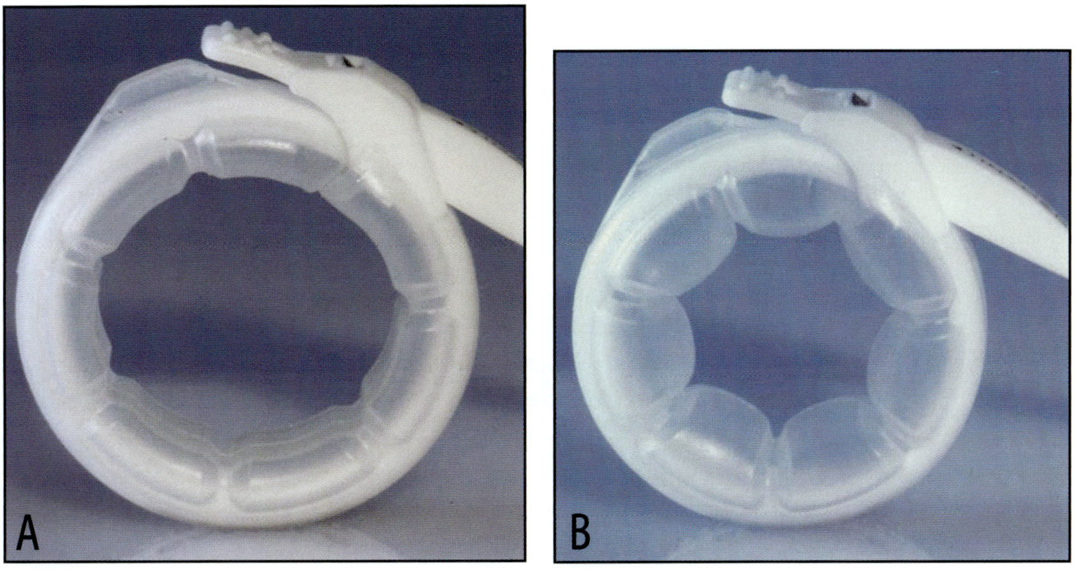

Figure 6-3. (A) Deflated gastric band. (B) Inflated gastric band. (Used with permission of Allergan.)

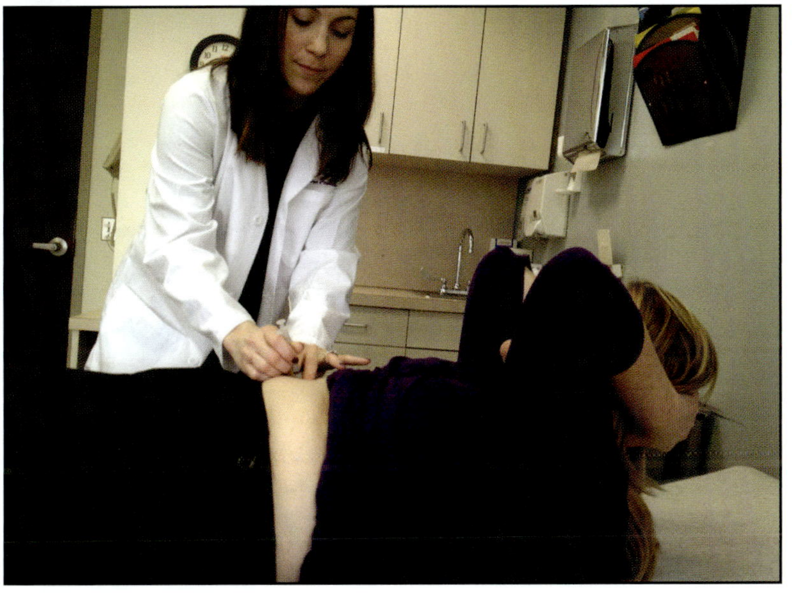

Figure 6-4. Patient position during band adjustment.

lie supine, with legs extended, with hands behind the head flexing forward (Figure 6-4). Another technique is to have the patient lie supine and "push" his or her abdomen out so that it appears distended. In patients who have a large hanging pannus, the standing position helps bring the pannus down away from the port using gravity. Once the port is located and stabilized with the nondominant hand, the noncoring Huber needle connected to a syringe in the dominant hand can puncture the skin into the membrane of the access port. Successful port access is confirmed by feeling the needle hit the metal base of the access port, and having free reflux of saline back into the syringe. Local anesthetic is unnecessary since oftentimes it creates more pain than the actual adjustment itself. Radiographic or ultrasound assistance may be needed to help localize and mark the port, particularly in patients who have a thick wall of subcutaneous fat. The learning curve for port localization using palpation is surprisingly long, and may take up to 50 cases. Real-time fluoroscopy is helpful in localizing and accessing the port; however, it can be time consuming and

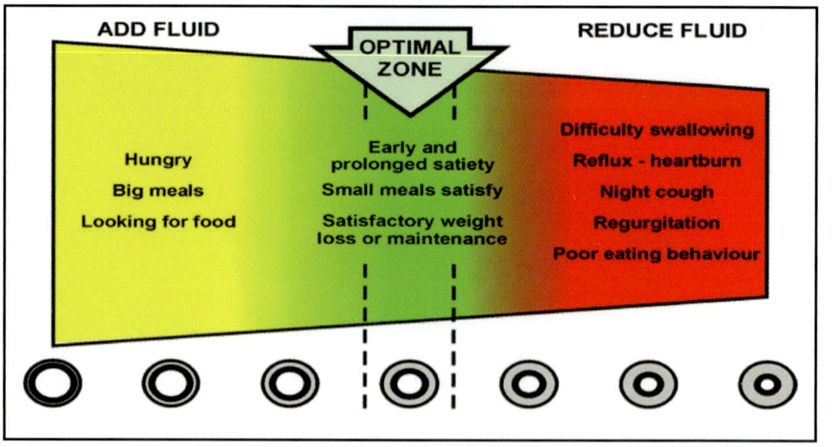

Figure 6-5. Green Zone chart. (Reprinted with permission from Dixon JB, Straznicky NE, Lambert EA, Schlaich MP, Lambert GW. Laparoscopic adjustable gastric banding and other devices for the management of obesity. *Circulation*. 2012;126[6]:774-785.)

expensive. Care must be taken to puncture the port using a noncoring Huber needle into the septum, rather than the neck of the port, which is not self-sealing. The septum is self-sealing only if a noncoring needle, such as a Huber needle, is used rather than a traditional hypodermic needle, otherwise the silicone of the membrane will be cored out, creating a leak of saline. The needle should be inserted into the membrane at 90 degrees (perpendicular) in order to ensure that the reservoir is successfully accessed. An obtuse approach will not reach the reservoir.

The Critical Role of After Care

It is most helpful to engage the patient in the decision-making process of whether to tighten or to loosen the band by introducing him or her to and using the Green Zone chart originally developed by Dixon[1] (Figure 6-5). The Green Zone chart describes 3 different states that the patient is in to help make the decision of how to manage the band. The yellow zone is when the patient feels hunger between meals, looks to snack in between meals, eats large portions, and is not losing weight. This signifies a band that is too loose and needs to be tightened. The green zone describes the patient as having good satiety with a small portion of food, not hungry between meals (typically 4 to 5 hours), and is losing weight. This signifies a patient whose band is just right and needs no adjustment. The red zone describes symptoms of heartburn, nighttime reflux or cough, and intolerance to most solid foods, with the patient resorting to soft or blended high-calorie foods. This typically necessitates for the band to be loosened. The actual amount of saline to inject or remove is more of an art rather than a science. The range of saline volume to inject is based on the type of band, its maximum recommended volume, and the average range of optimum volume that will put the patient in the green zone (Table 6-1).

After a patient receives an adjustment, it is prudent to have the patient drink a 6-ounce cup of water to ensure no obstruction of the band is present. The patient is then counseled to progress from a liquid to a solid meal gradually over the course of the next 4 days in order to acclimate to the new stoma outlet into the stomach that the band has created. The most important counseling that must be given to the patient is to slow down the pace of his or her eating and to chew each mouthful thoroughly. Behavior modification of this sort will lead to avoidance of obstructive symptoms, such as dysphagia, regurgitation, reflux, and vomiting. After the initial surgery, the first adjustment can be performed 1 month after surgery. Subsequently, it has been shown that regular follow-up visits of every 4 to 6 months in the first year improves weight loss outcomes when compared to those patients who come in less than 50% of the time. Patients who return more than 6 times in the first year after gastric banding lose on average of 20% more weight than those who

Table 6-1
Gastric Bands Available in the United States

BAND TYPE	MAXIMUM RECOMMENDED VOLUME (ML)	AVERAGE VOLUME RANGE (ML)
Apollo Endosurgery		
LAPBAND 9.75	4	2.5 to 3
LAPBAND 10	4	2.5 to 3
LAPBAND VG	11	9 to 10.5
LAPBAND APS	10	5.5 to 7.0
LAPBAND APL	14	8 to 10.5
Ethicon Endosurgery		
REALIZE	9	7.5 to 8.5
REALIZE-C	11	8.5 to 10.5

do not return as recommended.[3] Not only do the patients receive their adjustments in a timely manner and have their weight monitored, but each visit is an opportunity to reinforce behavior modification of their eating. The average number of adjustments that a typical patient requires to reach a stable green zone long term is 6 in the first year and 2 in the second year. After the second year, patients can be followed up annually or sooner if needed. If a patient is not losing weight, he or she must be encouraged and made to feel comfortable to return to his or her surgeon to investigate why it is happening. The interactive nature of the band as a tool allows it to be tightened if the patient is found to be in the yellow zone.

As mentioned earlier, a properly adjusted band allows the patient to achieve satiety with a smaller portion of food. However, which type of food (ie, caloric content) the patient ingests contributes to weight loss. High-calorie foods, which are typically high in sugar and/or fat content, although eaten in smaller quantities, will result in less weight loss when compared to lower calorie foods, which are typically proteins and vegetables. Therefore, patient collaboration is necessary for optimal weight loss outcomes, specifically maintaining healthy food choices. One misconception patients have is that the tighter the band is made, the more weight they will lose. This is true until a certain point, that point being when the patient is in the green zone. If the band is tightened further, then the outlet into the stomach is too small for well-chewed solid foods to pass through and the patient starts to experience greater frequency of regurgitation or vomiting. The patient will then naturally start to avoid foods such as vegetables and meats, and instead gravitate toward fat- or sugar-based foods, such as mashed potatoes, ice cream, or mayonnaise, because they are "easier" to eat. This is termed *maladaptive eating* and results in a converse weight gain. Often times these patients also experience heartburn or nighttime reflux and cough resulting from regurgitant esophagitis. These symptoms mean that the patient is in the red zone and needs to have the band loosened so that he or she can be able to eat solid healthier foods and/or relieve esophagitis. Patients are typically reluctant to have their band loosened for fear of gaining weight; however, by using the Green Zone chart and explaining the interactive nature of the band, they soon find that symptoms are immediately resolved with only a minor band loosening. Short-term sucralfate or proton pump inhibitors (PPIs) can be helpful in patients who have heartburn or reflux.

Device Maintenance

Although the band can be surgically removed, and therefore is "reversible," it does not mean that the band is removed upon the patient's reaching his or her goal weight. By removing, or even loosening, the band, appetite control and satiety disappear with return of hunger and lack of fullness. As a result, the patient invariably regains most if not all his or her weight back. Therefore, the band is kept in as long as possible, preferably for the patient's lifetime.

Since the gastric band is a device, it should undergo routine annual evaluation for placement. Oftentimes either patients are not symptomatic or do not realize that new symptoms are related to the band (eg, night cough). It is a good idea to have patients with an LAGB to be seen at least annually for an evaluation and a barium swallow esophagram. The esophagram is a simple noninvasive test that provides information on the following: band position, size of gastric pouch, outlet of band stoma, diameter, and general functionality of the esophagus. A normal esophagram (Figure 6-6A) means that the band is in a 2 o'clock-8 o'clock orientation, the height and width of the gastric band is not more than twice the length of the band itself, the barium is delayed but emptying through the band stoma outlet into the distal stomach, the esophagus is not wider than the width of the thoracic vertebrae, and the mucosal contour of the esophagus is smooth. Peristalsis may be seen on this as well. An abnormality in band positioning (Figure 6-6B) is representative of a band slippage where the lower stomach fundus pushes its way up through the band in a cephalad direction (see Complications). The band is oriented in a 10 o'clock-4 o'clock position. An abnormality in pouch size (Figure 6-6C) may be due to an overly tightened band or to excessive vomiting resulting in pouch dilation (see Complications) and may necessitate simple band loosening and behavioral counseling.

Outcomes

Weight Loss

Weight loss after LAGB is gradual and steady for up to 3 years after which a steady plateau of 45% to 55% excess weight loss (EWL) is maintained out to 15 years.[4] Weight loss after LAGB depends on several factors: proper surgical placement, properly adjusted band to achieve satiety and hunger control, and patient behavioral modification. Because so many variables are at stake, there can be a spectrum of weight loss outcomes. The healthier the food choices that are made and the more time spent in exercise, the greater the weight loss achieved. The converse is true. Although this may seem somewhat obvious to the clinician, many patients may mistakenly believe that some calories are not absorbed, or because their meals are smaller, patients underestimate the number of calories in beverages or snacks. Preoperative education is important to alert the patient of this reality, and postoperative counseling and reinforcement are helpful to motivated patients.

In addition, the patient must understand that no operation, including LAGB, is a guarantee of initial or long-term weight loss. It is merely a tool to allow for decreased portion intake; suboptimal weight loss or even weight gain can occur if the patient does not work with the band. The typical daily caloric intake typically is between 1000 and 1400 calories/day for women and 1200 to 1600 calories/day for men, thus resulting in a 1- to 2-lb/week weight loss achieved. This gradual weight loss limits the amount of weight lost from muscle mass, and rather targets fat mass.

Weight loss failure or regain most commonly occurs as a result of (1) maladaptive eating behavior secondary to gastric prolapse, dysphagia, or overtightening of the band, or (2) a nonrestricting band secondary to band erosion, tubing disconnection, leakage of saline from the system, or failure of the patient to return for adjustments. The most unfortunate, and soluble, reason for weight loss failure is insufficient adjustment of the band due to surgeon refusal, unavailability, or

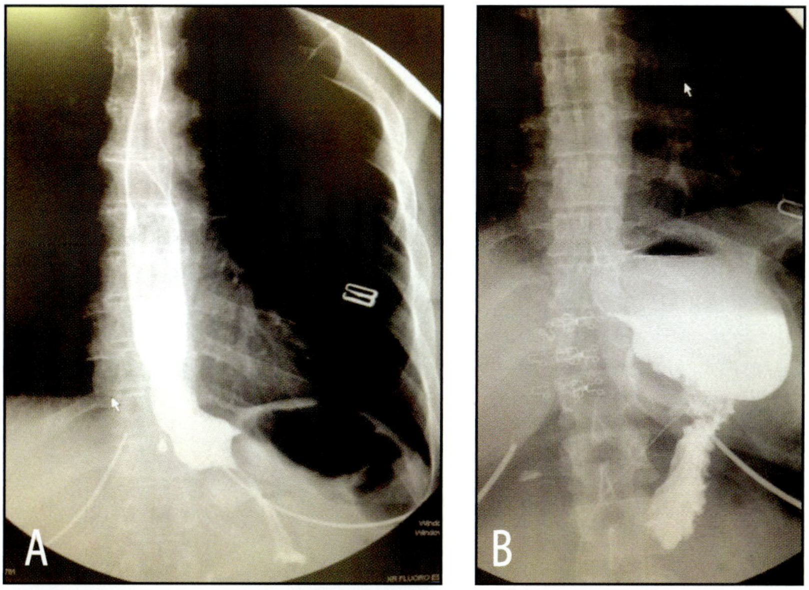

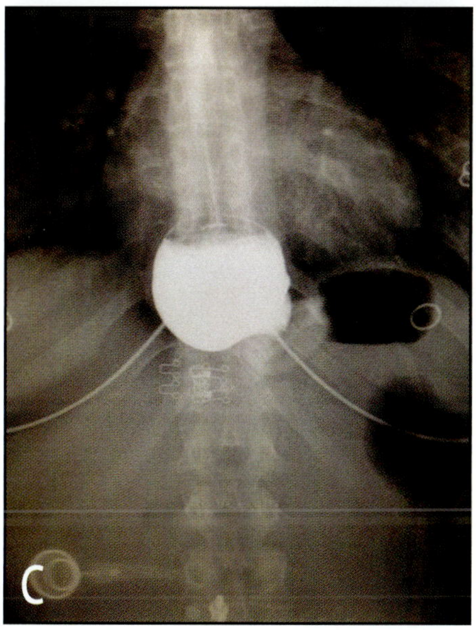

Figure 6-6. (A) Normal post-LAGB esophagram. (B) Esophagram depicting a band slippage. (C) Esophagram depicting pouch dilation.

undereducation. A nonrestricted band will not provide appetite suppression, satiety, or behavior modification, and therefore is nonfunctional. Mechanical problems require either port replacement, tubing reconnection, or band reposition. The number of patients achieving less than 25% EWL is 8% at 2 years and 4% at 3 years after initial LAGB surgery.[4]

Certainly not all patients will benefit from an LAGB. A functioning but ineffective band can be removed laparoscopically, and then be revised to a Roux-en-Y gastric bypass (RYGB), vertical sleeve gastrectomy, or a malabsorptive procedure. This has been most commonly performed for dysphagia, reflux, poor weight loss, or band erosion. O'Brien et al had an explantation rate of 5.6% in their 3227 patients.[4] Laparoscopic removal of gastric band by itself is a very simple straightforward procedure. The band creates very little scar tissue around it and therefore all that is involved is cutting of the band and sliding it away from the stomach without significant dissection of adhesions. It is removed out of the abdominal cavity, along with the subcutaneous access port.

Health Improvements

The majority of obesity-related illnesses are improved and often resolve after weight loss, particularly if it is kept off for many years. Illnesses that most commonly improve after weight loss from LAGB are obstructive sleep apnea, fatty liver (nonalcholic steatohepatitis), hypercholesterolemia, type 2 diabetes mellitus, asthma, cardiomyopathy, gastroesophageal reflux, and osteoarthritis pain.[5] Sultan et al found that in 95 LAGB patients with type 2 diabetes mellitus (oral hypoglycemics and/or insulin), there was over 50% EWL at 5 years with 80% improvement or complete normalization of lab values off medications.[6] In fact, weight loss after LAGB results in increased insulin sensitivity and increased pancreatic beta-cell function, particularly in those patients who are diabetic for less than 7 years.[7] Even if they do not improve, many illnesses can be stopped from progression. In addition, improvements in quality of life occur most significantly in mobility, exertional dyspnea, and self-esteem.

COMPLICATIONS

Early

The actual surgical procedure of LAGB implantation is safe, the safest of all available bariatric operations. The Australian Safety and Efficacy Register of New Interventional Procedures—Surgical (ASERNIP-S), a subcommittee of the Royal Australasian College of Surgeons, evaluated the LAGB against vertical banded gastroplasty and RYGB in terms of safety and efficacy.[8] The mortality is 0.1%, and if occurs is usually due to a cardiac event or pulmonary embolism. Early complication rates are low and most often involve nausea and dehydration. Rarely internal organ injury or bleeding can occur and must be considered if a patient returns soon afterward with pain or fever.[9]

Late

Gastric Pouch Enlargement

The gastric pouch refers to the region of the stomach above the gastric band. This should normally contain a volume of 15 to 30 mL and have a width and length of 3 to 4 cm. Therefore, the distance between the gastroesophageal junction and the band should be typically no more than 4 cm. If the pouch is larger in size and volume, the patient may experience heartburn, reflux, dysphagia, or food intolerance. The shape of the gastric pouch can be either concentric or asymmetric. A concentric gastric pouch is typically called pouch dilation (see Figure 6-6C). An asymmetric gastric pouch (see Figure 6-6B) is traditionally called a band slippage; either the medial or the lateral aspect of the pouch lies in a dependent position and therefore does not empty properly, and thus results in retained food in the gastric pouch, which can reflux into the esophagus. Both of these gastric pouch enlargements can present similarly; symptoms are most pronounced during sleep when the patient is lying supine, often causing heartburn, reflux, night cough, hoarseness, and aspiration pneumonia. Diagnosis is made by barium swallow esophagram. On occasion, esophagram is not diagnostic and an upper endoscopy may be helpful. Initial treatment involves loosening of the band and a course of PPI or sucralfate. Surgical revision and band repositioning is indicated in most cases. Other options include band removal alone and band removal with conversion to a different bariatric operation (RYGB, sleeve gastrectomy, malabsorptive operation).

Device Malfunction/Leak

Port and tubing problems include port migration, port infection, tubing disconnection, tubing kink, and port leak. These mechanical problems are not lethal, but rather impede the weight loss process, due to failure of the band adjustment mechanism. The incidence ranges from 0% to 7%. Port and tubing problems can be resolved with replacement or revision of the reservoir port in an outpatient setting. Port infections can be prevented with early antibiotic treatment, particularly in diabetic and sleep apnea patients.

Band Erosion

Band erosion occurs rarely (0% to 3%) and its etiology is unclear, usually occurring years after band implantation. The band burrows its way through the gastric wall into the lumen of the stomach over a period of time. Patients are not systemically ill due to the confinement of the gastric perforation by healing of the stomach over the band. Typical presentation is cellulitis overlying the access port or lack of restriction despite maximum band adjustment. Endoscopy confirms band erosion and necessitates band explantation.

Gastroesophageal Reflux Disease

Patients who have gastroesophageal reflux disease (GERD) prior to LAGB surgery typically have resolution, especially if it was associated with a hiatal hernia that was repaired simultaneously. Conversely, patients can develop GERD many months after their LAGB. There are 3 main reasons for post-LAGB GERD: esophagitis, pill esophagitis, and sliding hiatal hernia. All 3 entities result in exposure of the distal esophagus to acid leading to esophagitis, which decreases esophageal motility, specifically stripping waves, which clear saliva, particularly when the patient is supine. The patient typically complains of reflux, regurgitation, heartburn, or cough when sleeping, and as a result, sleeps with his or her head elevated. Patients rarely complain of GERD during the day, but may experience heartburn. Therefore, if an LAGB patient presents with new onset nocturnal GERD, the clinician should find out if the patient has had regurgitation or vomiting more than once a month or has been taking any pills larger than a Tic-Tac. Frequent regurgitation can be brought on if the band is too tight or if the patient is eating too fast or too much. Stress and variation in sex hormones (menses) can bring on esophageal spasm, which can lead to vomiting. Band loosening can relieve vomiting from esophageal spasm. Behavioral counseling will educate the patient who is eating too fast and subsequently regurgitating. Pill esophagitis is an underreported phenomenon and occurs more frequently in LAGB patients because of the narrow stoma outlet into the stomach created by the band, which is typically 10 mm in diameter or less. Therefore, any pills or capsules larger than a Tic-Tac should be either crushed and mixed into applesauce/yogurt or taken in a liquid/chewable form. The most common culprits of pill esophagitis are vitamins, antibiotics, and nonsteroidal medications. Pill esophagitis is treated with temporary band loosening, sucralfate, and adjustment of pill size. If the LAGB patient with GERD has neither regurgitation or pill esophagitis, the clinician should investigate for a hiatal hernia, which can be diagnosed on either barium swallow esophagram or upper endoscopy. Treatment can be conservative with band loosening and/or PPI or surgical hernia repair.

Esophageal Dilation

Esophageal dilation is usually reversible and occurs from an overinflated band or one that is placed too low. On esophagram, it is typically seen in association with gastric pouch dilation, is usually associated with dysphagia, and resolves with loosening of the band. Once the condition resolves, the band can be slowly retightened. On rare occasions, pseudoachalasia is seen, which does not resolve with complete loosening of the band. In these circumstances, the band should be removed, which typically resolves the condition.[10]

Summary

LAGB is a safe and effective treatment for morbid obesity that provides a satiety-inducing and appetite-curbing mechanism for weight loss that is adjustable with no malabsorption. Efficacy relies on a combination of surgical skill, band adjustments, and the recognition and treatment of complications. Failure of any of these 3 components will deem gastric banding futile. Durability of weight loss averages over 50% up to 15 years, with significant impact on comorbidity resolution. Weight loss failure or regain can be addressed by band explantation and revision to a different bariatric procedure.

References

1. Dixon JB, Straznicky NE, Lambert EA, Schlaich MP, Lambert GW. Laparoscopic adjustable gastric banding and other devices for the management of obesity. *Circulation.* 2012;126(6):774-785.
2. Dixon AF, Dixon JB, O'Brien PE. Laparoscopic adjustable gastric banding induces prolonged satiety: a randomized blind crossover study. *J Clin Endocrinol Metab.* 2005;90(2):813-819.
3. Shen R, Dugay G, Rajaram K, Cabrera I, Siegel N, Ren CJ. Impact of patient follow-up on weight loss after bariatric surgery. *Obes Surg.* 2004;14:514-519.
4. O'Brien PE, MacDonald L, Anderson M, Brennan L, Brown WA. Long-term outcomes after bariatric surgery: fifteen-year follow-up of adjustable gastric banding and a systematic review of the bariatric surgical literature. *Ann Surg.* 2013;257:87-94.
5. O'Brien PE, McPhail T, Chaston TB, Dixon JB. Systematic review of medium-term weight loss after bariatric operations. *Obes Surg.* 2006;16(8):1032-1040.
6. Sultan S, Gupta D, Parikh M, et al. Five-year outcomes of patients with type 2 diabetes who underwent laparoscopic adjustable gastric banding. *Surg Obes Relat Dis.* 2010;6(4):373-376.
7. Dixon J, O'Brien P. Improvements in insulin sensitivity and cell function (HOMA) with weight loss in the severely obese. *Diab Med.* 2003;20:127-134.
8. Chapman AE, Kiroff G, Game P, et al. Laparoscopic adjustable gastric banding in the treatment of obesity: a systematic literature review. *Surgery.* 2004;135:326-351.
9. Parikh MS, Laker S, Weiner M, Hajiseyedjavadi O, Ren CJ. Objective comparison of complications resulting from laparoscopic bariatric procedures. *J Am Coll Surg.* 2006;202:252-261.
10. Khan A, Ren-Fielding C, Traube M. Potentially reversible pseudoachalasia after laparoscopic adjustable gastric banding. *J Clin Gastroenterol.* 2011;45(9):775-779.

7

Sleeve Gastrectomy

Stacy A. Brethauer, MD and Philip R. Schauer, MD

How Has This Procedure Evolved?

Sleeve gastrectomy (SG), also referred to as vertical gastrectomy, has been used as a bariatric operation for several decades. Initially, SG was used as the restrictive component of the duodenal switch (DS) procedure. This partial gastrectomy provided early weight loss during the bowel adaption period of this malabsorptive procedure. Typically, the SG created during DS procedures was larger in caliber than the operation performed as a primary operation today. Several surgeons reported performing SG alone during a planned DS procedure. In these cases, intraoperative events required termination of the operation before the bypass portion of the procedure was completed. The postoperative course demonstrated significant weight loss with the SG alone and prompted others to begin using SG as a first-stage procedure for patients who were high risk or had a high body mass index (BMI). In this staged approach, patients' medical conditions improved in the 1 or 2 years after SG and many subsequently went on to a second-stage bypass procedure (gastric bypass or DS). In a study by Cottam and colleagues, 126 high-risk superobese patients with a mean preoperative BMI of 65.3 kg/m^2 underwent laparoscopic SG as a first-stage procedure. The mean excess weight loss at 1 year was 43%, and there were significant reductions in the number of comorbidities and ASA classification prior to the second-stage gastric bypass procedure.[1] In the past 10 years, SG has increasingly been used as a stand-alone primary bariatric procedure and has gained popularity among patients and bariatric surgeons. This operation has appeal to patients and surgeons because it is easy for patients to understand, the anatomy is not "rearranged," it is technically straightforward to perform, and there is no implantable device or adjustments required.

There has been rapid growth in the number of SGs performed in the past 5 years, and it currently comprises more than 40% of all bariatric operations performed worldwide[2] and has replaced gastric banding in many practices.

Forse RA, Apovian CM, eds.
Bariatric Surgery: What Every Provider Needs to Know (pp 89-100).

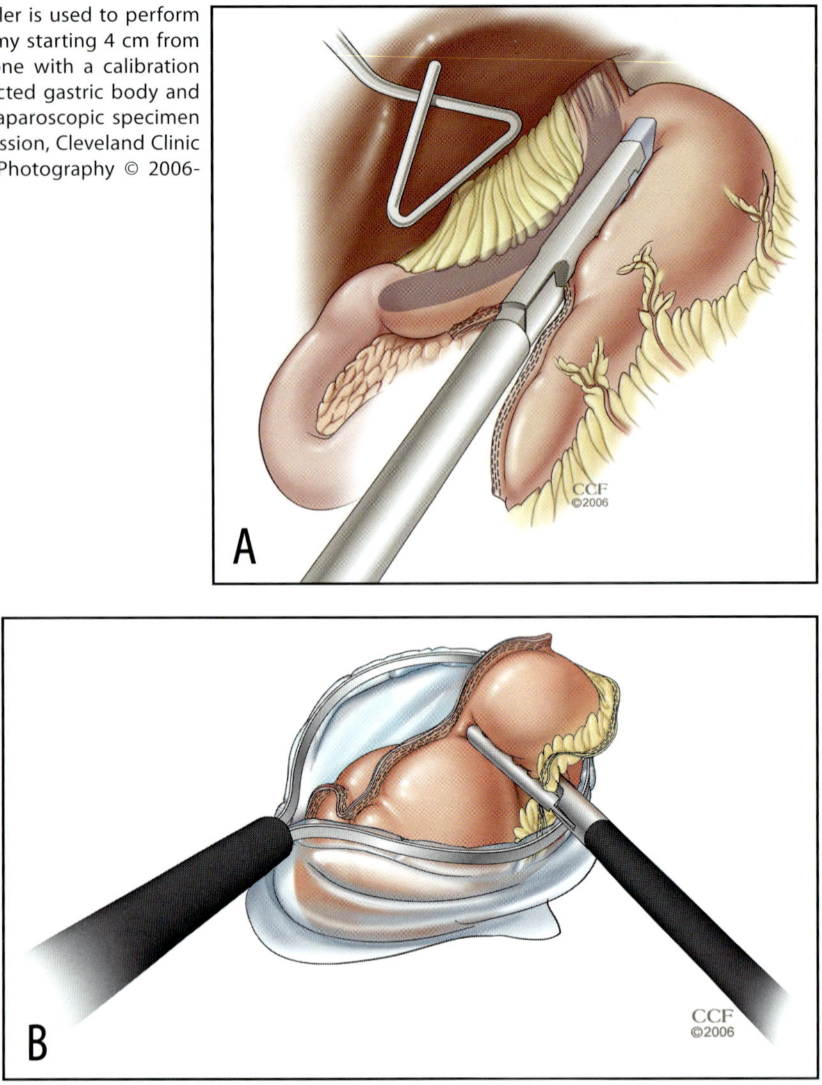

Figure 7-1. The linear stapler is used to perform a vertical sleeve gastrectomy starting 4 cm from the pylorus. (A) This is done with a calibration tube in place. (B) The resected gastric body and fundus are removed in a laparoscopic specimen bag. (Reprinted with permission, Cleveland Clinic Center for Medical Art & Photography © 2006-2013. All rights reserved.)

Technique and Postoperative Care

Laparoscopic SG involves a vertical gastrectomy that results in a narrow, tubular stomach. The concept of SG is relatively simple, but there are components of the operation that, if performed incorrectly, can result in serious complications. Typically, 4 or 5 ports are placed across the upper abdomen. The vascular attachments of the gastroepiploic arcade and the short gastric vessels are divided with ultrasonic shears and the greater curvature is fully mobilized. Once this dissection is complete, a calibration tube or endoscope is placed into the stomach to determine the diameter of the remaining stomach (usually 32 to 40 Fr.). Linear cutting staplers are then sequentially fired starting about 4 cm from the pylorus and continuing proximally to the angle of His (Figure 7-1). Some surgeons use absorbable staple line buttressing material to reinforce the staple line, others

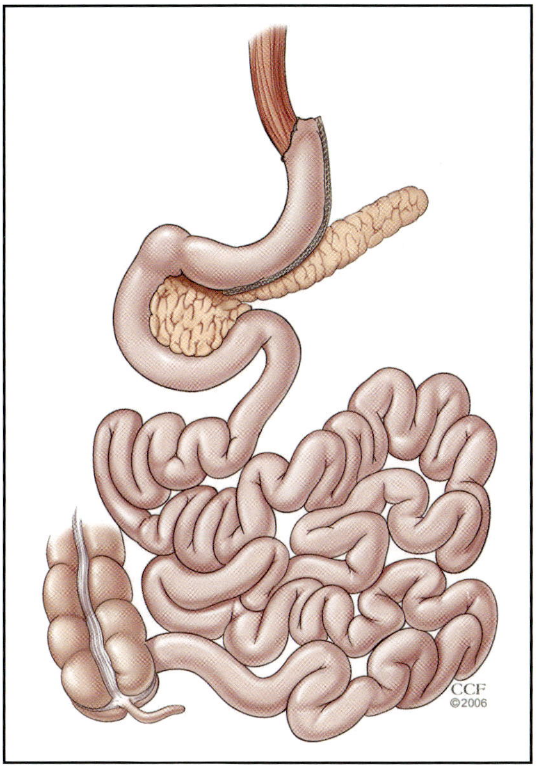

Figure 7-2. Completed sleeve gastrectomy. (Reprinted with permission, Cleveland Clinic Center for Medical Art & Photography © 2006-2013. All rights reserved.)

oversew the staple line, and others leave the staple line as is. There is no strong evidence to suggest any of these methods are superior in terms of staple line leak, and our practice is to oversew the staple line to ensure hemostasis and prevent leaks.

An intraoperative leak test is performed to ensure the integrity of the staple line, and this can be done with endoscopic insufflations or instillation of methylene blue dye via an orogastric tube. Figure 7-2 shows the completed SG. Some surgeons leave drainage tubes in the left upper quadrant after SG.

Postoperatively, patients are started on a clear liquid diet on postoperative day 1. Some surgeons perform routine upper gastrointestinal studies prior to initiation of a liquid diet. SG can be performed with 23-hour overnight stays for low-risk patients. Higher risk, older, or less mobile patients usually require 2 to 3 days to return to their baseline activity and advance their oral intake prior to discharge. After discharge, patients are seen in the office at 1 week and then at 1, 3, 6, 9, 12, and 18 months, followed by annual visits. Activity is advanced as tolerated and exercise can begin within weeks as soon as the patient feels ready to begin. Diet progression after discharge starts with 1 week of full liquids followed by weekly progression to puréed consistency, soft food, and then solid food 1 month after surgery. Some patients require antinausea medication for several weeks to facilitate their diet progression. Vitamin and micronutrient levels are checked at 6 months, 1 year, and then annually to monitor for deficiencies. There are currently limited data regarding long-term nutritional deficiencies after laparoscopic SG. Our practice is to supplement our SG patients with a daily multivitamin, vitamin B_{12}, iron, calcium citrate, and vitamin D to ensure that deficiencies are minimized due to decreased dietary intake.

Outcomes

Weight Loss

The weight loss outcomes after SG have varied according to the population studied, but when all the data are reviewed in aggregate, the average excess weight loss after SG is around 60%. The initial reports of SG utilized this operation as a way to downstage high-risk medical patients or superobese patients prior to a staged bypass procedure. Because many of these patients went on to have a planned second-stage procedure, most of the early reports of SG did not provide follow-up beyond 1 or 2 years. Ultimately, many surgeons found it to be an effective primary bariatric procedure for lower BMI patients, and the more recent literature represents this change. With this increasing experience over the past 5 years, longer term outcome data are now emerging.

A systematic review of 36 studies evaluated overall weight loss after SG and also assessed weight loss for the staged and primary patient groups.[3] The mean preoperative BMI for all patients included in the systematic review was 51.2 and this decreased to 37.1 during the reported follow-up periods, which were predominantly 3 years or less. The mean excess weight loss (EWL) after SG was reported in 24 studies (n = 1662) and ranged from 33% to 85% with an overall mean EWL of 55.4%. The mean preoperative BMI was 60.0 (range, 49.1 to 69.0) for the staged/high-risk patient group and 46.6 (range, 37.2 to 54.5) for the patients undergoing SG as a primary procedure. Reduction in BMI and the EWL reported after SG in these 2 groups is shown in Table 7-1.

There are several studies that compare SG to other bariatric procedures. Himpens et al conducted a randomized controlled trial comparing laparoscopic SG to laparoscopic adjustable gastric banding (AGB).[4] At 3 years, the authors reported greater EWL (66% vs 48%, p = .025), greater loss of hunger (46.7% of patients vs 2.9%), and greater loss of craving for sweets (23.3% of patients vs 2.9%) with laparoscopic SG. Two patients in that trial (5%) had insufficient weight loss 3 years after laparoscopic SG and underwent a DS. Another small randomized trial also demonstrated superior weight loss and decreased ghrelin levels 6 months after laparoscopic SG compared to laparoscopic AGB.[5]

There are also several studies that have compared laparoscopic SG to Roux-en-Y gastric bypass (RYGB). In a prospective, double-blind study with 16 patients in each group, Karamanakos et al reported better weight loss with laparoscopic SG at 1 year compared to RYGB (EWL 69.7% vs 60.5%, respectively, p = .05).[6] They attributed this difference to more pronounced changes in specific gut hormones after the sleeve resulting in decreased hunger. In a nonrandomized study by Vidal et al, laparoscopic SG (n = 39) and RYGB (n = 52) patients were matched for various diabetes parameters, and 1 year after surgery, weight loss was similar for the 2 groups (31% of initial weight).[7]

Despite being widely adopted in the past 5 years, the long-term durability of SG has remained a concern. The first publication reporting 5-year weight loss data was by Weiner and colleagues in 2007,[8] in which BMI decreased from 60.7 to 45.0. Since the publication of the systematic review in 2009,[3] there have been several important studies published that report longer term follow-up (Table 7-2). Himpens reported the long-term weight loss data on 41 patients who underwent SG intended as a primary procedure.[9] The median preoperative BMI in this study was 39 and after the sixth year of follow-up the mean EWL overall was 57.3%. Eleven patients underwent a second-stage DS procedure and improved their EWL to 70.8% at 6 years (mean BMI of 27). The stand-alone laparoscopic SG patient group (n = 30) had 53% EWL and a mean BMI of 31 at 6 years. This report demonstrates that some patients do regain weight long term after laparoscopic SG when it is used as a primary procedure and weight loss can be improved by performing a second-stage procedure in selected patients. Despite these issues, patient acceptance of the laparoscopic SG procedure remained good at 6+ years in this study.

Table 7-1
Outcomes of Sleeve Gastrectomy in High-Risk/Staged Patients vs Primary Procedure

	HIGH-RISK PATIENTS/ STAGED APPROACH	PRIMARY PROCEDURE
Number of studies* (number of patients)	13 (821)	24 (1749)
Preoperative BMI range (mean) kg/m^2	49.1 to 69.0 (60.0)	37.2 to 54.5 (46.6)
Postoperative BMI range (mean) kg/m^2	36.4 to 53.0 (44.9)	26.0 to 39.8 (32.2)
Follow-up	4 months to 5 years	3 months to 3 years
% excess weight loss range (mean)	33.0% to 61.4% (46.9) IVW mean = 46.6% (43.8% to 49.5%)	36.0% to 85.0% (60.4) IVW mean = 60.7% (55.1% to 66.3%)
Complication rate all studies (mean)	0 to 23.8% (9.4%)	0 to 21.7% (6.2%)
Studies with n > 100	3.3% to 15.3%	0 to 14.1%
Leaks**	8/686 (1.2%)	45/1681 (2.7%)+
Bleeding**	11/686 (1.6%)	17/1681 (1.0%)++
Strictures**	6/686 (0.9%)	9/1681 (0.5%)
Mortality	2/821 (0.24%)	3/1749 (0.17%)

*One study included clearly defined patients in both groups. **Includes studies with detailed complication data only. +p = .02 compared to high-risk group. ++p not significant compared to high-risk groups.

IVW = inverse variable weighted.

Table 7-2
Long-Term Results After Sleeve Gastrectomy

AUTHOR	PATIENTS (N)	PREOPERATIVE BMI	FOLLOW-UP	WEIGHT LOSS
Weiner et al[8]	8	62	5 years	-17 BMI
Himpens et al[9]	41	39	6 years	53% EWL
Bohdjalian et al[10]	26	48	5 years	55% EWL
Eid et al[11]	74	66	6 to 8 years	48% EWL
Sarela et al[12]	20	46	8 to 9 years	69% EWL
D'Hondt et al[13]	23	39	6 years	56% EWL

BMI = body mass index, EWL = excess weight loss.

Another report of long-term outcomes after SG was recently published by Bohdjalian et al.[10] The authors provide 5-year weight loss data for 26 patients who underwent SG. Mean BMI prior to surgery was 48.2 and one-third of the patients were superobese. Mean EWL at 5 years was 55%. Four patients (15%) underwent a second-stage gastric bypass for weight regain (n = 3) and gastroesophageal reflux (GERD) (n = 1).

The largest laparoscopic SG study reporting long-term follow-up to date is by Eid and colleagues.[11] Seventy-four patients with mean preoperative BMI of 66 underwent laparoscopic SG with a mean follow-up of 73 months (range, 38 to 95 months). The mean age was 50 years (range, 25 to 78 years), and the mean number of comorbidities was 9.6. Perioperative mortality (< 30 days) was zero, and the incidence of short- and long-term postoperative complications was 15%. Mean EWL at 72, 84, and 96 months after laparoscopic SG was 52%, 43%, and 46%, respectively, with an overall EWL of 48%. The mean BMI decreased from 66 (43 to 90) to 46 (22 to 73). Seventy-seven percent of the patients with diabetes showed improvement or remission of the disease. This study demonstrates that, even in superobese patients, weight loss and comorbidity reduction can be sustained long term after SG.

Comorbidity Improvement

Diabetes remission has been reported to different degrees after all of the currently performed bariatric procedures. A randomized controlled trial by Schauer et al evaluated the effects of intensive medical therapy (IMT), IMT plus laparoscopic SG, and IMT plus RYGB in patients with lower BMIs (27 to 42) and poorly controlled type 2 diabetes (mean hemoglobin A1c [HbA1c] 9.2%). At 1 year the proportion of patients with the primary endpoint (HbA1c < 6%) was 12% (5 of 41 patients) in the medical therapy group vs 42% (21 of 50 patients) in the gastric bypass group ($p = .002$) and 37% (18 of 49 patients) in the SG group ($p = .008$). Glycemic control improved in all 3 groups, with a mean glycated hemoglobin level of $7.5 \pm 1.8\%$ in the medical therapy group, $6.4 \pm 0.9\%$ in the gastric bypass group ($p < .001$), and $6.6 \pm 1.0\%$ in the SG group ($p = .003$). Weight loss was greater in the gastric bypass group and SG group (-29.4 ± 9.0 kg and -25.1 ± 8.5 kg, respectively) than in the medical therapy group (-5.4 ± 8.0 kg) ($p < .001$ for both comparisons).[14]

A randomized controlled trial by Lee and colleagues from Taiwan compared gastric bypass (n = 30) to SG (n = 30) for the treatment of type 2 diabetes (remission defined as fasting glucose < 126 mg/dL and HbA1c < 6.5% off glycemic therapy).[15] Laparoscopic SG resulted in remission of diabetes in 47% of patients at 1 year and was associated with an average 3% reduction in HbA1c levels. Gastric bypass, however, had more powerful effects on weight loss, waist circumference, the remission rate of type 2 diabetes (93%), and improvements in the metabolic syndrome in this study. In a matched, cohort analysis in which patients undergoing laparoscopic SG and RYGB were matched for severity and duration of diabetes, both groups had 84% remission of diabetes and comparable rates of resolution of the metabolic syndrome at 1 year (62% for SG, 67% for RYGB).[7]

A recent systematic review by Gill et al evaluated the rates of diabetes improvement after SG and found 28 studies that met their inclusion criteria.[16] The patient population included 673 patients with a mean preoperative BMI of 47.4. In this analysis, laparoscopic SG resulted in diabetes remission in 66.2% of patients. Of those studies that reported improvement and remission of diabetes, 97% of patients had either improvement or remission. The mean HbA1c decreased from 7.9 to 6.2 in the 11 studies that included this measure of glucose control.

Improvement in other major obesity-related comorbidities after laparoscopic SG are shown in Figure 7-3. In addition to improvements in the components of the metabolic syndrome, significant improvement or resolution of sleep apnea, joint pain, depression, and leg edema have been reported.[1,8,17-20]

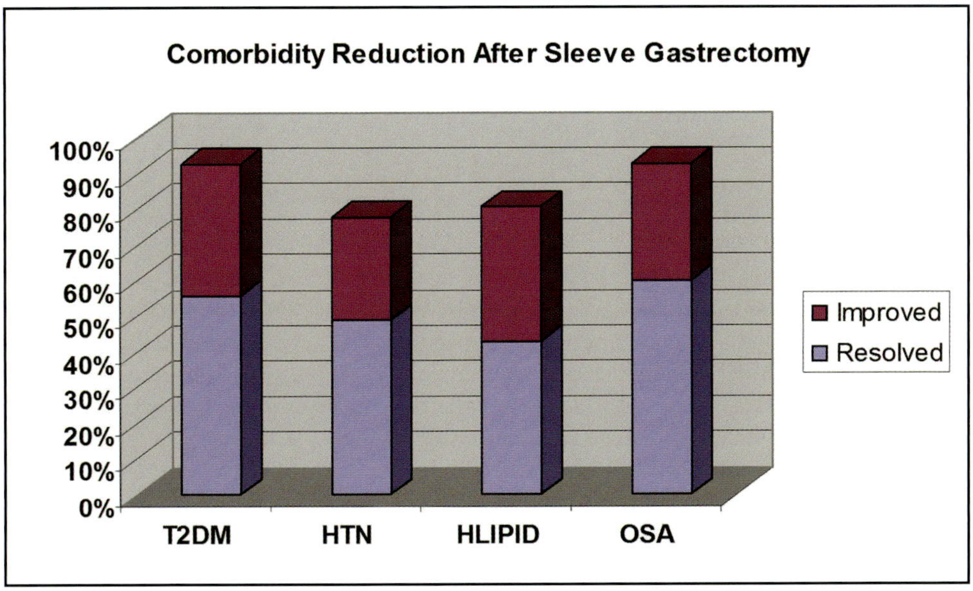

Figure 7-3. Improvement and remission rates of major comorbidities after sleeve gastrectomy (data from Brethauer et al[3]). HLIPID = hyperlipidemia, HTN = hypertension, OSA = obstructive sleep apnea, T2DM = type 2 diabetes mellitus.

Mechanisms of Action

The mechanisms of action by which SG produces early satiety, hunger control, and improvement in metabolic parameters is still not completely understood. Initially thought to be a purely restrictive operation, that concept has been challenged by studies reporting changes in gut hormones and the metabolic effects of this procedure. Ghrelin, an orexigenic hormone produced primarily in the gastric fundus, is significantly decreased after SG[5] and this decrease has been shown to persist 5 years after the procedure.[10] While ghrelin may affect changes in hunger, satiety, and even glucose metabolism after sleeve, it is unlikely to be the only mechanism that contributes to the long-term effects of this procedure. Rapid nutrient transit to the distal bowel is one of the mechanisms that is responsible for early satiety and improvements in glucose metabolism after gastric bypass. These effects are mediated by gut hormones (peptide $YY_{3\text{-}36}$ and glucagon-like peptide-1) produced in the L cells located in the distal bowel. There is evidence that nutrient transit is also increased after SG, likely due to the limited gastric capacity. Melissas et al demonstrated increased gastric emptying after SG and this rapid transit of solid food to the distal bowel may have similar effects on the L cell mass as the gastric bypass.[21] In a small randomized trial comparing RYGB to laparoscopic SG, Karamanakos and colleagues demonstrated similar increases in fasting and post-prandial peptide $YY_{3\text{-}36}$ after these 2 procedures. Weight loss was greater at 12 months after laparoscopic SG in this study (69.7% vs 60.5%, p = .05), however, and the authors attributed this to the lower ghrelin levels and decreased appetite seen after laparoscopic SG compared to RYGB. While further studies are needed to define the mechanisms of weight loss and diabetes remission after laparoscopic SG, early evidence suggests that this operation does have metabolic effects beyond weight loss.

Complications

The risks of laparoscopic SG are intermediate between those of AGB and gastric bypass. The Michigan Bariatric Surgery Collaborative (MBSC) evaluated 30-day complication rates for

62 bariatric surgeons in 25 hospitals and reported the risk of serious complication after laparoscopic SG to be 2.2% compared to 0.9% for laparoscopic AGB and 3.6% for RYGB.[22] Another publication from MBSC used a registry of 25,469 bariatric patients to develop a risk prediction model for serious complications after bariatric surgery and found the risk of SG to fall between laparoscopic AGB and RYGB.[23]

Staple line leaks are the most concerning early complication after SG. The most common site of a leak is near the angle of His or at the gastroesophageal junction. This may be due to placement of the final staple line too close to the gastroesophageal junction or distal esophagus with resultant staple line disruption. Another potential factor that can contribute to a proximal leak is mid-sleeve stenosis. This can be due to a truly stenotic lumen or, more commonly, twisting or kinking of the sleeve at the incisura that causes a functional obstruction. This relative downstream obstruction in the setting of a proximal leak can lead to a persistent fistula that does not resolve with conservative management. Leaks occur less than 2% of the time in most published series, and the leak rates associated with primary and staged SG are shown in Table 7-1. The higher leak rate reported in the lower BMI primary procedures may be related to some of the authors reporting their early experience with this procedure. (There were several multicenter studies in this group that included low case volumes with high complication rates.)

A high index of suspicion and early identification of leaks after laparoscopic SG are critical to achieving an acceptable outcome after this complication. Unexplained tachycardia, fevers, abdominal pain, or persistent hiccups after the procedure should alert the surgeon to investigate for a leak. If the surgeon becomes concerned about a leak and a drain was left in place at the time of surgery, the drain fluid can be sent for an amylase level. If the fluid amylase level is much higher than normal serum levels (in the 1000s), this suggests that saliva is entering the drain. Regardless of the drain amylase level, early imaging is warranted if there is clinical suspicion of a leak. Upper gastrointestinal contrast studies are often ordered first but computed tomography scans can provide more information about fluid collections in the left upper quadrant (Figure 7-4). Diagnostic laparoscopy or laparotomy is warranted if clinical suspicion of leak is high, even if imaging is not diagnostic.

The management of the leak depends on the patient's clinical condition. The surgeon managing this complication must have a clear treatment strategy or algorithm based on the patient's status, the duration of the leak, and the resources available.[24,25] If the leak presents as a well-defined abscess several days or weeks after surgery and the patient is clinically stable, percutaneous image-guided drainage, antibiotics, and nutritional support with parenteral nutrition or a nasojejunal tube is appropriate.[18] If drainage is adequate, endoluminal therapies can be employed to facilitate closure of the leak. This often includes placement of endoscopic clips, fibrin glue or bioabsorbable fistula plugs, and endoluminal stenting across the leak. Stenting has been shown to be effective in small series of selected cases,[18,26-28] but results can be variable depending on the size and duration of the leak. Prior to attempts at stenting, the extraluminal collection must be adequately addressed in all cases and surgical placement of drains with washout of the infected field is often warranted to promote closure of the leak.

A chronic gastrocutaneous fistula after laparoscopic SG is a challenging problem. If a leak or gastrocutaneous fistula persists for months despite adequate surgical drainage, endoluminal therapy, and nutritional support, reoperation may be the only solution.

Bleeding complications requiring transfusion or reoperation occur less than 2% of the time after laparoscopic SG. Common sites of bleeding include the sleeve staple line, short gastric vessels, the spleen, and omental vessels that have been divided during the dissection of the greater curvature. There is some evidence suggesting that the use of staple line buttressing can decrease intra- and postoperative blood loss after laparoscopic SG, but these studies include small numbers of patients and do not provide definitive evidence that staple line reinforcement is superior to oversewing or no reinforcement in terms of preventing postoperative complications.[29,30]

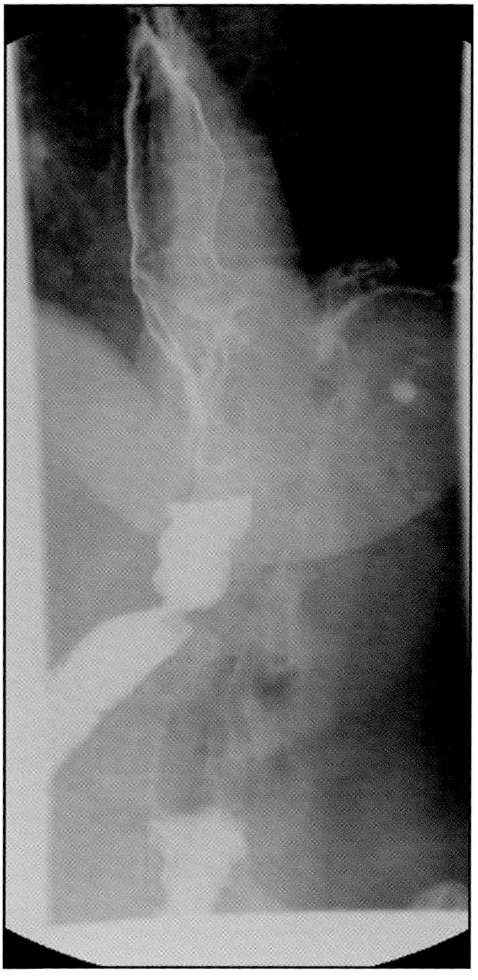

Figure 7-4. Upper gastrointestinal contrast study demonstrating extravasation of contrast from the upper stomach into the left subphrenic space.

Strictures requiring endoscopic dilation or surgical revision occur less than 1% of the time after SG. The most common site of lumenal narrowing is at the incisura. While true strictures can occur, this problem after laparoscopic SG is typically not a true mucosal or luminal stricture as much as it is an angulation or kinking of the stomach in this area (Figure 7-5). This functional obstruction presents as persistent dysphagia to solids and liquids with nausea and vomiting. When creating the SG initially, it is important to avoid this complication by avoiding sharp angulation of the staple line as well as allowing for adequate lumen size as the stapler approaches the incisura. Treatment includes symptom control with anti-emetics and repeated endoscopic balloon dilations of the area. Conversion to gastric bypass is occasionally necessary to alleviate the obstruction.

GERD remains a concern after SG, and the onset of severe refractory GERD after laparoscopic SG may be an indication to revise the procedure to gastric bypass. There is often early improvement in GERD symptoms after laparoscopic SG,[4] but late onset of GERD symptoms after laparoscopic SG has been reported. In Himpens' report with 6-year follow-up, the overall incidence of new onset GERD (defined as symptoms requiring proton pump inhibitor use) was 26%.[9] Additionally, after 5 years of follow-up in the study by Bohdjalian, 31% of patients were taking chronic acid suppression medication for GERD.[10] This long-term complication needs to be evaluated further with objective testing but the possibility of new or recurrent GERD symptoms should be considered when discussing this procedure with patients.

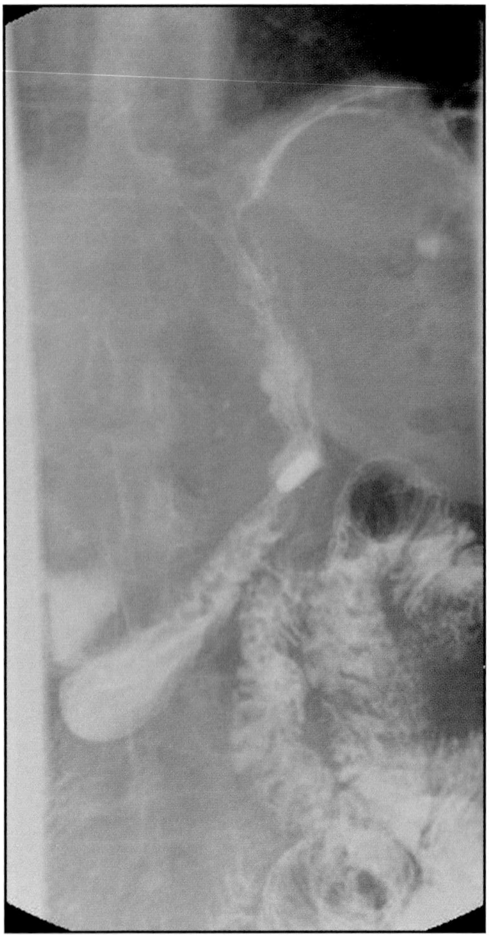

Figure 7-5. There is stenosis of the mid-portion of the sleeve where the barium tablet is lodged.

The overall 30-day mortality rate in the published literature (n = 2570 patients) includes 5 deaths for an overall mortality rate of 0.19%.[3] The mortality rates for the staged/high risk and primary groups are shown in Table 7-1.

Summary

Laparoscopic SG is an accepted bariatric procedure that can be used for many different patient populations. It has been effectively used as part of a staged risk management strategy for high-risk patients and has gained popularity as a primary bariatric procedure. The body of evidence supporting the safety and efficacy of SG continues to grow, and long-term data are emerging that report EWL above 50%. A second-stage gastric bypass or DS promotes further weight loss in selected patients with weight regain or inadequate weight loss after laparoscopic SG. Attractive features of laparoscopic SG are rapid weight loss and comorbidity reduction and avoidance of long-term complications of bypass procedures or implantable devices. Concerns remain regarding the risks of leak after laparoscopic SG, the long-term incidence of GERD symptoms, and weight loss durability beyond 5 years. Management of leaks after laparoscopic SG is a formidable challenge for the bariatric surgeon and early diagnosis followed by a multidisciplinary treatment strategy is key. The precise mechanism of sustained weight loss and diabetes remission after SG is unclear, but early evidence suggests that this is a metabolic procedure that affects nutrient transit, gut hormones, and the enteroinsular axis in a favorable way.

References

1. Cottam D, Qureshi FG, Mattar SG, et al. Laparoscopic sleeve gastrectomy as an initial weight-loss procedure for high-risk patients with morbid obesity. *Surg Endosc.* 2006;20(6):859-863.
2. Angrisani L, Santonicola A, Iovino P, Formisano G, Buchwald H, Scopinaro N. Bariatric surgery worldwide 2013. *Obes Surg.* 2015. Apr 4 Epub ahead of print.
3. Brethauer SA, Hammel JP, Schauer PR. Systematic review of sleeve gastrectomy as staging and primary bariatric procedure. *Surg Obes Relat Dis.* 2009;5(4):469-475.
4. Himpens J, Dapri G, Cadiere GB. A prospective randomized study between laparoscopic gastric banding and laparoscopic isolated sleeve gastrectomy: results after 1 and 3 years. *Obes Surg.* 2006;16(11):1450-1456.
5. Langer FB, Reza Hoda MA, Bohdjalian A, et al. Sleeve gastrectomy and gastric banding: effects on plasma ghrelin levels. *Obes Surg.* 2005;15(7):1024-1029.
6. Karamanakos SN, Vagenas K, Kalfarentzos F, Alexandrides TK. Weight loss, appetite suppression, and changes in fasting and postprandial ghrelin and peptide-YY levels after Roux-en-Y gastric bypass and sleeve gastrectomy: a prospective, double blind study. *Ann Surg.* 2008;247(3):401-407.
7. Vidal J, Ibarzabal A, Romero F, et al. Type 2 diabetes mellitus and the metabolic syndrome following sleeve gastrectomy in severely obese subjects. *Obes Surg.* 2008;18(9):1077-1082.
8. Weiner RA, Weiner S, Pomhoff I, et al. Laparoscopic sleeve gastrectomy: influence of sleeve size and resected gastric volume. *Obes Surg.* 2007;17(10):1297-1305.
9. Himpens J, Dobbeleir J, Peeters G. Long-term results of laparoscopic sleeve gastrectomy for obesity. *Ann Surg.* 2010;252(2):319-324.
10. Bohdjalian A, Langer FB, Shakeri-Leidenmuhler S, et al. Sleeve gastrectomy as sole and definitive bariatric procedure: 5-year results for weight loss and ghrelin. *Obes Surg.* 2010;20(5):535-540.
11. Eid GM, Brethauer S, Mattar SG, et al. Laparoscopic sleeve gastrectomy for super obese patients: forty-eight percent excess weight loss after 6 to 8 years with 93% follow-up. *Ann Surg.* 2012;256(2):262-265.
12. Sarela AI, Dexter SP, O'Kane M, et al. Long-term follow-up after laparoscopic sleeve gastrectomy: 8-9-year results. *Surg Obes Relat Dis.* 2012;8(6):679-684.
13. D'Hondt M, Vanneste S, Pottel H, et al. Laparoscopic sleeve gastrectomy as a single-stage procedure for the treatment of morbid obesity and the resulting quality of life, resolution of comorbidities, food tolerance, and 6-year weight loss. *Surg Endosc.* 2011;25(8):2498-2504.
14. Schauer PR, Kashyap SR, Wolski K, et al. Bariatric surgery versus intensive medical therapy in obese patients with diabetes. *N Engl J Med.* 2012;366(17):1567-1576.
15. Lee WJ, Chong K, Ser KH, et al. Gastric bypass vs sleeve gastrectomy for type 2 diabetes mellitus: a randomized controlled trial. *Arch Surg.* 2011;146(2):143-148.
16. Gill RS, Birch DW, Shi X, et al. Sleeve gastrectomy and type 2 diabetes mellitus: a systematic review. *Surg Obes Relat Dis.* 2010;6(6):707-713.
17. Moon Han S, Kim WW, Oh JH. Results of laparoscopic sleeve gastrectomy (LSG) at 1 year in morbidly obese Korean patients. *Obes Surg.* 2005;15(10):1469-1475.
18. Silecchia G, Boru C, Pecchia A, et al. Effectiveness of laparoscopic sleeve gastrectomy (first stage of biliopancreatic diversion with duodenal switch) on co-morbidities in super-obese high-risk patients. *Obes Surg.* 2006;16(9):1138-1144.
19. Ou Yang SO, Loi K, Jorgensen J, Talbot M. Hp25 laparoscopic sleeve gastrectomy for morbidly obese patients. *ANZ J Surg.* 2007;77(Suppl 1):A45.
20. Kasalicky M, Michalsky D, Housova J, et al. Laparoscopic sleeve gastrectomy without an over-sewing of the staple line. *Obes Surg.* 2008;18:1257-1262.
21. Melissas J, Koukouraki S, Askoxylakis J, et al. Sleeve gastrectomy: a restrictive procedure? *Obes Surg.* 2007;17(1):57-62.
22. Birkmeyer NJ, Dimick JB, Share D, et al. Hospital complication rates with bariatric surgery in Michigan. *JAMA.* 2010;304(4):435-442.
23. Finks JF, Kole KL, Yenumula PR, et al. Predicting risk for serious complications with bariatric surgery: results from the Michigan Bariatric Surgery Collaborative. *Ann Surg.* 2011;254(4):633-640.
24. Lalor PF, Tucker ON, Szomstein S, Rosenthal RJ. Complications after laparoscopic sleeve gastrectomy. *Surg Obes Relat Dis.* 2008;4(1):33-38.
25. Tan JT, Kariyawasam S, Wijeratne T, Chandraratna HS. Diagnosis and management of gastric leaks after laparoscopic sleeve gastrectomy for morbid obesity. *Obes Surg.* 2010;20(4):403-409.
26. de Aretxabala X, Leon J, Wiedmaier G, et al. Gastric leak after sleeve gastrectomy: analysis of its management. *Obes Surg.* 2011;21(8):1232-1237.
27. Nguyen NT, Nguyen XM, Dholakia C. The use of endoscopic stent in management of leaks after sleeve gastrectomy. *Obes Surg.* 2010;20(9):1289-1292.
28. Eubanks S, Edwards CA, Fearing NM, et al. Use of endoscopic stents to treat anastomotic complications after bariatric surgery. *J Am Coll Surg.* 2008;206(5):935-938; discussion 938-939.

29. Dapri G, Cadiere GB, Himpens J. Reinforcing the staple line during laparoscopic sleeve gastrectomy: prospective randomized clinical study comparing three different techniques. *Obes Surg.* 2010;20(4):462-467.
30. Consten EC, Gagner M, Pomp A, Inabnet WB. Decreased bleeding after laparoscopic sleeve gastrectomy with or without duodenal switch for morbid obesity using a stapled buttressed absorbable polymer membrane. *Obes Surg.* 2004;14(10):1360-1366.

8

Gastric Bypass

John Magaña Morton, MD, MPH, FACS, FASMBS and Natalia Leva, MD

Morbid obesity is the leading public health crisis of the industrialized world.[1,2] The prevalence of obesity in the United States continues to rise at an alarming rate with two-thirds of adults currently considered overweight, and half of whom are obese.[3] The etiology of obesity is complex and only partially understood. Genetic, environmental, and psychological factors are all involved to varying degrees in each individual. However, more simply stated, obesity is a disorder of energy imbalance wherein there is an increase in stored fat such that it compromises the patient's organ function, susceptibility to disease, and general health. Obesity has been shown to predispose to many diseases including cardiovascular disease, diabetes mellitus, sleep apnea, and osteoarthritis.

Overweight is defined by a body mass index (BMI) > 25 kg/m^2, obesity is > 30, morbid obesity is > 40, and supermorbid obesity is > 50. Rising rates of obesity are seen across the United States in men and women, and in all major racial, ethnic, and socioeconomic groups.[4] Morbid obesity reduces life expectancy by 5 to 20 years, and for the first time in history, it is predicted that the current generation may have a shorter life expectancy than the last.[5]

Energy intake and expenditure are finely regulated by neural and hormonal mechanisms. Key players in energy regulation include insulin, leptin, ghrelin, and peptide YY. Insulin, produced by the beta cells in the pancreas, is a potent anabolic hormone with multiple synthetic and growth-promoting effects. Adipose cells secrete leptin; it reduces food intake and increases the expenditure of energy. Leptin's counterpart, ghrelin, is secreted by the fundus of the stomach and induces hunger and stimulates anabolic circuits in the body. Endocrine cells in the ileum and colon secrete peptide YY post-prandially, and it is considered a signal of satiety.

Obesity is a complex disease with an array of root causes that vary for each patient. While it is often difficult to tease out the primary contributor in the obesity epidemic, in order for treatment to be sustainable, it must be administered in such a way that it addresses both environmental and psychological components. Weight loss may be achieved by employment of behavioral, medical, and surgical methods; however, combined with careful screening assessments and counseling, bariatric surgery is the most efficacious therapeutic option.[6] Weight loss surgery has changed significantly since its inception in the 1950s. Today, with increased efforts by the American College of Surgeons and American Society of Metabolic and Bariatric Surgery's new Metabolic Bariatric

Forse RA, Apovian CM, eds.
Bariatric Surgery: What Every Provider Needs to Know (pp 101-111).

Surgery Accreditation and Quality Improvement Program (MBSAQIP) to develop evidence-based recommendations, weight loss surgery has mortality rates comparable to routine general surgery procedures such as laparoscopic cholecystectomy or fundoplication.[7]

Surgeon and hospital experience can mitigate the risks associated with weight loss surgery. In the United States, a volume outcome effect has been recognized by the Centers for Medicare and Medicaid Services such that Medicare patients are required to undergo surgery only at Bariatric Surgery Centers of Excellence.[8] Numerous criteria enable a Bariatric Surgery Center of Excellence, but the primary current conditions are a surgeon volume of more than 50 cases and hospital volume exceeding 125 cases annually with a potential change to 25 stapled cases for surgeons and 50 for hospitals. The best demonstrated and most protective effect against complications is an experienced surgeon and hospital.[8-11]

The Roux-en-Y gastric bypass (RYGB) surgery induces sustained weight loss by altering metabolic processes through fundamental changes in appetite, energy regulation, satiety, and metabolism. The mechanisms of its effects are incompletely understood; however, long-term follow-up studies have shown that the RYGB impacts patients' overall health by reversing some of the metabolic consequences of morbid obesity. RYGB is capable of reducing mortality by improving lipid levels, diabetes, hypertension, obstructive sleep apnea, and cardiovascular events such as myocardial infarction.[12]

We are still discovering new benefits of bariatric surgery, but it has already been demonstrated that bariatric surgery is superior to medical therapy for weight loss, survival, and treatment of comorbidities. The number of weight loss surgeries has increased by 800% between 1996 and 2004.[13] While there is no single "best" operation, one of the more common methods is gastric bypass surgery, which will be the topic of discussion in this chapter. The following discussion will include indications for surgery, preoperative evaluation, surgical techniques, peri- and postoperative complications, postoperative care, and outcomes and safety.

Evaluation and Selection of Bypass Surgery Candidates

To qualify for bariatric surgery, patients must meet the 1991 National Institutes of Health consensus criteria, which include having a BMI ≥ 40 or a BMI ≥ 35 with obesity-related comorbidities, and at least 6 months of documented, medically supervised weight loss attempts.[14] Obesity-related comorbidities include hypertension, diabetes mellitus, hyperlipidemia, gastroesophageal reflux disease, arthritis, irritable bowel syndrome, obstructive sleep apnea, and nonalcoholic steatohepatitis. Substantial preoperative workup should attempt to uncover potential occult comorbidities such as coronary artery disease, sleep apnea, and obesity hypoventilation syndrome (Pickwickian syndrome). Because of the complexity of the preoperative evaluation, a multidisciplinary approach is necessary. The team should include a nutritionist, psychologists, anesthesiologists, bariatric surgeons, and other subspecialists who can address any cardiovascular, pulmonary, or endocrine-related issues. Family and social support should not be underestimated, and are an integral part of the team as well.[15] Additionally, patient education is paramount to successful outcomes after bariatric surgery. Educational sessions with dieticians, specialized nurses, and the bariatric surgeon detailing pre- and postoperative diet and lifestyle modifications, as well as preparing patients for what to expect after surgery, should be routine.

Some bariatric surgeons require patients to lose additional weight through diet and exercise between the time of initial bariatric surgery consultation and the date of operation. Preoperative weight loss is a method for "downstaging," acting in the same manner as preoperative chemoradiation therapy does for cancer. This additional required preoperative weight loss is not correlated with comorbidity resolution or complication rates[16,17]; however, it is associated with shorter operative times, a smaller liver, and greater weight loss at 1 year after the surgery. Therefore, it may be encouraged in all patients while balancing access to care for patients.[16] In order to achieve weight loss prior to surgery, our team recommends that the patient follow a liquid diet beginning 2 weeks before the surgery is scheduled.

Bariatric surgery candidates in particular benefit from preoperative nutrition evaluation and counseling. After RYGB, patients are instructed to consume a progression of diets, first full liquid, followed by pureéd, soft foods, and finally regularly textured foods. This restricted progression of food consistencies allows the stomach pouch and anastomoses to heal. All diets are designed to maximize protein intake and minimize carbohydrates and fats. Practicing healthy eating behaviors is equally important and should begin prior to surgery. Patients are counseled to eat only at regularly scheduled times, to eat slowly and chew carefully, have protein first, and measure portion sizes. Patients should strive for 60 to 80 g of protein per day. Patients should also be reminded that gastric bypass is a restrictive procedure, and therefore smaller, more frequent meals are most appropriate.[18]

Contraindications to RYGB include psychiatric conditions, such as schizophrenia, developmental delay, active substance abuse, recent major depression with hospitalization or suicidal attempts, and severe bipolar disease. Other contraindications include severe cardiac disease that would prohibit safe and effective anesthesia, severe coagulopathy, or inability to comply with rigorous postoperative nutritional requirements including life-long vitamin replacement. RYGB in patients over 65 or younger than 18 years old is controversial, but age is not a contraindication in patients with severe comorbidities.[19]

Prior to surgery, patients must complete an extensive screening process including consultation with a surgeon, psychological evaluation, nutrition consultation, chest roentgenogram, electrocardiogram, and an esophagogastroduodenoscopy (EGD).

The EGD is recommended by the European Association for Endoscopic Surgery to detect and treat any upper gastrointestinal lesions that may cause postoperative complications or influence the decision of which type of bariatric surgery should be performed.[20] In a study of 272 gastric bypass patients who underwent preoperative EGD, 12% of patients had clinically significant preoperative findings, which included erosive esophagitis (3.7%), Barrett's esophagus (3.7%), gastric ulcer (2.9%), erosive gastritis (1.8%), duodenal ulcer (0.7%), and gastric carcinoid (0.3%); 1.1% had more than one lesion. Given that 12% of these patients who eventually underwent RYGB had clinically significant preoperative findings, but only 67% of those patients had upper gastrointestinal symptoms, it is important to perform EGD preoperatively because the excluded distal stomach cannot be evaluated easily after an RYGB procedure.[21]

Medical evaluations of cardiovascular disease, respiratory illness, and diabetes should be completed prior to surgery. Cardiovascular evaluation should include a recent history of chest pain and assessment of exercise tolerance. Patients with a history of a deep vein thrombosis or venous stasis disease may require temporary inferior vena cava filter placement prior to surgery to prevent venous thromboembolism.[22] It is also important to identify occult obstructive sleep apnea so that the anesthesiologist may anticipate and combat periods of hypoxia in the immediate postoperative period when it may be compounded by narcotic pain medications and postoperative fluid shifts.[23] Additionally, diabetes must be well controlled preoperatively in order to reduce the incidence of perioperative morbidity such as wound infection.[23]

Techniques

The gastric bypass employs both restrictive and hormonal mechanisms to limit food intake and its absorption. It was first performed by Mason and Ito in 1967 and has since been modified twice to incorporate a Roux limb rather than a loop gastrojejunostomy, and in 1994 to be primarily laparoscopic.[24]

The laparoscopic approach is superior to the open approach with its increasing availability and considerably lower complications. There is reduced mortality, wound infections, pulmonary complications, thromboembolic complications, reduced rates of incisional hernias, and decreased hospitalization time to an average of about 2 days.[25] It should be noted that there are no differences in excess weight loss (EWL), resolution of comorbidities, or improvement in quality of life between the open and laparoscopic approaches. There are many variations of the laparoscopic RYGB surgery techniques; however, the essential components include construction of a gastric pouch, attaching the pouch to the jejunum, and rerouting the digestive enzymes such that they do not contact food for digestion until it reaches the jejunojejunostomy.[7]

At the time of surgery, care is taken to appropriately position the patient to facilitate intubation and prevent nerve compression and skin breakdown. In order to prevent postoperative nausea and vomiting, several strategies are employed including intravenous hydration, a small steroid dose, and Zofran (ondansetron). An orogastric tube is placed to prevent any gastric distension or aspiration. Prophylactic 5000 units of subcutaneous heparin, sequential compression devices, and 2 g of cefoxitin should be administered prior to incision. In the operating room, special equipment such as a gastroscope and longer instruments should be available.

Surgery is begun by placing an index trocar at 18 cm below the xiphoid in the midline after the Veress needle has been introduced to establish pneumoperitoneum. After remaining trocars are placed, laparoscopic exploration of the abdomen is conducted. The greater omentum is elevated and the ligament of Treitz is identified. The jejunum is divided into a biliopancreatic and Roux limbs at 20 cm distal to the ligament of Treitz. Next, the jejunojejunostomy is performed after a 75- to 150-cm Roux limb is run. The Roux limb may be passed toward the proximal gastric pouch through the transverse mesocolon (retrocolic) or in front of the colon (antecolic) pathway, and the retrocolic method may either take a retrogastric or antegastric route. Any mesenteric defects between loops of bowel are a potential hernia site and are thus closed with permanent running suture. Subsequently, the liver retractor is placed so that the gastric pouch can be fashioned. The gastric pouch should be between 15 to 30 mL in size, and is constructed based on the lesser curve, begun horizontally at the second vascular arcade, and finished vertically up to the angle of His. Finally, the gastrojejunostomy is constructed either through circular-stapled, linear-stapled, or hand-sewn techniques and a surgical drain may be placed.

Potential pitfalls that may occur include bleeding, inability for the Roux limb to reach the gastric pouch without tension, and unexpected anatomy such as malrotation, enlarged liver, excessive omentum, or thick abdominal wall. Though rare, unexpected findings during a laparoscopic gastric bypass may influence the operative course. For example, previous surgery may yield tenacious adhesions requiring lysis, malrotation of the ligament of Trietz necessitating a mirror image approach to the technique, hernia findings requiring a change in port placement, a gastrointestinal stromal tumor that may not have been revealed with preoperative assessment may be resected in its entirety and the gastric bypass completed, or cirrhosis that may require biopsy or even aborting the case if ascites or varices are noted.

Surgical Complications

The average mortality rate for gastric bypass is 0.2%.[26] Complications can be divided into 3 categories: intraoperative, early postoperative (within 30 days of surgery), and late postoperative (>30 days after surgery). Nonmodifiable risk factors for all complications are male gender and age over 65 years. Significant progress has been made to monitor outcomes and detail evidence-based guidelines of criteria and benchmarks that determine safe practices. As mentioned previously, complication rates are directly related to surgeon and hospital experience.

Complications of bariatric procedures include anastomotic leak or stenosis, pulmonary embolus and deep vein thrombosis, gastrointestinal bleeding, nutritional deficiencies, wound complications, bowel obstructions, ulcers, hernias, and respiratory and cardiovascular-related complications. Among the different surgical procedures, the rate of complications is proportional to the amount of weight loss produced by each operation: banding (7%), gastroplasty (18%), gastric bypass (17%), and biliopancreatic diversion (38%).[26,27]

Intraoperative complications include trocar injury during placement of the Veress needle or ports while the pneumoperitoneum is established. Splenic injury, most commonly capsule tear, typically occurs if there is excess traction on the short gastric vessels; splenectomy is very uncommon. Bowel ischemia may occur during division of the mesentery, due to a twisted Roux limb or internal herniation.[28] Signs of intestinal ischemia are severe abdominal pain, hematochezia, and an acute abdomen in a prior bariatric surgery patient.

Early postoperative complications include leaks, deep venous thrombosis, pulmonary embolism, cardiovascular complications, pulmonary complications, and mortality. Anastomotic, gastric pouch, or duodenal leak occurs with 2.2% of RYGB, 1.0% of vertical banded gastroplasty, and 1.8% of biliopancreatic diversion.[26] Anastomotic leak, most commonly from the gastrojejunostomy, is an independent risk factor for mortality.[29] It has been demonstrated that a surgeon's experience has significant influence on the leak rate, with a rate of 1% to 2% in experienced hands and up to 5% in surgeons earlier in their careers.[30] Pulmonary embolism accounts for 50% of deaths in the perioperative period. Currently, as mentioned in the Techniques section, a combination of anticoagulants and sequential compression devices are used for prophylaxis. For patients who are at the highest risk for deep vein thrombosis or pulmonary embolism, including those who have a history of a venous thrombotic event, venous stasis, poor ambulation, pulmonary hypertension, severe sleep apnea, or BMI > 60, an inferior vena cava filter may be temporarily placed preoperatively.[31] It was shown to decrease risk of pulmonary embolism from 2.94% to 0.63% in a series of 330 patients with such high-risk qualities.[31] Cardiovascular complications such as myocardial infarction are also a significant cause of death in the early postoperative period. For this reason, it is important to perform a careful preoperative cardiac evaluation and to involve a cardiologist in high-risk patients. Pulmonary complications are more likely in patients who are on Medicare, have chronic lung disease, are over the age of 50, or are male.[10] Persistent vomiting due to stomal stenosis increases the risk of aspiration pneumonia. After laparoscopic RYGB, atelectasis occurs at a rate of 8.4%; therefore, early ambulation after surgery is essential.[28]

Late postoperative complications, or those occurring more than 30 days after the surgery, include stenosis or anastomotic stricture, gallstone formation, nutrition deficiencies, bowel obstruction, intussusception, marginal ulcers or ulcers in the remnant stomach and duodenum, fistula, dumping syndrome, and hypoglycemia. Stenosis of the gastrojejunostomy has been reported between 2% and 14% of patients. Stenosis often manifests 4 to 6 weeks postoperatively as vomit ing and progressive intolerance first to solids and subsequently liquids.[32] A high incidence of gallstone formation has been well documented when morbidly obese patients undergo rapid surgically induced weight loss.[33] Cholelithiasis can develop in up to 38% of patients after RYGB; however, if a patient has gallstones preoperatively, the surgeon may perform a concomitant cholecystectomy, though this is less common with the laparoscopic approach.[34] Gallstone formation occurs secondary to a combination of vagus nerve damage, altered enteric nerve stimulation, decreased gallbladder emptying, and changes in calcium concentration and in the bile salt/cholesterol ratio.[28] It has been shown in a double-blind, randomized placebo-controlled trial that a daily dose of 600 mg ursodiol for the first 6 months after surgery reduces the incidence of gallstones to 2%.[33] Therefore, in order to prevent this complication, surgeons recommend a 6-month course of ursodiol for patients who keep their gallbladder in order to reduce the incidence of cholelithiasis.[33] Nutritional deficiencies can be extensive, related to both the changes in anatomy and postoperative sequelae such as persistent vomiting, and will be discussed in detail in the Nutritional Deficiencies section. Bowel obstruction occurs in between 0.2% and 7% of RYGB patients; the range varies depending on the surgical technique. For example, if the Roux limb is passed in a retrocolic fashion, there are 3 potential hernia sites.[15] The majority of bowel obstructions develop between 6 and 24 months postoperatively; however, they can occur earlier due to technical errors secondary to mesenteric defects. Bowel obstructions that occur early usually require a bowel resection to prevent retrograde distention of the biliopancreatic limb and distal part of the stomach, which could result in rupture of the distal gastric staple line, and consequently peritonitis.[15] In later bowel obstructions, surgical intervention is only required after failure of nasogastric decompression, intravenous fluid resuscitation, and nothing-by-mouth status. Intussusception ensues when the bowel telescopes into itself. This complication usually occurs years after surgery; patients with the highest risk of developing intussusception are those who have lost greater than 90% of their excess weight.[28]

Marginal ulcers are ulcers located in the jejunum near the anastomotic site. They are estimated to occur in 1% to 16% of gastric bypass patients.[35,36] Perforated marginal ulcers occur in 1% of RYGB patients. Ulcer perforation is linked to smoking and use of nonsteroidal anti-inflammatory drugs or glucocorticoids.[37] The use of nonabsorbable sutures, as opposed to absorbable sutures, for the inner layer of the gastrojejunal anastomosis is associated with increased ulcer incidence.[38] The presence of *Helicobacter pylori* also increases risk for marginal ulcers.[39] It is common practice for bariatric surgeons to introduce a 6-month postoperative course of proton pump inhibition. If a marginal ulcer is recalcitrant to medical therapy, the possibility of a gastric-gastric fistula must be entertained. If a gastric-gastric fistula is present with a marginal ulcer, then surgical correction is mandated. The remnant stomach maintains a pH of 2 to 3 and still responds to vagal and hormonal stimulation; therefore, ulcers may also occur in the gastric remnant and duodenum years after surgery and independent of *H pylori* status. Endoscopic evaluation of the gastric pouch is challenging given the divided stomach, thus unstable patients require surgical exploration.[28] Fistulas occur rarely, and often concurrently with a marginal ulcer.[28] They form most commonly between the gastric pouch and gastric remnant, secondary to a gastrointestinal leak.[40] Large, undiagnosed gastrogastric fistulas may result in weight regain.[15] Fistulas require elective surgical repair.

Dumping syndrome occurs in up to 20% of RYGB patients[41]; it is classified as early or late depending on how soon it develops after a meal. Early dumping ensues 15 to 30 minutes after eating and is thought to be secondary to the rapid entry of hyperosmotic foods into the jejunem. Symptoms include crampy abdominal pain, voluminous diarrhea, bloating, dizziness, nausea, flushing, and tachycardia and are due to a combination of hypovolemia and a subsequent sympathetic response.[28] Dumping syndrome is triggered by consumption of simple sugars, acidic foods, and nutrient-rich drinks such as sport drinks.[41] Foods high in protein and fiber should be consumed to avoid this uncomfortable syndrome. Additionally, behavior modifications include smaller, frequent meals and avoiding very hot and very cold foods.[15] Early dumping is usually self-limited and resolves between 7 and 12 weeks. Late dumping syndrome occurs 2 to 3 hours after a meal. It is secondary to rapid glucose absorption, subsequent hyperglycemia, and release of glucagon-like peptide-1 and gastric inhibitory peptide. An exaggerated insulin response ensues, leading to hypoglycemia and hypokalemia. Patients present with diaphoresis, weakness, fatigue, and dizziness.[41] The same modifications suggested for early dumping syndrome should also ameliorate the symptoms of late dumping syndrome.[28] Treatment includes dietary and medical interventions to control serum glucose levels.[28]

Gastrointestinal bleeding can occur postoperatively in 2.0% of RYGB, 0.7% of vertical banded gastroplasty, 0.3% of laparoscopic adjustable gastric banding (AGB), and 0.2% of biliopancreatic diversion. In RYGB patients, postoperative dysphagia is not significantly worse than the patient's matched preoperative symptoms.[42]

Beyond the type of procedure, there are identified risk factors for complications after bariatric surgery including older age, male gender, greater BMI, comorbidities, and Medicare insurance status.[43-46] The increased risk for Medicare patients is beyond age given that eligibility for Medicare is disability, which may affect outcomes. Although patients with the most risk factors carry the highest risk for surgery, they also may derive the most benefit from bariatric surgery given the disease burden they carry.[11] Of note, complications may not affect long-term weight loss, which is the outcome that best predicts long-term mortality risk.[16]

Nutritional Deficiencies

Nutritional and vitamin deficiencies and electrolyte abnormalities occur in 16.9% of RYGB patients.[26] Patients who do not take daily vitamins postoperatively or patients who experience frequent vomiting are at an increased risk of developing such deficiencies, most common of which are protein, iron, vitamin B_{12}, folate, calcium, and the fat-soluble vitamins A, D, E, and K.[47]

Prolonged vomiting may result in thiamine (vitamin B_1) deficiency, which can lead to Wernicke's encephalopathy, a syndrome of confusion, ataxia, ophthalmoplegia, and impaired short-term memory. This neurologic deficit is preventable with appropriate administration of thiamine. If thiamine deficiency is suspected, the patient should be given intravenous or intramuscular thiamine immediately in order to increase the chances of symptom resolution.[48] Early treatment is imperative because if symptoms become significant, they may not be reversible despite delayed administration of thiamine.

The parietal cells of the stomach produce intrinsic factor, which is necessary for vitamin B_{12} absorption in the terminal ileum. Patients who undergo RYGB may develop B_{12} deficiency because RYGB separates the parietal cells in the fundus of the stomach from the smaller gastric pouch. There is, therefore, no contact between ingested food and intrinsic factor until the intersection of the Roux limb in the jejeneum.[49,50] In addition, often following RYGB the parietal cells of the stomach cease to produce intrinsic factor altogether, presumably because the fundus no longer has any contact with food.[51] It has been shown that restrictive bariatric surgery does not cause vitamin B_{12} deficiency because the parietal cells in the fundus of the stomach remain attached.[52]

Calcium, iron, and folate deficiency can occur because they are absorbed in the duodenum and proximal jejunum. These segments of the digestive track are commonly bypassed in gastric bypass surgery. Moreover, the fat-soluble vitamin D is necessary for calcium absorption, and so vitamin D deficiency will further contribute to any calcium deficiency.[47]

Outcomes

The steep rise in bariatric surgery utilization can be attributed to its proven efficacy as a treatment for morbid obesity. Two meta-analyses have provided strong validation that bariatric surgery leads to successful weight loss and mortality reduction.[6,26] A meta-analysis by Buchwald that included 22,094 patients found the mean percentage of EWL for all patients to be 61.2%.[6] EWL was highest for vertical banded gastroplasty (68.2%), RYGB (61.6%), and lowest for laparoscopic AGB (47.5%). Maggard's meta-analysis found similar weight loss trends at 3 years or more postoperatively, with the greatest weight loss achieved after the malabsorptive procedures of biliopancreatic diversion (53 kg) and RYGB (42 kg), and less weight loss after the restrictive laparoscopic AGB (35 kg) and gastroplasty (32 kg).[26]

Such substantial weight loss is associated with a clear reduction in long-term mortality. A retrospective cohort study of 9949 RYGB patients matched to 9628 severely obese controls found that having RYGB surgery reduced the adjusted long-term mortality from any cause of death by 40%.[53] Among RYGB patients, mortality was decreased 56% from coronary artery disease, 92% from diabetes, and 60% from cancer. The decrease in cancer mortality was shown in an additional study to be related to a 14% decrease in cancer incidence among patients who underwent RYGB. The biggest reductions in cancer incidence were seen among types of cancers that are considered obesity related, including esophageal adenocarcinomas (2% reduction); colorectal (30%); postmenopausal breast (4%); corpus and uterine (78%); renal, non-Hodgkin lymphoma (27%); and multiple myeloma (54%).[54] The lower cancer risk of patient's post-RYGB was presumably due to weight loss, which has been shown in many studies to reduce cancer incidence. Furthermore, once patients with obesity lose weight, they may have better access to needed health surveillance like

Pap smears and colonoscopy. Finally, given that increased BMI leads to worse surgical oncologic outcomes, it may be surmised that with weight loss a better surgical outcome may be anticipated.

Overall, bariatric surgery dramatically improves survival and decreases mortality from all disease-related causes of death. Only the rate of deaths not caused by disease, including deaths resulting from accidents and suicide, increased after bariatric surgery and were 58% higher in the RYGB patients.[53] One speculation as to why accidents and suicides were higher in the surgical group was higher is perhaps alcohol abuse. One study demonstrated altered alcohol metabolism after gastric bypass surgery perhaps accounting for a propensity for alcohol abuse.[55] One study of bariatric surgery candidates found that 9% reported attempted suicide and 19% reported alcohol abuse preoperatively.[56] There is concern that this vulnerable patient population has additional difficulty with the psychological adjustments to weight loss, which further supports the need for psychological counseling before and after surgery.[57,58]

In addition to benefiting from a decreased mortality, bariatric patients benefit from decreased morbidity. Morbidly obese patients suffer from more intense gastrointestinal symptoms (eg, abdominal pain, heartburn) and sleep disturbances than do normal-weight patients. By 6 months after their RYGB, however, the frequency and severity of gastrointestinal symptoms many morbidly obese patients have reduced to levels seen in normal-weight patients. The only gastrointestinal symptom that is worse following RYGB is dysphasia, which is common in morbidly obese patients who all experience increased intra-abdominal pressure. Dysphasia may worsen following surgery from further increased esophageal pressure due to overeating and overfilling of the restrictive small gastric pouch, underscoring the need for pre- and postoperative education regarding diet.[42]

Recently, there have been a number of clinical trials that demonstrated the dramatic effect of bariatric surgery on glycemic control in patients with type 2 diabetes, such that the need for medical therapy was decreased or eliminated. Moreover, in a prospective nonrandomized case-matched Swedish trial, type 2 diabetes was significantly less likely to develop in obese participants who underwent a bariatric procedure than in their controlled counterparts.[59] While this is not an indication that bariatric surgery should be used for the purpose of preventing development of type 2 diabetes in obese patients nor serve as a replacement for medical therapy, it does suggest that the mechanisms by which bariatric surgery prevent progression from abnormalities in glucose metabolism to frank diabetes is an area that should be further explored.[59]

The effects of obesity are not merely physiologic. Patients who are obese have difficulty completing functions of daily living. Walking around a grocery store is painful, riding on an airplane requires seatbelt extenders, and negative stigma around obesity affects work opportunities and job promotions. The validated Short Form 36 (SF-36) survey assesses quality of life by evaluating the following domains: vitality; physical functioning; bodily pain; general health perceptions; physical, emotional, and social role functioning; and mental health. Administration of the SF-36 survey shows that quality of life improves greatly after RYGB surgery. Preoperatively, morbidly obese patients score significantly lower than US population norms in the categories of general health, vitality, physical functioning, bodily pain, and emotional and social functioning. As soon as 3 months following RYGB, these same patients score no differently than US norms in these categories.[60]

Summary

Obesity in the United States is often unfairly stigmatized and attributed to careless eating habits or lack of exercise. In reality, causes of obesity are multifactorial with issues including genetics, physiology, socioeconomic status, level of education, access to healthy foods, and awareness of how food directly impacts health. However, there is increasing cognizance on a national level of how policy can affect public health. While such policies make a public impression and are a step in the right direction, the rapid growth of the obesity epidemic must be addressed in such a way as to achieve more immediate outcomes. Surgical treatment of morbid obesity is safer and more effective than ever. Bariatric surgery has become a routine component of general surgery training, and it currently represents the fastest growing area in the field.[22] Gastric bypass is an effective procedure that results in significant long-term weight loss, improvement and often remission of comorbidities, and increased life expectancy. There are greater than 150,000 weight loss operations performed annually and thus health care providers across all fields will likely find themselves caring for a post-bariatric surgery patient. Health care providers must work together to optimally support and care for this population, whether they are working independently to lose weight, considering weight loss surgery, or have undergone weight loss surgery.

References

1. Ogden CL, Carroll MD, Curtin LR, McDowell MA, Tabak CJ, Flegal KM. Prevalence of overweight and obesity in the United States, 1999-2004. *JAMA*. 2006;295(13):1549-1555.
2. Yoon KH, Lee JH, Kim JW, et al. Epidemic obesity and type 2 diabetes in Asia. *Lancet*. 2006;368(9548):1681-1688.
3. Parikh NI, Pencina MJ, Wang TJ, et al. Increasing trends in incidence of overweight and obesity over 5 decades. *Am J Med*. 2007;120(3):242-250.
4. Mokdad AH, Bowman B, Ford ES, Vinicor F, Marks JS, Koplan JP. The continuing epidemics of obesity and diabetes in the United States. *JAMA*. 2001;286(10):1195-1200.
5. Fontaine KR, Redden D, Wang C, Westfall AO, Allison DB. Years of life lost due to obesity. *JAMA*. 2003;289(2):187-193.
6. Buchwald H, Avidor Y, Braunwald E, et al. Bariatric surgery: a systematic review and meta-analysis. *JAMA*. 2004;292(14):1724-1737.
7. Longitudinal Assessment of Bariatric Surgery (LABS) Consortium. Perioperative safety in the longitudinal assessment of bariatric surgery. *N Engl J Med*. 2009;361:445-454.
8. Nguyen NT, Mahbod P, Stevens CM, Mavandadi S, Zainabadi K, Wilson SE. The relationship between hospital volume and outcome in bariatric surgery at academic medical centers. *Ann Surg*. 2004;240(4):586-593; discussion 593-584.
9. Livingston EH, Ko C. Assessing the relative contribution of individual risk factors on surgical outcome for gastric bypass surgery: a baseline probability analysis. *J Surg Res*. 2002;105(1):48-52.
10. Poulose BK, Griffin M, Zhu Y, et al. National analysis of adverse patient safety for events in bariatric surgery. *Am Surg*. 2005;71(5):406-413.
11. Wolfe BM, Morton J. Weighing in on bariatric surgery: procedure use, readmission rates, and mortality. *JAMA*. 2005;294(15):1960-1963.
12. Sjostrom L, Lindroos A, Peltonen M, et al. Lifestyle, diabetes, and cardiovascular risk factors 10 years after bariatric surgery. *N Engl J Med*. 2004;351(26):2683-2693.
13. Zhao Y, Encinosa W. *Bariatric surgery utilization and outcomes in 1998 and 2004*. Rockville, MD: Agency for Health Care Policy and Research (US); 2006-2007.
14. National Institutes of Health. NIH consensus statement covers treatment of obesity. *Am Fam Physician*. 1991;44(1):305-306.
15. Fischer JE. *Fischer's Mastery of Surgery*. 6th ed. Philadelphia, PA: Wolters Kluwer Health/Lippincott Williams & Wilkins; 2012.
16. Alvarado R, Alami R, Hsu G, et al. The impact of preoperative weight loss in patients undergoing laparoscopic Roux-en-Y gastric bypass. *Obes Surg*. 2005;15(9):1282-1286.
17. Harnisch MC, Portenier D, Pryor AD, Prince-Petersen R, Grant JP, DeMaria EJ. Preoperative weight gain does not predict failure of weight loss or co-morbidity resolution of laparoscopic Roux-en-Y gastric bypass for morbid obesity. *Surg Obes Relat Dis*. 2008;4(3):445-450.
18. Flancbaum L, Belsley D, Drake V, Colarusso T, Tayler E. Preoperative nutritional status of patients undergoing Roux-en-Y gastric bypass for morbid obesity. *J Gastrointest Surg*. 2006;10(7):1033-1037.
19. Yermilov IM, McGory M, Shekelle PW, Ko CY, Maggard MA. Appropriateness criteria for bariatric surgery: beyond the NIH guidelines. *Obesity*. 2009;7(8):1521.
20. Sauerland S, Angrisani L, Belachew M, et al. Obesity surgery: evidence-based guidelines of the European Association for Endoscopic Surgery (EAES). *Surg Endosc*. 2005;19(2):200-221.
21. Mong C, Van Dam J, Morton J, Gerson L, Curet M, Banerjee S. Preoperative endoscopic screening for laparoscopic Roux-en-Y gastric bypass has a low yield for anatomic findings. *Obes Surg*. 2008;18(9):1067-1073.
22. Schuster R, Hagedorn J, Morton JM. Retrievable inferior vena cava filters may be safely applied in gastric bypass surgery. *Surg Endosc*. 2007;21(12):2277-2279.

23. Richards WO. Morbid obesity. In: Beauchamp R, Evers, MB, Mattox KL, Sabiston DC, Townsend CM, eds. *Sabiston Textbook of Surgery: The Biological Basis of Modern Surgical Practice.* 19th ed. Philadelphia, PA: Elsevier Saunders; 2012.
24. Szomstein S, Tucker ON. Outcomes of laparoscopic gastric bypass. In: Nguyen N, DeMaria, EJ, Ikramuddin, S, Hutter, MM, eds. *The SAGES Manual: A Practical Guide to Bariatric Surgery.* New York, NY: Springer; 2008:145-151.
25. Lancaster RT, Hutter M. Bands and bypasses: 30-day morbidity and mortality of bariatric surgical procedures as assessed by prospective multi-center, risk adjusted ACS-NSQIP data. *Surg Endosc.* 2008;22:2554-2563.
26. Maggard MA, Shugarman L, Suttorp M, et al. Meta-analysis: surgical treatment of obesity. *Ann Intern Med.* 2005;142(7):547-559.
27. Inge TH, Krebs N, Garcia VF, et al. Bariatric surgery for severely overweight adolescents: concerns and recommendations. *Pediatrics.* 2004;114(1):217-223.
28. Lim RB, Blackburn GL, Jones DB. Benchmarking best practices in weight loss surgery. *Current Problems in Surgery.* 2010;47(2):79-174.
29. Gonzalez RM, Murr M. Anastomotic leaks following gastric bypass surgery. In: Jones DB, Rosenthal R, eds. *Weight Loss Surgery: A Multidisciplinary Approach.* Edgemont, PA: Matrix Medical Communications; 2008.
30. Sekhar N, Torquati A, Lufti R, Richards WO. Endoscopic evaluation of the gastrojejunostomy in laparoscopic gastric bypass. A series of 340 patients without postoperative leak. *Surg Endosc.* 2006;20(2):199-201.
31. Lehman Center Wight Loss Surgery Expert Panel. Commonwealth of Massachusetts: Betsy Lehman Center for Patient Safety and Medical Error Reduction. *Expert Panel on Weight Loss Surgery: executive report update.* 2009;17.
32. Pitt TB, Brethauer S, Schauer P. Laparoscopic gastric bypass. In: Jones SB, Jones D, eds. *Obesity Surgery: Patient Safety and Best Practices.* Chapter 40. Woodbury, CT: Cine-Med, Inc; 2008.
33. Sugerman HJ, Brewer W, Shiffman ML, et al. A multicenter, placebo-controlled, randomized, double-blind, prospective trial of prophylactic ursodiol for the prevention of gallstone formation following gastric-bypass-induced rapid weight loss. *Am J Surg.* 1995;169(1):91-96; discussion 96-97.
34. Schneider B, Villegas L, Blackburn GL, Mun EC, Critchlow JF, Jones DB. Laparoscopic gastric bypass surgery: outcomes. *J Laparoendosc Adv Surg Tech A.* 2003;12:247-255.
35. Dallal RM, Bailey L. Ulcer disease after gastric bypass surgery. *Surg Obes Relat Dis.* 2006;2(4):455-459.
36. Higa KD, Boone K, Ho T. Complications of the laparoscopic Roux-en-Y gastric bypass: 1,040 patients: what have we learned? *Obes Surg.* 2000;10(6):509-513.
37. Felix EL, Kettelle J, Mobley E, Swartz D. Perforated marginal ulcers after laparoscopic gastric bypass. *Surg Endosc.* 2008;22(10):2128-2132.
38. Sacks BC, Mattar S, Qureshi FG, et al. Incidence of marginal ulcers and the use of absorbable anastomotic sutures in laparoscopic Roux-en-Y gastric bypass. *Surg Obes Relat Dis.* 2006;2(1):11-16.
39. Rasmussen JJ, Fuller W, Ali MR. Marginal ulceration after laparoscopic gastric bypass: an analysis of predisposing factors in 260 patients. *Surg Endosc.* 2007;21(7):1090-1094.
40. Gumbs A, Duffy AJ, Bell RL. Incidence and management of marginal ulceration after laparoscopic Roux-en-Y gastric bypass. *Surg Obes Relat. Dis.* 2006;2:92-97.
41. Ukleja A. Dumping syndrome: pathophysiology and treatment. *Nutr Clin Pract.* 2005;20:517-525.
42. Clements RH, Gonzalez Q, Foster A, et al. Gastrointestinal symptoms are more intense in morbidly obese patients and are improved with laparoscopic Roux-en-Y gastric bypass. *Obes Surg.* 2003;13(4):610-614.
43. Benotti PN, Wood G, Rodriguez H, Carnevale N, Liriano E. Perioperative outcomes and risk factors in gastric surgery for morbid obesity: a 9-year experience. *Surgery.* 2006;139(3):340-346.
44. Livingston EH, Huerta S, Arthur D, Lee S, De Shields S, Heber D. Male gender is a predictor of morbidity and age a predictor of mortality for patients undergoing gastric bypass surgery. *Ann Surg.* 2002;236(5):576-582.
45. Morton J, Hagedorn J, Encarnacion B, et al. *Post-operative gastric bypass complications do not affect weight loss.* 11th Annual IFSO Meeting Sydney, Australia, August 2006.
46. Williams DB, Hagedorn J, Lawson EH, et al. Gastric bypass reduces biochemical cardiac risk factors. *Surg Obes Relat Dis.* 2007;3(1):8-13.
47. Bloomberg RD, Fleishman A, Nalle JE, Herron DM, Kini S. Nutritional deficiencies following bariatric surgery: what have we learned? *Obes Surg.* 2005;15(2):145-154.
48. Aasheim ET. Wernicke encephalopathy after bariatric surgery: a systematic review. *Ann Surg.* 2008;248(5):714-720.
49. Coupaye M, Puchaux K, Bogard C. Nutritional consequences of adjustable gastric banding and gastric bypass: a 1-year prospective study. *Obes Surg.* 2009;19(1):56-65.
50. Skroubis G, Sakellaropoulos G, Pouggouras K, Mead N, Nikiforidis G, Kalfarentzos F. Comparison of nutritional deficiencies after Roux-en-Y gastric bypass and after biliopancreatic diversion with Roux-en-Y gastric bypass. *Obes Surg.* 2002;12(4):551-558.
51. Marcuard SP, Sinar D, Swanson MS, Silverman JF, Levine JS. Absence of luminal intrinsic factor after gastric bypass surgery for morbid obesity. *Dig Dis Sci.* 1989;34(8):1238-1242.

52. Cooper PL, Brearley L, Jamieson AC, Ball MJ. Nutritional consequences of modified vertical gastroplasty in obese subjects. *Int J Obes Relat Metab Disord.* 1999;23(4):382-388.
53. Adams TD, Gress R, Smith SC, et al. Long-term mortality after gastric bypass surgery. *N Engl J Med.* 2007;357(8):753-761.
54. Adams TD, Stroup AM, Gress RE, et al. Cancer incidence and mortality after gastric bypass surgery. *Obesity.* 2009;17(4):796-802.
55. Hagedorn JC, Encarnacion B, Brat GA, Morton JM. Does gastric bypass alter alcohol metabolism? *Surg Obes Relat Dis.* 2007;3(5):543-548; discussion 548.
56. Sansone RA, Wiederman M, Schumacher DF, Routsong-Weichers L. The prevalence of self-harm behaviors among a sample of gastric surgery candidates. *J Psychosom Res.* 2008;65(5):441-444.
57. Hsu LK, Benotti P, Dwyer J, et al. Nonsurgical factors that influence the outcome of bariatric surgery: a review. *Psychosom Med.* 1998;60(3):338-346.
58. Waters GS, Pories W, Swanson MS, Meelheim HD, Flickinger EG, May HJ. Long-term studies of mental health after the Greenville gastric bypass operation for morbid obesity. *Am J Surg.* 1991;161(1):154-157; discussion 157-158.
59. Carlsson LMS, Peltonen M, Ahlin S, et al. Bariatric surgery and prevention of type 2 diabetes in Swedish obese subjects. *N Engl J Med.* 2012;367(8):695-704.
60. Nguyen NT, Goldman C, Rosenquist CJ, et al. Laparoscopic versus open gastric bypass: a randomized study of outcomes, quality of life, and costs. *Ann Surg.* 2001;234(3):279-289; discussion 289-291.

9

Biliopancreatic Diversion With Duodenal Switch

Mustafa Hussain, MD and Alfons Pomp, MD, FACS, FRCSC

Despite the efforts of the medical community and public health agencies, the obesity epidemic continues to be a significant challenge in the developed and developing world. While the rapid rate of increase in obesity seems to have plateaued in recent years, the absolute numbers of individuals with obesity remain staggering, with an estimated 60% of the US population being overweight and 30% being classified as obese.[1] Obesity, of course, is immediately linked with several health conditions, in particular cardiovascular disease that shortens individual life expectancy and burdens the health care system. Those who are severely obese (with a body mass index [BMI] > 35 kg/m^2) are at particular risk of developing significant health problems, such as diabetes. For these individuals diet and exercise, while the cornerstone of lifestyle intervention, is often not successful. Weight loss is generally modest (10% of total body weight) and generally short lived. Most individuals regain weight, and some with interest.[2]

Bariatric surgery, on the other hand, is a proven and effective means of significant and sustained weight loss in severely obese individuals. The magnitude of weight loss is generally 2 to 4 times higher than with medical weight loss. In addition, weight loss can be more durable, with surgical patients reported sustained results for 20 to 30 years after surgery. More significantly, perhaps, is that weight loss surgery often results in resolution of many medical conditions that contribute to the morbidity and mortality of patients who are severely obese. Many times the effect on medical conditions is more pronounced than with lifestyle modification alone. This is particularly seen with diabetes, and may suggest that there is more to weight loss surgery than losing weight.[2]

The focus of this chapter will be to highlight a particular weight loss procedure that results in the most dramatic weight loss and resolution of comorbidities: the biliopancreatic diversion with duodenal switch (BPD-DS). This procedure combines a vertical gastrectomy procedure with a significant intestinal rearrangement resulting in only 50 to 100 cm of bowel exposed to both ingested food and the digestive enzymes from the liver and pancreas. It is not a common procedure performed, representing less than 5% of bariatric procedures performed in the United States. The procedure requires significant technical skill, perioperative clinical and nutritional support, and appropriate patient selection. These factors lead to the perception of greater risk incurred by the practitioner and patient. Nevertheless, there are particular patients who may benefit from this

Forse RA, Apovian CM, eds.
Bariatric Surgery: What Every Provider Needs to Know (pp 113-122).

procedure, and its implementation will likely increase in the years to come. For this reason, all practitioners should become familiar with it, and be aware of potential complications that may arise.

What Is the Procedure and How Did It Come to Be?

Intestinal rearrangement resulting in malabsorption is not a new intervention for the treatment of obesity. The most dramatic example of this was the jejunoileal bypass (JIB). This now-abandoned procedure bypassed the majority of the intestine with surgeons dividing the proximal jejunum, leaving a blind end, and reconnecting it to the terminal ileum. While weight loss from this was dramatic, significant side effects from protein and micronutrient malabsorption occurred. In addition, the intestinal blind extremity resulted in significant bacterial overgrowth, causing a multitude of side effects, the most severe of which was liver cirrhosis.

Nicola Scopinaro is credited for addressing the issue of bacterial overgrowth, by eliminating the blind end of intestine, while creating an intestinal rearrangement that results in significant fat malabsorption.[3] He performed a hemigastrectomy, and connected the ileum to the remaining stomach, followed by reestablishing continuity of the bowel in a Roux-en-Y configuration with a 50-cm common channel that allowed food and digestive secretions to comingle. The procedure is known as the BPD or Scopinaro procedure. The constant flow of bile and pancreatic juices through the biliopancreatic limb decreases the chances of bacterial overgrowth, and therefore reduces the complications associated with the JIB. This procedure continues to be performed, particularly in Europe, and has dramatic, sustained weight loss results. Scopinaro's report of his 15-year data has greater than 70% excess weight loss (EWL), with remarkable longevity.[4]

Despite the improvement over the JIB, Scopinaro's BPD carries the risk of certain significant side effects. These are generally related to the partial post-gastrectomy syndromes that result in dumping, diarrhea, and marginal ulceration. Several of these side effects are thought to be due to the elimination of the pylorus that regulates the release of gastric contents into the small bowel. Preserving the pylorus, theoretically, allows for more physiologic release of gastric contents into the small bowel. Marceau from Canada is first credited for combining DeMeester's concept of pylorus preservation with Scopinaro's BPD. Hess and Hess soon after reported on a further modification by completely dividing the duodenum just proximal to the ampulla of Vater. These modifications collectively gave rise to the current BPD-DS. In 1998, Marceau et al reported similar weight loss as with the Scopinaro procedure, but with significantly less dumping, diarrhea, and marginal ulceration.[5]

The operation has traditionally been performed through an "open" technique via a midline laparotomy and continues to be performed this way in several centers. In 2000, however, Gagner's group from New York first reported on a totally laparoscopic or minimally invasive BPD-DS.[6] This was a technically daunting and impressive achievement. The minimally invasive technique reduces pulmonary and infectious morbidities over the open technique, and allows patients to return to normal routines sooner, while maintaining the excellent weight loss. The procedure can be performed through 6 to 7 laparoscopic keyholes ranging from 0.5 to 15 mm. Several modifications to the technique have been reported, including the incorporation of robotic technology and variations on methods of rejoining the intestines (hand-sewn, stapled, etc). Common features of the current BPD-DS include a vertical sleeve gastrectomy (VSG) over a 40- to 60-Fr. bougie, 200- to 250-cm alimentary limb, and 50- to 100-cm common channels (Figure 9-1). There is no blind limb, as with JIB. It is important to recognize these subtle differences as they can result in significant nutritional and lifestyle consequences for the patient.

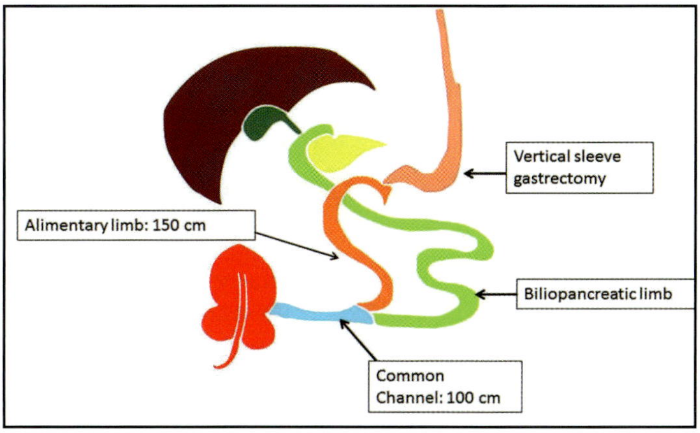

Figure 9-1. Schematic for biliopancreatic diversion/duodenal switch.

How Does It Work?

The traditional mechanisms of action of weight loss procedures are thought to be related to caloric restriction, malabsorption, or some combination of the two. Indeed, this at least serves as a partial explanation. In the BPD-DS, the VSG limits the amount of ingested food and increases the sensation of satiety. The intestinal rearrangement results in a 100-cm common channel where ingested food and biliopancreatic juices can comingle, and is the main area of fat emulsification and digestion. This results in limiting the amount of fat that can be absorbed by the intestine.

More recent studies of the hormonal changes that occur as a result of bariatric surgery speak to other mechanisms that contribute to weight loss and maintenance. Production of ghrelin, which regulates hunger and satiety, is altered, as a result of the sleeve gastrectomy component of the BPD-DS. The VSG component of the surgery also serves other physiologic mechanisms. Reduction of acid-producing gastric mucosa reduces the chances of marginal ulceration. The configuration also results in rapid gastric emptying, speaking against the purely restrictive mechanism of the surgery.

Rapid gastric emptying together with shorter alimentary distances results in more rapid delivery of undigested nutrients to the terminal ileum. This results in a more enhanced secretion of a variety of peptide hormones such as peptide YY and glucagon-like peptide-1, which affect satiety and glucose metabolism. These hormonal alterations enhance weight loss, appetite, satiety, and metabolism in a mechanism far more complex than restriction and malabsorption alone.[7]

These mechanisms are not unique to BPD-DS, but are also seen in Roux-en-Y gastric bypass (RYGB). The magnitude of these effects are likely much more pronounced in BPD-DS as a result of the shorter alimentary limb and significant biliopancreatic limb exclusion.

The superiority of the BPD-DS in terms of the magnitude and longevity of weight loss most likely comes from the handling of fatty acids. Fat malabsorption alters the circulating lipid profile. This results in depletion of fats as an intracellular energy source from the liver and muscle, which enhances mobilization from peripheral fat stores. Indeed our work has demonstrated that BPD-DS patients lose more fat mass than comparable patients with other bariatric procedures.[8,9]

How Effective Is It?

In 2004, Buchwald et al reported a landmark meta-analysis on the outcomes obesity surgery, which was a summation of 136 studies with more than 22,000 patients.[10,11] At the time, the study established that all weight loss procedures (gastric banding, gastroplasty, gastric bypass, and BPD-DS) resulted in impressive weight loss that was far superior to any medical intervention for obesity.

BPD-DS, however, demonstrated to be the most effective for reducing weight, yielding an average of 70% EWL. Moreover, the resolution of comorbidities was also noted to be significantly higher with BPD-DS, with near resolution of diabetes and hypertension in nearly all patients. These findings are at times even more noteworthy in large individual series from high-volume centers. When examining BPD without DS, Scopinaro has reported 77% EWL at 10 years in a large series of 2241 patients.[4] His experience clearly demonstrates one that is among the largest in the world. Hess et al, who modified Scopinaro's BPD to a divided DS, similarly reported 75% EWL with more than 10 years of follow-up.[12]

The Canadian experience, published by Marceau et al, reported on nearly 1500 patients with up to 15 years of follow-up. This group achieved an average of 73% EWL, with greater than 80% of patients achieving greater than 50% EWL, making the results of the procedure fairly homogeneous. Moreover, the procedure "cured morbid obesity" (ie, induced a BMI < 40 for those with starting BMI > 50 or BMI < 35 for a starting BMI < 50) in 83% and 92% of each group, respectively.[13]

When Is Biliopancreatic Diversion With Duodenal Switch an Appropriate Procedure of Choice?

Despite the effectiveness of BPD-DS, the procedure has significant short- and long-term risks, which we will discuss later in this chapter. This has led to the general unpopularity and limited implementation. Nevertheless, there are some clinical scenarios where BPD-DS has clear superiority and should be considered.

Supermorbid Obesity (BMI > 50)

The proportion of individuals with obesity has been dramatically rising over the past few decades. But what is more staggering is the severity of obesity is also increasing with the highest prevalence of supermorbid obese ever seen. These individuals present a distinct problem as they are most at risk from obesity-related comorbidities, but have the fewest options available to them. Morbidity and mortality is clearly higher in this group as a result of surgery, with those whose BMI is > 60 suffering the highest rates.[14]

No doubt the superobese population has the most to gain from surgical weight loss, and it is these patients who are frequently referred to surgery by their medical doctors. Unfortunately, this group experiences less weight loss than their non-superobese counterparts when undergoing more commonly performed weight loss procedures such as gastric banding and gastric bypass.

Average weight loss with laparoscopic adjustable banding is reported in wide ranges, but when taking into account Buchwald's large meta-analysis, average EWL is generally considered to be a modest 47%. Gastric banding is at times considered an attractive option in superobesity, due to its simplicity and relatively low perioperative complication rate. Indeed, when looking at short-term data, it would appear that banding maybe a good option. Parikh et al reported on a cohort of more than 300 patients, with a mean BMI of 55, undergoing banding, gastric bypass, and BPD-DS. In this study with 3-year follow-up, it appeared that banding was at least as effective as gastric bypass (EWL about 50%), with significantly fewer complications. BPD-DS had the more efficacy, with EWL averaging about 70%, but had significantly higher operative times, lengths of stay, and conversions to open surgery. The authors concluded that gastric banding was a suitable strategy in the superobese.[15] Longer term data, with up to 10-year follow-up, is not as promising.[16] In a cohort of nearly 200 superobese patients, more than 50% of patients had their band removed due to complication or intolerance. On average, they were still morbidly obese (BMI > 40), and 22% had not achieved even 25% EWL.

Gastric bypass is similarly less effective in the superobese population. Christou et al reported on a large cohort of patients with over 10-year follow-up.[17] At 10 years, nearly 60% of patients with a starting BMI > 50 failed to reach a BMI < 35 (not severely obese), as compared to 20% with a starting BMI < 50. This difference was also seen as early as 5 years, with 43% of superobese patients still being severely obese as compared to 9% of those whose starting BMI was < 50.

In studies that compare BPD-DS to gastric bypass, BPD-DS generally fairs better. Prachand et al reported on 350 supermorbidly obese patients undergoing either gastric bypass or BPD-DS. BPD-DS more frequently induced patients to have a BMI < 35 (ie, no longer severely obese.) Importantly, there was no significant increase in morbidity with BPD-DS.[18]

BPD-DS has also shown superiority to RYGB in a randomized study of superobese patients. At 1 year, the mean change in BMI in the DS group was 75% vs 54% with gastric bypass. In a 2-year follow-up study, the superior effectiveness of DS was maintained. DS was also more effective in reducing plasma lipid levels in the superobese patient. Both operations had comparable perioperative risk, though surgical time and hospital stay are longer with DS.[19]

Redo Weight Loss Surgery

As weight loss surgery becomes more prevalent, the population of patients that either fail to lose sufficient weight after surgery or regain weight after surgery continues to grow. There are complex reasons for this and speaks to our poor understanding of the causes and treatments of morbid obesity. Generally speaking, procedures that cause more fat malabsorption can result in more weight loss and more durable weight loss than restrictive procedures. Several groups have reported conversions from primary laparoscopic adjustable banding, vertical banded gastroplasty (VBG), and RYGB to BPD-DS.

Revisional or conversional surgery can have significant associated risks, and, in addition to procedure choice, expert surgical technique and patient selection are important to this undertaking.

Keshishian et al reported on from VBG and RYGB to BPD-DS via an open approach. At the time of the conversion to BPD-DS, the mean BMI was 49. At 30-month follow-up, the EWL was 75%, with the mean BMI being 29.2. There were no perioperative deaths in the cohort, and complication rate was 8.5%, which included 4 leaks.[20]

Gagner et al reported on a series of patients with inadequate weight loss after RYGB that were converted to BPD-DS using minimally invasive techniques. At the time of conversion, mean BMI was 40.7, with total EWL at 42.3% after the initial procedure. At 11-month follow-up, the group had an additional 63% EWL, resulting in a total of 79% EWL.[21]

Weight loss failure after adjustable banding may be more prevalent than after RYGB. Other complications, such as band intolerance, reflux, esophageal dilation, erosion, and band slippage, may require removal of the device and that a secondary weight loss procedure be performed. It would appear that BPD-DS after laparoscopic adjustable gastric banding would result in greater weight loss, however, this conversion may carry unacceptable risks, and RYGB may be a better option. In a report of 53 patients having conversion from laparoscopic adjustable gastric banding to RYGB or BPD-DS, DS did result in greater weight loss, but is associated with increased complications, particularly leaks occurring at the site of the previous band. Importantly, this cohort was not on average superobese. This perhaps diminished any advantage that BPD-DS might have over RYGB after conversion.[22]

Revisonal surgery for weight loss after VSG is a special category. The initial intention of the VSG was to stage the BPD-DS in higher risk patients who could not tolerate the extent of the full BPD-DS in one sitting. Indeed, this strategy reduced the morbidity of the operation, particularly for the super-superobese. Interestingly, however, some patients were able to sufficiently lose enough weight with VSG alone, and did not need the second stage of the procedure.[23]

Himpens et al published data on sleeve gastrectomy as a stand-alone procedure with 6-year follow-up. At 3 years EWL was 73%, but was 57% at 6 years. The authors use 50% EWL procedure success. When using this criterion, sleeve gastrectomy alone results in 47% failure rate at 3 years, and 64% failure at 6 years. Eleven patients underwent second-stage BPD-DS, and went on to have an EWL of 70.8% at 6 years compared to 53% EWL of those that had sleeve gastrectomy alone. This suggests that sleeve gastrectomy alone is effective in inducing weight loss, but may have a significant long-term failure or weight regain rate. These patients can be successfully managed by conversion to BPD-DS.[24]

Diabetes

In addition to superior weight loss, BPD-DS also has a greater impact on resolution of diabetes. This was noted in Buchwald's meta-analysis of surgical weight loss interventions, where BPD with or without DS improved or resolved diabetes 98% of the time, compared to 84% of the time with RYGB. While this may be a small increment of benefit, there may be populations of patients who may warrant the more extensive BPD-DS to impact their diabetes. Prachand et al noted that the superobese is one such group where BPD-DS was able to free patients of diabetes medications. On the other hand, superobese patients with diabetes who underwent gastric bypass still required medication 40% of the time.[25]

In the randomized study for the treatment of morbidly obese patients who were diabetic for 5 years or greater, medical therapy was compared to surgery where the surgical intervention was either BPD or RYGB. In this cohort with significant diabetes, BPD induced remission (or medication-free state) in 95% of patients as compared to 75% with RYGB and 0% with medical therapy.[26]

The reasons for improved diabetes remission after DS are unclear and, again, are likely due to enterohormal changes as a result of bypassing a greater portion of small intestine, and the resultant fat malabsorption with depletion of intracellular energy stores.

What Are the Specific Surgical Risks of Biliopancreatic Diversion With Duodenal Switch?

BPD-DS, particularly when performed laparosocopically, is the most complex bariatric procedure. It requires significant technical skill and clinical support to execute safely. The reported rates of morbidity and mortality are higher than that reported for gastric bypass: 15% to 38% and 0.9% to 8%, respectively. BPD-DS is generally performed in higher BMI patients, and this certainly adds to the reported complication rates. When looking at studies that directly compare DS to RYGB in matched patients, differences in morbidity and mortality are lower, though operative times and lengths of stay are generally universally longer for DS. Reports from centers with a high volume of DS also tend to have the lowest level of complications and deaths.[7]

Surgical complications such as bleeding, anastomotic leak, infection, hernia, and bowel obstruction are all possible after DS. Close observation and follow-up with the surgeon is important to identify signs and symptoms of surgical complications.

Two areas that are unique to BPD-DS and require attention by a surgeon who is familiar with post-DS anatomy are bowel obstruction and complications from biliary disease. Bowel obstruction in a patient who is status-post DS can be a life-threatening emergency. Due to the bowel reconstruction after DS, a closed-loop obstruction can quickly develop, without the usual prodrome of nausea and vomiting that can be seen in patients with normal anatomy. Because a significant portion of bowel is not in continuity with the stomach and mouth, ischemia and perforation can be precipitous. Therefore, it is important to have a high degree of suspicion and workup any abdominal pain in post-DS patients. Computed tomography scanning is generally adequate, and can identify obstruction either from adhesions, kinking of bowel, or internal hernias that occur due to rearrangement of bowel. It is important to note that false negatives can occur in up to 15% of series, and surgical exploration should be performed in patients with unexplained abdominal pain.

Biliary disease from cholelithiasis can occur in 50% of post-bariatric patients with massive weight loss. Treating patients with ursodiol during the period of weight loss can reduce the incidence to fewer than 10%. If complications of gallstone disease, such as pancreatitis, choledocholithiais, and cholangitis, occur, then it is important to know that endoscopic retrograde cholangiopancreatography (ERCP) is not feasible in these patients. If exploration of the common bile duct or ampulla needs to occur, then surgical exploration or transhepatic intervention will be necessary. ERCP may be performed in a surgically assisted fashion, but can be challenging even for talented operators.

What Are the Long-Term Nutritional Risks Associated With Biliopancreatic Diversion With Duodenal Switch?

Fear of severe malnutrition after extensive intestinal bypass is a frequently cited reason for many practitioners to caution against bariatric surgery. Many of these fears are generally based on complications from the now historic JIB. While this was a very effective weight loss operation, derangements in iron, calcium, fat, and protein metabolism were frequent. In addition, bacterial overgrowth added to the problem in JIB. BPD and BPD-DS have tremendously improved nutritional and metabolic profiles compared with JIB, and fears of severe nutritional dysfunction are likely overestimated. Nevertheless, without adequate patient education and follow-up, significant micronutrient and protein deficiencies can develop, warranting reversal of the procedure in some cases.

Knowing the sites of absorption of various nutrients helps the provider predict possible nutritional deficiencies that may develop in these patients. Patients after BPD-DS have reduced gastric mass, bypass of the duodenum and jejunum, and have a limited area of ileum that is exposed to both ingested items and biliopancreatic secretions. Reduced gastric mass and surface area restrict the amount of ingested globally, and serves as the primary factor for inadequate nutrition. Difficulty ingesting sufficient protein mainly contributes to protein calorie malnutrition and resultant hypoalbuminemia. In addition, reduced gastric cell mass results in reduced acidification, thought to be important for iron metabolism, and reduced intrinsic factor important for B_{12} absorption. The duodenum, the majority of which is excluded in the BPD-DS, is the primary site of iron and calcium absorption. The terminal ileum is the primary site of B_{12} and folate absorption. The decreased time emulsification is allowed to occur after BPD-DS means decreased availability of the fat-soluble vitamins A, D, E, and K. Not surprisingly, deficiencies in all these have been reported in BPD-DS (as well as other bariatric procedures).[27,28]

Specialized centers may have lower rates of nutritional deficiencies seen, partly due to experience in patient selection, follow-up, and surgical technique. In the large Canadian series with long-term follow-up, the majority of patients had normal levels of serum protein levels. Hyperalimentation for deficiency was necessary in less than 1% of the cohort. Surgical revision for malnutrition (requiring limb lengthening) was rarely indicated. This is possibly due to the preferential use of a 100-cm common channel as opposed to 50-cm described elsewhere. When examining the hemoglobin levels, as a surrogate of iron, B_{12}, and folate metabolism, mean hemoglobin levels were decreased compared to the general population, but less than 1% of patients had a hemoglobin < 10 g/dL. In terms of the fat-soluble vitamins, only data on vitamin A levels were available. Frank deficiency was noted in 2% of the population, but 21% had low levels. Vitamin D levels were not routinely measured throughout the study period so data are difficult to interpret. Looking at calcium as a surrogate, one-fifth had low levels of serum calcium with about 1% being deficient, and nearly half the patients had elevated levels of parathyroid hormone. Bone density data were available on 87 patients and slightly decreased as compared to a nonsurgical control group.[13]

No doubt these patients require life-long vitamin supplementation, and this may avoid the development of deficiencies. Topart et al reported on a small group of patients followed for 5 years. Patients were found to only be deficient in vitamin D, with increasing levels of parathyroid hormone over time. The patients in this study received baseline supplementation with 50,000 IU of vitamin A, 2000 mg of calcium, 1600 IU of vitamin D, 160 mg of iron, and a multivitamin. Additional supplementation, including intramuscular dosing of vitamins, was administered when appropriate. There were no cases of protein deficiency, though 2 patients required limb lengthening from 100 to 150 cm for diarrhea.[29]

Still other groups report higher rates of nutritional deficiencies, speaking to the heterogeneity of center practices and available data. A British study of 121 patients reported 12% deficiency in vitamin A at the end of 4 years and 40% deficiency in vitamin D. Hypoalbuminemia was infrequent but did require hyperalimentation in 6 patients. Four patients with vitamin A deficiency developed night blindness. This tended to occur years after surgery, emphasizing the need for long-term follow-up.[30]

As previously stated, the relationship between common channel length and nutritional status, though not precise, is reported in the literature. Gracia et al reported protein deficiency in 11% of patients with a common channel of 50 cm but 3% of those with a common channel of 75 cm. Revisional surgery requiring limb lengthening was necessary in 3% of patient with 50-cm common channels. Iron deficiency also increased in prevalence with shorter common channels. Shorter channels may also be associated with more frequent bowel movements and potentially impair quality of life. Most centers in the United States use common channels of about 100 cm.[31]

When looking at the data from the Scandinavian randomized trial comparing gastric bypass to BPD-DS in superobese patients, BPD-DS indeed carried more risk of developing nutritional complications, even with the short follow-up of 1 year. Patients with BPD-DS were found to have lower levels of vitamins A and D and a steeper decline in thiamine. Lower levels of hemoglobin were also noted in the BPD-DS group. Fourteen percent of BPD-DS patients had low albumin levels, as compared to none in the RYGB group. Overall, the BPD-DS group required more intense supplementation than the RYGB group and more frequent monitoring. Total parenteral nutrition, iron infusion, and the notation of night blindness were all reported in the BPD-DS group. It should be noted that in this study, the BPD-DS group had a smaller gastric reservoir compared to what is usually done. This may certainly add to the higher incidence of malnutrition.[32]

Despite the heterogeneity of the data, it is clear BPD-DS does carry additional nutritional risk. Routine measuring of nutrient levels should be undertaken along with daily life-long vitamin supplementation. Supplementation can incur a financial burden to the patient, as insurance may not cover the cost of $20 to $40/month. Currently, there is no evidence-based consensus regarding optimal supplementation. Our protocol includes (1) multivitamin with iron, (2) calcium citrate (carbonate is not well absorbed) with added vitamin D (1000 to 1200 mg + 800 U/d) in 2 doses, (3) a B-complex vitamin (without additional herbal products), (4) vitamin A (dry) 10,000 IU daily, and (5) vitamin D (dry) 10,000 IU daily in 2 divided doses. Gel-based and enteric-coated vitamins should be avoided.

These issues must be addressed with each patient prior to surgery, and their understanding of the risk should be included in the decision making to proceed with surgery. Clearly there is no litmus test to predict patient compliance, but patients with limited understanding of the risks, those with a history of noncompliance, or those with limited financial resources are generally poor candidates.

How Are Bowel Habits Altered After Surgery?

Another barrier to the routine employment of BPD-DS is the conception that patients will suffer from very frequent and uncontrollable bowel movements after surgery due to steatorrhea. This is generally exaggerated. Indeed it follows that due to more rapid intestinal transit, an alimentary limb of 250 cm, and a reduced surface area where fat can be absorbed, more bowel movements are expected. But studies comparing BPD-DS to gastric bypass generally have found that while patients do have more bowel movements, the differences are not often statistically significant. In addition, the average absolute number of bowel moments is generally around 3 per day. Incontinence may be more frequent with BPD-DS as well, but also not statistically significant. Many times, these problems can be controlled with diet modification, education, and occasionally the use of medication.[33,34]

Summary

Morbid obesity is a prevalent complex condition that is challenging to treat. Bariatric surgery is currently the most effective modality to treat this condition. Of the available surgical options, BPD-DS results in the most weight loss and the highest frequency of resolution of many comorbidities. It may be the preferred surgical option in the superobese, those with severe diabetes, and in cases of weight regain after previous weight loss surgery. It is not, however, a frequently performed procedure for several factors, which include the technical complexity, patient selection, and perception of more frequent complications and change in bowel habits. But with proper expertise, this operation can be performed safely and effectively. Providers who come across patients who have had this procedure should be aware of their unique anatomy and the consequences it may have.

References

1. Ogden CL, Carroll MD, Kit BK, Flegal KM. Prevalence of obesity in the United States, 2009-2010. *NCHS Data Brief.* 2012(82):1-8.
2. Sjostrom L, Narbro K, Sjostrom CD, et al. Effects of bariatric surgery on mortality in Swedish obese subjects. *N Engl J Med.* 2007;357:741-752.
3. Scopinaro N, Gianetta E, Civalleri D, Bonalumi U, Bachi V. Bilio-pancreatic bypass for obesity: II. Initial experience in man. *Br J Surg.* 1979;66(9):618-620.
4. Scopinaro N. Biliopancreatic diversion: mechanisms of action and long-term results. *Obes Surg.* 2006;16(6):683-689.
5. Marceau P, Hould F, Simard S, et al. Biliopancreatic diversion with a duodenal switch. *World J Surg.* 1998;22:947-954.
6. Ren CJ, Patterson E, Gagner M. Early results of laparoscopic biliopancreatic diversion with duodenal switch: a case series of 40 consecutive patients. *Obes Surg.* 2000;10:514-523.
7. Sudan R, Jacobs DO. Biliopancreatic diversion with duodenal switch. *Surg Clin North Am.* 2011;91(6):1281-1293, ix.
8. Scopinaro N, Marinari G, Camerini GB, et al. Specific effect of biliopancreatic diversion on the major components of metabolic syndrom: a long-term follow-up study. *Diabetes Care.* 2005;28:2406-2411.
9. Strain GW, Gagner M, Pomp A, Dakin G, Inabnet WB, Saif T. Comparison of fat-free mass in super obesity (BMI >/= 50 kg/m^2) and morbid obesity (BMI < 50 kg/m^2) in response to different weight loss surgeries. *Surg Obes Relat Dis.* 2012;8(3):255-259.
10. Buchwald H, Avidor Y, Braunwald E, et al. Bariatric surgery: a systematic review and meta-analysis. *JAMA.* 2004;292(14):1724-1737.
11. Buchwald H, Estok R, Fahrbach K, et al. Weight and type 2 diabetes after bariatric surgery: systematic review and meta-analysis. *Am J Med.* 2009;122(3):248-256.
12. Hess DS, Hess DW, Oakley RS. The biliopancreatic diversion with the duodenal switch: results beyond 10 years. *Obes Surg.* 2005;15(3):408-416.

13. Marceau P, Biron S, Hould FS, et al. Duodenal switch: long-term results. *Obes Surg.* 2007;17(11):1421-1430.
14. Longitudinal Assessment of Bariatric Surgery Consortium. Perioperative safety in the longitudinal assessment of bariatric surgery. *N Engl J Med.* 2009;361:445-454.
15. Parikh MS, Fielding GA, Ren CJ. U.S. experience with 749 laparoscopic adjustable gastric bands: intermediate outcomes. *Surg Endosc.* 2005;19(12):1631-1635.
16. Arapis K, Chosidow D, Lehmann M, et al. Long-term results of adjustable gastric banding in a cohort of 186 super-obese patients with a BMI >/= 50 kg/m². *J Visc Surg.* 2012;149(2):e143-e152.
17. Christou NV, Look D, Maclean LD. Weight gain after short- and long-limb gastric bypass in patients followed for longer than 10 years. *Ann Surg.* 2006;244(5):734-740. PMCID: 1856611.
18. Prachand VN, Davee R, Alverdy JC. Duodenal switch provides superior weight loss in the super-obese (BMI > 50 kg/m²) compared with gastric bypass. *Ann Surg.* 2006;244:611.
19. Sovik TT, Taha O, Aasheim ET, et al. Randomized clinical trial of laparoscopic gastric bypass versus laparoscopic duodenal switch for super obesity. *Br J Surg.* 2010;97:160.
20. Keshishian A, Zahriya K, Hartoonian T, Ayagian C. Duodenal switch is a safe operation for patients who have failed other bariatric operations. *Obes Surg.* 2004;14(9):1187-1192.
21. Parikh M, Pomp A, Gagner M. Laparoscopic conversion of failed gastric bypass to duodenal switch: technical considerations and preliminary outcomes. *Surg Obes Relat Dis.* 2007;3(6):611-618.
22. Dapri G, Cadiere GB, Himpens J. Laparoscopic conversion of adjustable gastric banding and vertical banded gastroplasty to duodenal switch. *Surg Obes Relat Dis.* 2009;5(6):678-683.
23. Deitel M, Crosby RD, Gagner M. The First International Consensus Summit for Sleeve Gastrectomy (SG), New York City, October 25-27, 2007. *Obes Surg.* 2008;18(5):487-496.
24. Himpens J, Dobbeleir J, Peeters G. Long-term results of laparoscopic sleeve gastrectomy for obesity. *Ann Surg.* 2010;252(2):319-324.
25. Prachand VN, Ward M, Alverdy JC. Duodenal switch provides superior resolution of metabolic comorbidities independent of wieight loss in the super-obese (BMI > 50 kg/m²) compared with gastric bypass. *J Gastrointest Surg.* 2010;14:211-220.
26. Mingrone G, Panunzi S, De Gaetano A, et al. Bariatric surgery versus conventional medical therapy for type 2 diabetes. *N Engl J Med.* 2012;366(17):1577-1585.
27. Pournaras DJ, le Roux CW. After bariatric surgery, what vitamins should be measured and what supplements should be given? *Clin Endocrinol (Oxf).* 2009;71(3):322-325.
28. Shankar P, Boylan M, Sriram K. Micronutrient deficiencies after bariatric surgery. *Nutrition.* 2010;26(11-12):1031-1037.
29. Topart P, Becouarn G, Salle A. Five-year follow-up after biliopancreatic diversion with duodenal switch. *Surg Obes Relat Dis.* 2010;7(2):199-205.
30. Magee CJ, Barry J, Brocklehurst J, Javed S, Macadam R, Kerrigan DD. Outcome of laparoscopic duodenal switch for morbid obesity. *Br J Surg.* 2011;98(1):79-84.
31. Gracia JA, Martinez M, Elia M, et al. Obesity surgery results depending on technique performed: long-term outcome. *Obes Surg.* 2009;19(4):432-438.
32. Aasheim ET, Bjorkman S, Sovik TT, et al. Vitamin status after bariatric surgery: a randomized study of gastric bypass and duodenal switch. *Am J Clin Nutr.* 2009;90(1):15-22.
33. Sovik TT, Karlsson J, Aasheim ET, et al. Gastrointestinal function and eating behavior after gastric bypass and duodenal switch. *Surg Obes Relat Dis.* 2012;9(5):641-647.
34. Wasserberg N, Hamoui N, Petrone P, Crookes PF, Kaufman HS. Bowel habits after gastric bypass versus the duodenal switch operation. *Obes Surg.* 2008;18(12):1563-1566.

10

Other Surgical Procedures

Jaisa Olasky, MD and Daniel B. Jones, MD, MS, FACS

Innovative Procedures

Advances in endocrinology have improved our understanding of the physiology behind bariatric surgery and introduced new concepts in the surgical treatment of obesity and diabetes. In fact, the inclusion criteria for bariatric surgery have been expanded to include patients with lower body mass index (BMI) if they have type 2 diabetes or prediabetes. As a result of this, several of the new procedures described below have been specifically developed and trialed on patients with lower BMI (30 to 40 kg/m^2) who also have type 2 diabetes.

Laparoscopic Ileal Interposition Associated With Sleeve Gastrectomy

An ileal interposition can be created as an addition to a sleeve gastrectomy. This procedure is gaining popularity as a treatment option for patients with lower BMI and type 2 diabetes. The procedure begins with the creation of the sleeve in the usual fashion as described in a previous chapter in this book. When the sleeve is complete, the jejunum is stapled and divided 25 cm beyond the ligament of Treitz. The terminal ileum is then divided in 2 places, at 30 and 200 cm proximal to the terminal ileum to make a free-floating segment. The first anastomosis is made between the distal end of the long segment of jejunum/ileum to the terminal ileum. The 170-cm segment of ileum is then connected to the most proximal jejunal end, the piece that was previously measured to be 25 cm distal to the ligament of Treitz. The last anastomosis is created between the distal end of the ileal segment and the proximal end of the jejunum, in a stapled side-to-side fashion. Finally, all of the mesenteric defects are closed.[1]

The laparoscopic ileal interposition associated with sleeve gastrectomy (LII-SG) was studied by DePaula et al, who found that in 120 patients with BMI of 43, 15.8% of which had type 2 diabetes, the mean postoperative BMI at 38 months after the ileal interposition was 25.7. Type 2 diabetes resolved in 84.2%.[2] The same group evaluated 454 patients with a mean BMI of 29.7 and

Forse RA, Apovian CM, eds.
Bariatric Surgery: What Every Provider Needs to Know (pp 123-130).

type 2 diabetes for at least 3 years. The mean preoperative fasting glucose and post-prandial plasma glucose were 198 and 262, respectively. The mean postoperative BMI, fasting glucose, and post-prandial glucose were 25.8, 101, and 128, respectively. As described earlier, the LII-SG creates 3 anastomoses and a gastric staple line, all of which are at risk for leaking. Despite this risk, the overall mortality was only 0.4%.[1]

Surgical Gastric Pacer

Implantable gastric pacemakers (IGP) have traditionally been used to treat gastroparesis but by altering the pulse width and frequency controls they can be set to induce a feeling of early satiety. This was initially proven on pigs and later used to treat more than 500 obese patients.[3,4] The earliest large trial on gastric pacers for weight loss was performed from 2002 to 2003 in Europe. Investigators found that at 2 years the excess weight loss (EWL) was 25%.[5,6] These results were not reproducible in the 2004 US-based randomized controlled Screened Health Assessment and Pacer Evaluation (SHAPE) trial. In the SHAPE trial there was no significant difference between the treatment and control groups at 12 months.[7] Although the efficacy results are mixed, the morbidity and mortality is extremely low, making ongoing investigations of IGP attractive.

IntraPace has recently developed the Abiliti device that sends signals to the stomach, creating a full sensation with any oral intake.[8] This device is also able to create an electronic log of the patient's intake, essentially providing the patient with a food diary that helps the patient and his or her provider track the patient's progress. It was approved in Europe in 2011 but is still several years away from completing the Food and Drug Administration approval process in the United States. A randomized controlled trial that was completed in 2013 found that after 1 year the mean EWL was 28.7% and after 2 years it remained high at 27.5%.[9]

Although the implantation of the pacer is a short and low-risk procedure, there are complications that can occur during the surgery, such as gastric perforation. In the postoperative period there are rarely reports of complications, although in some cases the leads were found to be partially or completely dislodged, resulting in limited or no pacer function.[3]

Vagal Nerve Stimulation

Along similar lines to the gastric pacers, other nerve stimulators have been developed to target the vagus nerve specifically. One example of this is the vBloc device (EnteroMedics) (Figure 10-1). The vBloc neuroregulator device is placed in the subcutaneous tissue. The leads are placed laparoscopically at the vagal nerve trunks near the gastroesophageal junction and intermittently block the nerve signals. This is different from the permanent vagal disruption that occurs after surgical vagotomy. After permanent vagotomy some patients develop afferent reinnervation of the stomach, resulting in treatment failure. Since the vBloc only intermittently blocks the nerves, they are less likely to reestablish gastric innervation. Although animal and human trials showed an average of 20% EWL along with decreased weight savings, further research will be needed prior to its widespread adoption of this procedure.[10,11]

Brain Stimulators

There has been recent interest in the possibility of using brain stimulators to modulate appetite and satiety. Evidence shows that deep brain stimulation or transcranial brain stimulation may be a useful weight loss intervention in the future. A National Institutes of Health randomized controlled clinical trial in Arizona is studying the effects of dorsolateral prefrontal cortex stimulation over a period of 4 weeks. The outcome measures will be subjective satiety and weight loss. This study is set to be completed in 2015.[12]

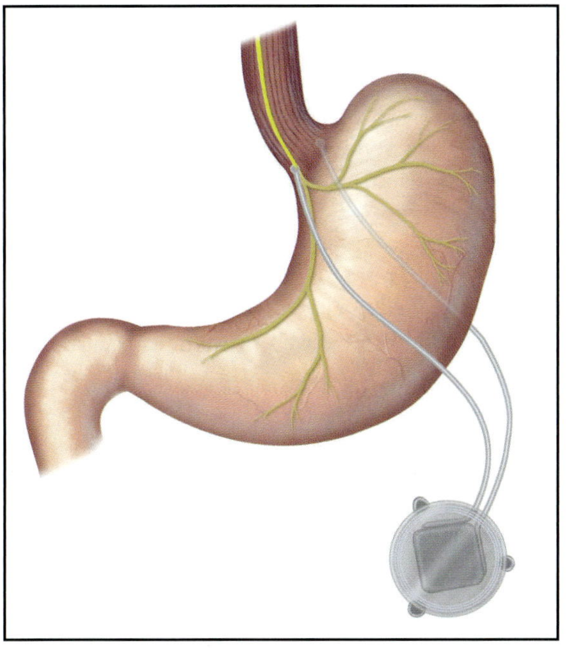

Figure 10-1. The vBloc device. (Reprinted with permission, Ciné-Med Publishing, Inc. Adapted from *Atlas of Metabolic and Weight Loss Surgery*, Copyright © 2010.)

Endoscopic Procedures

Endoscopic Intragastric Balloon

A variety of intragastric weight loss devices have been developed over the past 20 years. Currently indications for the intragastric balloon are BMI $\geq$ 35 with resistance to clinical treatment and refusal or contraindication to surgical treatment and BMI $<$ 35 with comorbidities and resistance to clinical treatment. Absolute contraindications are severe, active esophagitis; gastric or duodenal ulceration; inflammatory bowel disease; cancer; gastrointestinal bleeding; and alcoholism or drug addiction. In addition, caution should be used for patients with hiatal hernia larger than 5 cm, prior gastric surgery, those who are on anticoagulants or gastric irritants, and those with psychiatric disorders.[3]

Serious complications have been reported with intragastric balloons, such as esophagitis (1.27%), gastric outlet obstruction (0.76%), balloon rupture (0.36%), gastric perforation (0.21%), gastric ulcer (0.2%), and death (0.07%).[3,12] In addition, complete weight regain is not rare after balloon deflation. As a result of these adverse outcomes, industry standards were created at a 1987 conference. The guidelines state that any future intragastric devices should be effective at promoting weight loss, filled with liquid and not air, be capable of size adjustment, have a smooth surface (thus decreasing risk of ulcers and obstructions), contain a radio-opaque marker that allows proper follow-up of the device if it deflates, and be constructed of durable materials that do not leak.[13]

Several intragastric devices exist that fulfill this criteria, including the BioEnterics Intragastric Balloon ([BIB] Inamed Health), Heliosphere (Helioscopie), Silimed Gastric Balloon, and Semstationary Antral Balloon (JP Industria Farmaceutica). Of these, the BIB is the most studied.

The BIB intragastric balloon is currently only approved to be used as part of a trial in the United States.[10] The BIB is a spherical, saline-filled silicone device that can be filled with up to 700 mL. The minimal recommended fill volume is 400 mL. It has a smooth surface without external seams, thus fulfilling the above criteria and decreasing the risk of irritation of the gastric mucosa.

Methylene blue (10 mL) is added to the sterile saline so that the provider will be alerted to any balloon leakage.

The device is placed under endoscopic guidance through the esophagus into the stomach. The patient is sedated as per the standard of care for endoscopy at the institution. At most centers, this is monitored anesthesia care, with one agent for sedation and one for pain control (eg, Versed [midazolam] and fentanyl), with the patient breathing on his or her own. Radio-opaque markers allow the provider to monitor the balloon orientation during insertion. Once in place, the balloon is filled with a special catheter that is removed after the fill is complete. According to the manufacturers, the BIB can be kept in place for 6 months. At time of removal, a special endoscopic needle is used to deflate the balloon. After it is deflated it can be removed easily with an endoscopic grasper.

The early models of intragastric weight loss devices did not fare well in randomized studies. However, BIB had promising results in a randomized controlled crossover study. The patients had an average BMI of 43.7 and were planning for traditional bariatric procedures. Half of the 32 participants started with BIB and half with sham. After 3 months, the groups were crossed over. During the first period, the BIB group lost 5.5 BMI points as compared to only 0.5 BMI points for the sham group. During the second period, the group that crossed from sham to BIB lost 4.3 BMI points. These results correlate to a roughly 25% EWL.[14] In an additional study performed by the same group, at 6-month follow-up the average percent EWL was 33.9.[15] Further studies and long-term data are still needed before this is considered a standard bariatric procedure.

An alternative method of occupying gastric space with even less risk than the intragastric balloon is currently under development. The Elipse (Allurion Techonologies) is an intragastric device that does not require endoscopic placement, thus eliminating the risk of esophageal injury or complications from anesthesia. The device is swallowed by the patient while attached to a small catheter. Body temperature water is instilled until the balloon is filled. It will dissolve and be passed with the stool 3 months later. A multicenter human clinical trial began in Europe in 2014 and is still ongoing.

Endoscopic Intraluminal Gastric Stapling

In the era of natural orifice surgery, the use of endoscopic gastric stapling or suturing devices is no longer considered novel. There has been an unsurprising progression to the use of these tools to decrease the intraluminal volume of the stomach. The decrease in gastric lumen size after the endoscopic gastroplasty would be expected to lead to weight loss in the same way as the more commonly performed sleeve gastrectomy. However, any hormonal benefits one might get from removing the greater curve stomach tissue as with the sleeve would not be expected from endoscopic gastroplasty.

At present time the available instruments for endoluminal gastroplasty are the EndoCinch Suturing System (CR Bard) and the Transoral Gastroplasty System ([TOGA] Satiety, Inc). The TOGA system is a stapling device that narrows the stomach by stapling a full-thickness area of the lesser curve that has been suctioned into its jaws. After several firings of the stapler, spanning roughly 2 cm, a narrow stomach is created. A second device, the TOGA restrictor, is then used to make pleats with the outflow track, creating a narrowing at the distal end of the sleeve. The most commonly reported adverse events for TOGA are dysphagia immediately after the procedure, vomiting, and nausea. Patients who fail TOGA remain candidates for more invasive bariatric procedures.[16]

In a study from Rome, TOGA was compared to Roux-en-Y gastric bypass (RYGB) and biliopancreatic diversion. In the TOGA group, 59% of patients with an initial BMI < 45 reached a BMI < 35 postoperatively as compared to only 48% overall for all of the patients BMI < 45 combined from each arm. These results indicated that TOGA might be indicated for patients with lower BMI.[17]

Endoscopic Duodenal-Jejunal Endoluminal Sleeve

As a mounting body of evidence suggested that RYGB improved weight loss and diabetes beyond what could be explained from decreased caloric intake alone, scientists and surgeons began to perform rat experiments to identify the areas of the gastrointestinal tract that produced the most weight loss and diabetes-promoting hormones. The result was the creation of the duodenal-jejunal endoluminal sleeve. The sleeve is designed to block the absorption of food for the entire 60-cm length of the device. The device is designed to primarily cause weight loss from malabsorption and delayed mixing of food with biliopancreatic fluids but is also expected to cause a change in gastrointestinal hormonal release that will improve diabetes.[11]

The endoluminal device that has been studied the most thus far in humans is a form of the duodenojejunal bypass sleeve known as the EndoBarrier Gastrointestinal Liner (GI Dynamics Inc). It has been approved for sale in Europe and Australia and in August 2012 was approved for clinical trial in the United States on patients who have a BMI > 30 and type 2 diabetes. The device is placed under direct visualization during endoscopy. In trials the procedure lasted roughly 30 minutes. The proximal end is attached to the duodenal bulb to prevent migration. Once deployed it covers the duodenum and part of the jejunum. According to the manufacturer it can be left in for 12 months.[18] The EndoBarrier is removed endoscopically with the aid of a drawstring, similar to esophageal stents. It should be removed under an overtube to protect the esophagus and mouth.[6]

Studies conducted outside of the United States report a 19% mean EWL after 3 months.[19] These results have been corroborated by other studies. In a trial investigating the effect of the EndoBarrier on metabolic syndrome, over a period of 52 weeks there was a significant decrease in waist circumference, blood pressure, cholesterol, triglycerides, and fasting glucose. In one study, the EndoBarrier significantly lowered fasting blood glucose, fasting insulin, and hemoglobin A1c.[20]

As with other endoscopic bariatric procedures, the risks of the EndoBarrier are generally lower than that of surgery. In some patients, the procedure was aborted due to a short duodenal bulb that precluded device deployment. The device was removed early in some patients due to migration, gastrointestinal bleeding, or abdominal pain. Other known adverse reactions are back pain, pharyngeal tears, nausea, and vomiting.[21] While the future of endoluminal liners appears promising, their fate in the United States will be determined by data pending completion of the clinical trial.

Procedures of Historical Interest

Vertical Band Gastroplasty

Vertical band gastroplasty (VBG) (Figure 10-2) is a procedure now considered to be of historic interest only as the risks outweigh the benefits. It is an important subject to discuss as the nonsurgeon practitioner is the most likely physician to encounter a patient who has had this procedure.

Mason described VBG in its most popular form in a case series report in 1982.[22] The idea was to create an effective weight loss procedure that minimized the risk of intestinal leak that was present with the gastric bypass. In the Mason version of the VBG an end-to-end anastomosis stapling device is used to staple a circle of full-thickness stomach 5 cm past the gastroesophageal junction. This is done with a 32 Fr. bougie in place. A linear stapler is then applied from the lateral edge of the circular staple line across and up to the angle of His, completely transecting the tissue lateral to the circular staple line. A band is then placed from the right, through the gastrohepatic ligament, secured around the remaining gastric pouch, and sewn into place. Some surgeons also reinforce the staple lines with suture.[23]

Figure 10-2. Vertical band gastroplasty with conversion to a gastric bypass. (Reprinted with permission, Ciné-Med Publishing, Inc. Adapted from *Atlas of Metabolic and Weight Loss Surgery*, Copyright © 2010.)

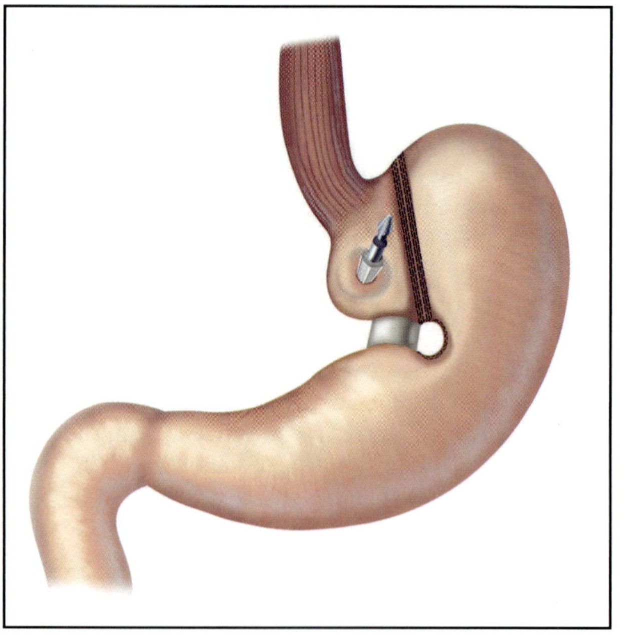

Although the perioperative complication rate was low, with a reported morbidity of 10% and mortality of 0.24%, the VBG has fallen out of favor due to a high rate of long-term complications and weight regain. During the first postoperative year, a 35% to 60% EWL was commonly achieved. However, if the transverse staple line were to break down, the resulting gastrogastric fistula usually leads to a complete weight regain. Weight is also regained due to pouch dilation. Other long-term complications include marginal ulcerations, stomal stenosis, severe reflux, and band slippage. Many of these patients have gone on to have a conversion procedure to RYGB or band removal alone. These procedures are notoriously long and arduous due to significant scarring around the staple line and band.[24,25]

Jejunoileal Bypass

Before the advent of the RYGB, the first malabsorptive obesity operation to receive widespread attention was the jejunoileal bypass (JIB) (Figure 10-3). The procedure was developed in the 1950s. After several permutations of the JIB, the most commonly performed version was developed. In this procedure the jejunum is transected 35.5 cm past the ligament of Treitz. The proximal end is anastomosed to the terminal ileum, roughly 10 cm before the ileocecal valve. The resulting anatomy leaves the patient with less than 50 cm of functional small bowel. The expected EWL was 50%.

The JIB maintained its popularity in the bariatric surgery world until the 1980s when the severe malabsorptive side effects led to its demise. Most commonly the patients presented with dehydration, severe diarrhea, protein malnutrition, dangerous electrolyte abnormalities, anemia, liver failure, oxalate urolithiasis, and immune complex arthritis. The majority of the estimated 100,000 procedures performed have been revised or reversed.[26]

Banded Bypass

The banded bypass is a modification of gastric bypass designed to keep the gastric pouch small by placement of a silastic band around the gastric bypass stomach. This technique was popularized by Dr. Fobi in 1986 and revised by him in 1992 with the addition of stomach transection, essentially adding a gastric band to the modern-day version of the RYGB. In Fobi's data, at 2 years

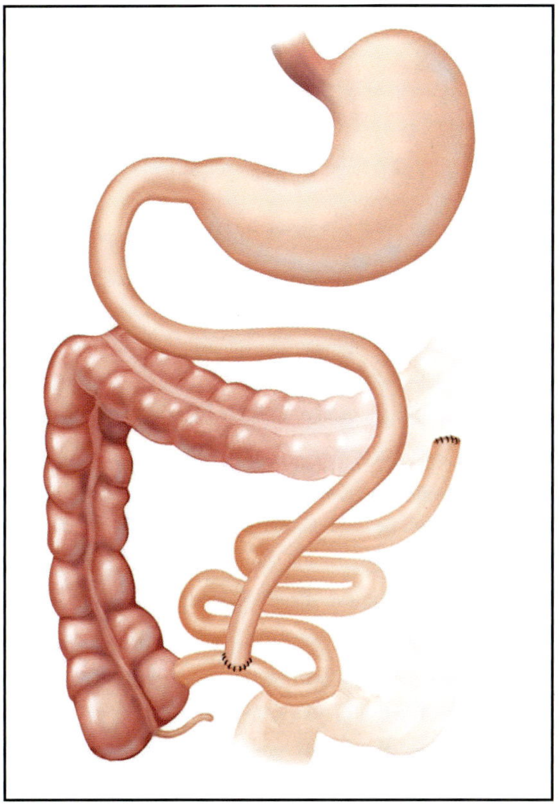

Figure 10-3. The jejunoileal bypass. (Reprinted with permission, Ciné-Med Publishing, Inc. Adapted from *Atlas of Metabolic and Weight Loss Surgery*, Copyright © 2010.)

postoperative complications included all of the known adverse events from gastric bypass, such as staple line breakdown, ulcers, dumping, and nutritional deficiencies, but with increased risk of outlet stenosis and band erosion. Unlike in the nonbanded bypass, the outlet stenosis usually does not respond to endoscopic dilation and instead requires band removal. Given the increased complications, some question whether placing the band is necessary at the time of the initial surgery or if instead the procedure should be reserved for salvage in a prior gastric bypass patient suffering from weight regain.[27]

References

1. DePaula AL, Stival AR, Halpern A, Vencio S. Thirty-day morbidity and mortality of the laparoscopic ileal interposition associated with sleeve gastrectomy for the treatment of type 2 diabetic patients with BMI < 35: an analysis of 454 consecutive patients. *World J Surg.* 2011;35:102-108.
2. DePaula AL, Stival AR, Halpern A, Vencio S. Surgical treatment of morbid obesity: mid-term outcomes of the laparoscopic ileal interposition associated to a sleeve gastrectomy in 120 patients. *Obes Surg.* 2011;5:668-675.
3. Stimaca D, Majanoviccb SK. Endoscopic approaches to obesity. *Dig Dis.* 2012;30:187-195.
4. Cigaina VV, Saggioro A, Rigo V, Pinato GP, Ischia S. Long-term effects of gastric pacing to reduce feed intake in swine. *Obes Surg.* 1996;6:250-253.
5. De Luca M, Segato G, Busetto L, et al. Progress in implantable gastric stimulation: summary of results of the European multi-center study. *Obes Surg.* 2004;(Suppl 1):S33-S39.
6. Miller K, Hoeller E, Aigner F. The implantable gastric stimulator for obesity: an update of the European experience in the LOSS (Laparoscopic Obesity Stimulation Survey) study. *Treat Endocrinol.* 2006;5:53-58.
7. Shikora SA, Bergenstal R, Bessler M, et al. Implantable gastric stimulation for the treatment of clinically severe obesity: results of the SHAPE trial. *Surg Obes Relat Dis.* 2009:5:31-37.
8. IntraPace. http://www.abiliti.com/en/for_physicians. Published 2012. Accessed December 1, 2012.

9. Horbach T, Thalheimer A, Seyfried F, et al. Abiliti® closed-loop gastric electrical stimulation system for treatment of obesity: clinical results with a 27-month follow-up. *Obes Surg.* 2015 Mar 15. [Epub ahead of print]
10. Verdam FJ, Schouten R, Greve JW. An update on less invasive and endoscopic techniques mimicking the effect of bariatric surgery. *J Obes.* 2012;2012:597871.
11. Nguyen NT, De Maria EJ, Ikramuddin S, Hutter MM. *The SAGES Manual: A Practical Guide to Bariatric Surgery.* New York, NY: Springer Science and Business Media, LLC; 2008.
12. National Institute of Diabetes and Digestive and Kidney Diseases (NIDDK). http://clinicaltrials.gov/ct2/show/NCT00739362. Updated December 6, 2012. Accessed December 7, 2012.
13. Dumonceau JM. Evidence-based review of the Bioenterics intragastric balloon for weight loss. *Obes Surg.* 2008;18:1611-1617.
14. Schapiro M, Benjamin S, Blackburn G, et al. Obesity and the gastric balloon: a comprehensive workshop. *Gastrointest Endosc.* 1987;334:323-327.
15. Genco A, Cipriano M, Bacci V, et al. BioEnterics® Intra-gastric Balloon (BIB®): a short-term, double-blind, randomised, controlled, crossover study on weight reduction in morbidly obese patients. *Int J Obes.* 2006;30:129-133.
16. Genco A, Bruni T, Doldi SB, et al. BioEnterics intragastric balloon: the Italian experience with 2,515 patients. *Obes Surg.* 2005;15:1161-1164.
17. Moreno C, Closset J, Dugardeyn S, et al. Transoral gastroplasty is safe, feasible, and induces significant weight loss in morbidly obese patients: results of the second human pilot study. *Endoscopy.* 2008;40:406-413.
18. Nanni G, Familiari P, Mor A, et al. Effectiveness of the Transoral Endoscopic Vertical Gastroplasty (TOGa®): a good balance between weight loss and complications, if compared with gastric bypass and biliopancreatic diversion. *Obes Surg.* 2012;22:1897-1902.
19. GI Dynamics. http://www.gidynamics.com/media/GI-Dynamics-Corporate-Fact-Sheet.pdf. Published Winter 2012. Accessed December 2, 2012.
20. Schouten R, Rijs CS, Bouvy ND, et al. A multicenter, randomized efficacy study of the EndoBarrier Gastrointestinal Liner for presurgical weight loss prior to bariatric surgery. *Ann Surg.* 2010;251:236-243.
21. Escalona A, Pimentel F, Sharp A, et al. Weight loss and metabolic improvement in morbidly obese subjects implanted for 1 year with an endoscopic duodenal-jejunal bypass liner. *Ann Surg.* 2012;255:1080-1085.
22. Mason EE. Vertical banded gastroplasty for obesity. *Arch Surg.* 1982;117:701-706.
23. De Moura E, Martins BC, Lopes GS, et al. Metabolic improvements in obese type 2 diabetes subjects implanted for 1 year with an endoscopically deployed duodenal-jejunal bypass liner. *Diabetes Technology and Therapeutics.* 2012;14(2):183-189.
24. Champion JK, Williams M. Laparoscopic vertical banded gastroplasty. *Curr Surg.* 2003;60:37-39.
25. Champion JK. Laparoscopic vertical banded gastroplasty. In: Schauer PR, Schirmer BD, Brethauer SA, eds. *Minimally Invasive Bariatric Surgery.* New York, NJ: Springer; 2007:165-172.
26. Fronza JS, Prystowsky JB, Hungness ES, Nagle AP. Revisional bariatric surgery at a single institution. *Am J Surg.* 2010;200:651-654.
27. Jejunoileal bypass. In: Jones DB, Schneider BE, Olbers T, eds. *Atlas of Metabolic and Weight Loss Surgery.* Woodbury, CT: Cine-Med Publishing; 2010:302-303.

11

Preoperative Evaluation of the Patient Undergoing Bariatric Surgery

Andrew S. Wu, MD and Daniel M. Herron, MD

Bariatric surgical procedures are performed in a high-risk population with many comorbid conditions and can be challenging and complex. Both the American College of Surgeons and the American Society for Metabolic and Bariatric Surgery (ASMBS) require established preoperative pathways as an essential component of designation as a certified bariatric center. Guidelines addressing preoperative patient evaluation were published in the SAGES guideline of March 2008 on the clinical application of laparoscopic bariatric surgery.[1] A substantial focus of these guidelines was on psychological and nutritional aspects of the patient in the preoperative setting, leaving the medical and surgical evaluation to the judgment of the operating surgeon. When reviewing the practice of preoperative evaluation, it is important to recognize that preoperative assessment protocols may be institution specific and may vary from region to region.

In this chapter, we provide an overview of the necessary components of a thorough preoperative bariatric evaluation, starting with initial assessment and patient selection. Although we briefly review choice of operation this will not be a focus, as it is addressed in-depth in a separate chapter. We also discuss the necessary medical assessments that are to be performed in the following categories: gastrointestinal, nutritional, psychological, cardiovascular, pulmonary, hepatic function, metabolic/endocrine, hematologic, renal function, and anesthesia.

The First Encounter: Overall Assessment

A major purpose of the preoperative evaluation is to identify and address issues that affect the patient's surgical and anesthetic risk. Medical consultants are thus important not only for the preoperative workup, but during the inpatient stay and after discharge, assisting with postoperative follow-up for the long term. In addition, the preoperative process serves to inform and educate the patient about the risks and benefits of the surgical procedure and nonsurgical alternatives.

The initial evaluation starts with a complete medical history and physical exam. The patient should be evaluated for signs and symptoms of comorbid conditions commonly associated with obesity, including sleep apnea, stress urinary incontinence, degenerative joint disease, venous

Forse RA, Apovian CM, eds.
Bariatric Surgery: What Every Provider Needs to Know (pp 131-139).

Table 11-1
Laboratory Tests Typically Ordered for the Preoperative Evaluation of the Bariatric Patient

- Chemistry panel, calcium, magnesium, phosphorus
- Liver function tests
- Complete blood count
- Coagulation profile
- Glucose level, hemoglobin A1c
- Iron level, total iron binding capacity
- Vitamin B_{12}, folate, thiamine, vitamin D
- Lipid panel

stasis disease, and skin infections, all of which may be easily overlooked in this patient population. A history of substance abuse or eating disorder such as bulimia may be a relative contraindication to surgery. A history of previous hospitalization for psychiatric illness including depression or suicidal ideation is an indication for a more thorough psychiatric evaluation and assessment.

The physical exam may reveal significant underlying problems requiring more extensive preoperative testing. Patients with a history of arrhythmia or signs of cardiac disease such as pedal edema will likely require cardiology evaluation including preoperative stress testing. Neck exam for thyroid nodules or enlargement is often difficult due to neck size. Skin problems such as fungal infection are also commonly found on exam.[2] Initial laboratory tests need to be performed during the initial assessment. A list of commonly ordered labs is given in Table 11-1 and discussed in-depth later in this chapter.

Patient Selection and Indications for Surgery

While surgical intervention is the only proven treatment for long-term weight management in the severely obese, appropriate patient selection is critical for a successful operation and outcome.[3] The National Institutes of Health consensus conference in 1991 established guidelines and indications for surgical management of severe obesity, which included a body mass index (BMI) ≥ 40 kg/m^2 or BMI ≥ 35 with significant comorbidity. Patients must also have demonstrated dietary attempts at weight loss that have been ineffective.[4] In February 2011, the US Food and Drug Administration did allow patients with a BMI ≥ 30 to be considered for an adjustable laparoscopic gastric band.[5]

Many insurance companies require evidence of ineffective dietary attempts at weight loss. This is inconsistent with data from many studies showing that patients with obesity fail to sustain long-term weight loss after dieting and that nearly all patients will regain all of their lost weight within 2 years.[3] Age as a criterion for patient selection is controversial at the extremes. Whereas there is a general agreement that ages 18 to 65 are appropriate, there is no consensus about younger teenagers and older patients. There has been recent interest and an upswing of media attention toward teenagers undergoing weight loss surgery given the tremendous rise of adolescent obesity. Concern regarding ongoing physical and mental development has led some medical and surgical care providers to argue that surgery should not be considered until after puberty. Others, however, argue that fighting adolescent obesity via surgical intervention provides a longer lasting effect in overall future health and reduced physical and psychological morbidity.

Specific criteria and recommendations of a particular type of bariatric surgery for each patient will be addressed in other chapters of this book. Although surgical treatment of obesity has been shown to improve or lead to complete resolution of many associated comorbidities, these medical conditions may complicate perioperative management. Identification and optimal treatment of all identified significant comorbidities may improve safety of surgery in this high-risk group of patients. In the remaining sections of this chapter, preoperative medical assessment will be discussed.

Preoperative Medical Assessment

Gastrointestinal

The bariatric patient with a history suggestive of symptomatic cholelithiasis should be screened with abdominal ultrasound. It has been shown that loss of more than 50 lb in 3 months is associated with an increased incidence of gallstone formation. The incidence of stone or sludge formation after gastric bypass has been shown to be above 30%.[6] The incidence of ultrasound-proven gallstones in the preoperative population planning to undergo bariatric surgery is approximately 20%. Of note, the management of cholelithiasis during bariatric surgery is controversial. While most bariatric surgeons would strongly consider concomitant cholecystectomy for patients with symptomatic cholelithiasis, a minority advocate prophylactic cholecystectomy for asymptomatic gallstones. The practice of performing prophylactic cholecystectomy on patients with a normal gallbladder was not uncommon in the era of open surgery but is now rare. Performing laparoscopic cholecystectomy in addition to laparoscopic gastric bypass will typically add approximately 30 minutes of additional operative time and subjects the patient to increased risks, including that of common bile duct injury.[6]

Routine use of upper endoscopy in the preoperative evaluation is also controversial. Many bariatric surgeons feel it is necessary due to the high prevalence of upper gastrointestinal pathology in patients with obesity, reported to be as high as 80%.[7] In the setting of gastric bypass surgery, evidence suggests an association between preexisting gastritis and infection with *Helicobacter pylori* and an increased risk of marginal ulceration postoperatively.[7] Gastroesophageal reflux disease (GERD) is common in patients with obesity, possibly due to increased intra-abdominal pressure and poor lower esophageal sphincter function. Most surgeons feel that preoperative upper endoscopy is indicated for patients with GERD symptoms. Upper endoscopy also serves to rule out the presence of Barrett's esophagus and is useful for screening the lower stomach and duodenum in patients undergoing gastric bypass because these areas will be excluded from endoscopic visualization postoperatively.

Routine preoperative upper gastrointestinal series is generally unnecessary since the diagnostic yield of this is low and results rarely influence the planned surgical approach. A study by Ghassemian et al analyzed 57 preoperative upper gastrointestinal studies in bariatric patients. Although more than 40% showed some anomaly, such as reflux or hiatal hernia, none resulted in delay of surgery. The authors also noted a significant cost reduction when eliminating the upper gastrointestinal series from the preoperative evaluation protocol.[8] There is thus an emerging consensus that upper gastrointestinal contrast swallow studies are not a necessary component of the routine preoperative evaluation for bariatric surgery.

Nutritional Assessment

Registered dieticians educate patients regarding the new diet that will be required both before and after bariatric surgery. By establishing a relationship preoperatively, the dietician can best prepare the bariatric patient for surgery and introduce him or her to healthy eating habits. This process will hopefully pave the way for success at initiating and maintaining weight loss throughout the patient's bariatric surgery journey. In addition, nutritionists help prepare bariatric patients for the postoperative diet changes by teaching about portion control and maintenance of adequate postoperative nutrition. Without such education, patients may tend to eat more fat and consume an unhealthy, unbalanced diet.[9]

Preoperative Weight Loss

Many insurance companies mandate that candidates for bariatric surgery participate in a 3- to 6-month medically supervised weight management program as a prerequisite for approving surgery, although there is no defined specific amount of weight loss required. One randomized trial showed that a 10% weight loss preoperatively decreased operative time by 23 minutes. In addition, the presence of preoperative weight loss correlated with an increased excess weight loss of 5% 1-year postopatively.[9]

A 10% absolute weight loss will immediately translate into a reduction of visceral, central, and abdominal fat. This may also improve the cardiovascular and thromboembolic risk factors, reduce chronic proinflammatory mediators associated with obesity, and improve the patient's respiratory mechanics.[10] When this weight loss occurs in the months prior to surgery, a decrease in liver volume has been observed during surgery, which has been confirmed using ultrasound or computed tomography imaging. Preoperative weight loss has also been shown to decrease visceral fat volume, omentum thickness, and the thickness of the abdominal wall.[11] These are factors that may aid in the technical portions of the surgery, with less surgical time and a lower incidence of intraoperative complications.[11]

There are different approaches to preoperative weight loss, and no single method has been shown to be optimal. Commercially available liquid diets may be helpful for preoperative weight loss. Many published studies have recommended a low-calorie diet consisting of 800 to 1200 kcal/day, or a very low calorie diet of only 600 kcal/day. Some surgeons have advocated placement of an intragastric balloon for preoperative weight loss, although this device is not approved for use in the United States. No single method has been shown to be significantly more successful.[12]

Many surgeons feel that preoperative weight loss of up to 10% of initial body weight should be recommended for morbidly obese patients at least 2 to 4 weeks before bariatric surgery, especially in patients with BMI > 50. However, patients unable to attain this goal should not be denied surgical intervention unless the surgeon feels that it may reduce the safety of the operation.

Psychological Evaluation

The mental and emotional aspects of obesity, weight loss, and weight loss surgery are an important consideration in the care of bariatric patients. Most weight loss programs in the United States require that a patient undergo a mental health evaluation prior to undergoing surgery. In fact, many insurance companies require such psychological evaluation prior to granting precertification for a bariatric procedure. It is important to address inadequately treated psychological disorders prior to surgery in order to increase the likelihood of a positive outcome for bariatric patients.

The primary goal of preoperative psychological evaluation is to ensure that the patient does not have any active psychological issues that need to be addressed before surgery. It is also a means for educating and introducing a patient to the expectations of his or her journey ahead as he or she proceeds with surgery.[13] Social history, life stressors, dietary and weight loss history, and eating disorders should be evaluated. Most centers assess for stability or adequate treatment of these conditions and may suggest deferring surgery until they are adequately addressed. Relative contraindications vary from institution to institution but may include behaviors such as smoking, significant alcohol intake, and other substance abuse. Other behaviors that may lead to poor long-term success include being consistently abusive to staff, missing multiple appointments, and significantly gaining weight while in the preoperative evaluation process.[14] Patients referred for bariatric surgery are more likely than the overall population to have psychopathology such as somatization, social phobia, obsessive-compulsive disorder, substance abuse/dependency, binge eating disorder, post traumatic stress disorder, generalized anxiety disorder, and depression.[15] For reasons that remain unclear, a higher rate of suicide after bariatric surgery has been documented when compared to the general population.[16]

Cardiovascular

Major cardiovascular causes of death in the morbidly obese include myocardial infarction, stroke, congestive heart failure, and arrhythmia. Morbidly obese patients often suffer from multiple cardiovascular risk factors, including hypertension, diabetes, and hyperlipidemia. These patients often develop left ventricular hypertrophy (LVH) as a result of hemodynamic overload from an increased blood volume and cardiac output demands of their increased body mass and hypertension. LVH is a risk factor for cardiac arrhythmias and sudden death, which has a 5- to 6-fold increase in incidence compared to patients without LVH.[2] Left-sided heart failure is also increased in the setting of hypertension and diabetes. Patients with a history of hypertension or coronary artery disease along with diabetes should be carefully assessed preoperatively for cardiac function. Other indicators for preoperative cardiac evaluation include a strong family history of heart disease or risk factor history for coronary artery disease.

It is frequently helpful to have the preoperative evaluation be guided by the expertise of a cardiologist. The patient workup should always include an assessment of the patient's history, functional status, and physical exam. Many patients will also require electrocardiogram and some form of echocardiogram or stress testing. Stress testing is frequently advisable and may include dobutamine or exercise stress with electrocardiogram or echocardiogram. Dobutamine-stress perfusion studies may be necessary for those patients unable to exercise. Patients who show signs of ischemia during stress testing typically require further evaluation including cardiac catheterization for possible stenting or bypass.

With the recent increase in the cardiac stenting, the surgeon must be aware of the types of stents used. Perioperative management of antiplatelet therapy will depend upon whether drug eluting or bare metal stents have been used. It has been suggested, although not formally studied, that bariatric surgery be avoided within 1 year of the placement of coronary tents, and aspirin and clopidogrel should be discontinued 5 to 7 days prior to surgery. Low-dose aspirin (81 mg) can be continued up to the date of surgery.[17]

Numerous studies have shown the benefit of starting medications such as statins and beta-blockers in the preoperative setting to reduce cardiac risk.[18] The perioperative use of beta-blockers has been shown to reduce the incidence of postoperative myocardial ischemia, myocardial infarction, and cardiac mortality by decreasing myocardial oxygen consumption and workload, although this has not been studied specifically in the morbidly obese population. The perioperative use of beta-blockers in high-risk patients undergoing major noncardiac surgery is supported by the published data. However, studies have questioned the benefits of this approach in moderate-risk patients and report that the potential harm in low-risk groups might outweigh the benefit, stressing the importance of patient selection.[17]

Deep venous thrombosis (DVT) prophylaxis is another major concern in the morbidly obese. Those with history of DVT are at high risk of developing pulmonary embolism especially after surgery with published rates exceeding 1%. Although bariatric surgery has been proven effective in reducing the morbidity and mortality of obesity and associated health care costs, it is elective and risk must be minimized. No dosing guidelines exist for pharmacologic prophylaxis in patients with obesity who are already at increased risk for these events. Although the current ASMBS and *CHEST* guidelines recommend preoperative pharmacologic prophylaxis against thromboembolic events, no standard dosing protocols exist for the obese population.[19] Low-molecular-weight heparin and unfractionated heparin are both effective in reducing the risk, along with calf compressive devices and early mobilization. In patients with a BMI > 60, pulmonary hypertension, obstructive sleep apnea, and history of DVT or pulmonary embolus, the placement of a prophylactic inferior vena cava (IVC) filter may be considered. There are insertion-related complications with IVC filter placement, and insertion of IVC filters in superobese patients can pose a technical challenge for the interventionalist. There are no data on the long-term safety of IVC filters and no strong data comparing permanent vs retrievable filters.

Pulmonary

Many bariatric patients have impaired lung function including decreased functional reserve capacity. Patients with obesity also commonly suffer from obstructive sleep apnea and are at risk for early desaturation when at rest or in the postoperative setting.

Obstructive sleep apnea is defined as the presence of an apnea-hypopnea index (AHI) of more than 5 events per hour of sleep. The estimated prevalence is about 24% in men and 9% in women and can reach rates of greater than 30% in obese participants.[20] It is caused by increased upper airway pressures from relaxation and collapse of the pharyngeal musculature during sleep and worsened if a patient has a short neck or increased fatty tissue. Oxygen levels will fall and carbon dioxide levels rise during apneic episodes until patient arousal results in airway opening. Patients ultimately develop pulmonary vasoconstriction and right heart strain with sustained chronic hypoxia and hypercarbia progressing toward pulmonary hypertension.[3] One of the benefits of weight loss surgery is a resolution of sleep apnea, but in the early postoperative period, many factors may exacerbate apnea, in which the medical and surgical team should be aware. Such factors include placing the patient in the flat supine position and administering general anesthesia and narcotics.

Patients with sleep apnea will often use their own custom-fitted continuous positive airway pressure (CPAP) face mask. It is advisable that patients bring their fitted and customized mask with them during their inpatient hospital stay rather than using a generic hospital mask that may not be as comfortable.

An entity known as obesity hypoventilation syndrome occurs in patients who have shortness of breath and heart failure. This is diagnosed in patients with an arterial oxygen of 55 mm Hg or less and arterial carbon dioxide of 47 mm Hg or greater. These patients tend to have pulmonary hypertension as elevations in pulmonary pressures are necessary to maintain an adequate cardiac output. Many of these patients also have polycythemia, which is a risk factor for thromboembolism. It has been suggested that patients with a BMI > 60 with the combination of severe pulmonary hypertension and polycythemia be considered for a preoperative vena cava filter to decrease the risk of pulmonary embolus, although this recommendation is not well supported by rigorous data.[3]

Hepatic Function

Hepatic function should be assessed preoperatively, especially in patients with known hepatitis or steatosis. Any patient with elevated liver function tests suggestive of advanced cirrhosis should be considered to be at excessive risk for a bariatric surgical intervention. If a patient with known nonalcoholic steatotic hepatitis (NASH) and elevated transaminases has normal hepatic synthetic function, it is recommended that these patients undergo weight reduction surgery if no other contraindications exist.[21] Anesthesiologists should avoid potentially hepatotoxic anesthetic agents or other medications during surgery. Because these livers may be quite engorged or quite fatty, liver retractor placement and injury may occur. Some bariatric surgeons have instituted a preoperative "liver reduction" protocol in which patients are placed on short-term preoperative low-carbohydrate diets in order to decrease the stored triglyceride content in the liver and decrease liver size. One study had shown a 43.8% decrease in the left lateral segment of the liver with a 4-week program of drinking a low-carbohydrate nutritional supplement.[22]

Many patients evaluated for bariatric surgery have NASH. Studies from routine liver biopsies performed during gastric bypass show that the incidence of steatosis was as high as 83%.[21] The importance of NASH in the obesity population cannot be disregarded as its incidence has been significantly rising in the past decade. A 2012 report cited NASH as having overtaken hepatitis C in the United States as the primary indication for liver transplantation.[23] The presence of diabetes was shown to increase the odds of a patient having NASH by 128 times and fibrosis by 75 times over the nondiabetic patient.[24] Most patients with biopsy-proven NASH were asymptomatic preoperatively, and there have not been any major increases in perioperative mortality. However, there may be a benefit in having high-risk patients with a combination of diabetes, hypertension, and elevated liver function tests undergo a liver biopsy intraoperatively.

Metabolic/Endocrine

Type 2 diabetes mellitus is a disease commonly associated with morbid obesity. Mortality is in the range of 5% per year in morbidly obese patients with diabetes. Preoperative testing typically includes fasting glucose and serum hemoglobin A1c (HbA1c). Poor glucose control has been associated with poor wound healing, increased perioperative infections, and increased mortality in critically ill patients. Thus, making sure to maintain normal glucose levels along with keeping HbA1c less than 8 preoperatively may decrease postoperative complications and mortality.[3] In general, patients with diabetes undergoing surgery are instructed to withhold or reduce insulin the morning of surgery to avoid the risk of hypoglycemia. Most patients having undergone bariatric surgery will have a marked reduction of insulin requirements postoperatively. We also recommend seeking the consultation of an endocrinologist to follow these patients both preoperatively and postoperatively to aid in establishing and maintaining normal glucose levels.

Hematologic Testing/Coagulation

A history of anemia or bleeding is an important component of a preoperative assessment. Preoperative coagulation studies have been consistently shown by many studies to be an insufficient screen for potential perioperative bleeding problems.[2] A careful history includes inquiring about any previous bleeding after surgery, any history of trauma, and any family history of bleeding. When asking these specific questions, the surgeon is much more likely to pick up undiagnosed coagulopathy disorders.

Preoperative lab testing can be selected based on the type of surgery that is planned. For restrictive bariatric surgery such as gastric banding, a normal hemoglobin or hematocrit to preoperatively confirm the absence of an existing anemia may be all that is needed. For those patients undergoing a Roux-en-Y gastric bypass, it is appropriate to obtain a baseline complete blood count and preoperative iron, B_{12}, and folate levels. Iron, B_{12}, and folate levels are useful to compare with postoperative levels as a marker for vitamin level alterations associated with surgery. These patients are at risk of becoming deficient after gastric bypass with about 15% incidence of B_{12} deficiency and up to 40% incidence of iron deficiency being observed after a bypass.[25] Some surgeons feel that it is informative to order a full set of nutritional labs on all preoperative bariatric patients, even those undergoing a restrictive procedure such as banding or sleeve gastrectomy; such information allows for any deficiencies to be identified and appropriately treated before surgery.

If patients are found to have iron deficiency anemias preoperatively, they should be give oral supplements to correct the deficiencies prior to surgery. They should also undergo a thorough investigation to potential sources of blood loss such as gastrointestinal bleeding or occult malignancy.

Renal Function

There is no absolute contraindication in performing bariatric surgery in someone with renal insufficiency or even renal failure. These patients must be evaluated thoroughly for the etiology of their renal insufficiency or failure and the associated comorbidities. Many patients undergoing bariatric surgery have diabetes, which may be accompanied with renal insufficiency. Diabetic nephropathy suggests a long-standing severe case of diabetes accompanying vascular pathology, which must be evaluated.

Anesthesia

Many bariatric patients have one or more comorbidities, such as sleep apnea or cardiovascular disease, that may significantly impact their response to general anesthesia. The anesthesiologist must be fully cognizant of this in the preoperative anesthetic risk assessment and intraoperative management. Specific concerns include the airway exam and potential for difficult intravenous access. As a morbidly obese patient can present a very difficult airway to manage, the anesthesia team must be cognizant of these challenges and be prepared to use advanced intubation techniques such as video laryngoscopy or away fiber-optic intubation if required. Insertion of a central line and/or an arterial line may be additional components necessary for safe intraoperative patient monitoring. A separate chapter in this book details in-depth the preoperative anesthetic considerations in the bariatric patient.

Summary

Bariatric surgical procedures are performed in a high-risk population with many comorbid conditions. With the increase in obesity over the past decade, more and more patients are seeking surgery to achieve durable weight loss and improved overall health. The preoperative evaluation is critical to the outcomes of bariatric surgery. A thorough assessment of all medical problems must take place well in advance, and this must integrate a team of medical care providers and support groups for patients. The surgeons who best prepare their patients for surgery with a comprehensive preoperative assessment of existing comorbid medical conditions will reap the benefits of these efforts and enjoy the most successful postoperative outcomes.

References

1. SAGES guideline for clinical application of laparoscopic bariatric surgery. *Surg Obes Relat Dis.* 2009;5:387-405.
2. Schirmer BD, Scott JR. Preoperative evaluation and assessment of medical problems. In: Inabnet WB, Demaria EJ, Ikramuddin S, eds. *Laparoscopic Bariatric Surgery.* Philadelphia, PA: Lippincott Williams & Wilkins; 2005:38-46.
3. Davis DG, Bessler M. Patient selection and preoperative assesment. In: Inabnet WB, Demaria EJ, Ikramuddin S, eds. *Laparoscopic Bariatric Surgery.* Philadelphia, PA: Lippincott Williams & Wilkins; 2005:36.
4. NIH Conference: Gastrointestinal surgery for severe obesity. *Consensus Development Conference Statement.* 1991;9(1).
5. FDA News Release, February 16, 2011. FDA expands use of banding system for weight loss. http://www.fda.gov/NewsEvents/Newsroom/PressAnnouncements/ucm245617.htm. Accessed September 2, 2015.
6. Shiffman ML, Sugerman HJ, Kellum JM. Gallstone formation after rapid weight loss: a prospective study in patients undergoing bypass surgery for treatment of morbid obesity. *Am J Gastroenterol.* 1991;86:1000-1005.

7. Eldar S, Heneghan HM, Brethauer S, Schauer PR. A focus on surgical preoperative evaluation of the bariatric patient—the Cleveland Clinic protocol and review of the literature. *The Surgeon.* 2011;9:273-277.
8. Ghassemian AJ, MacDonald KG, Cunningham PG, Swanson M, Brown BM, Morris PG. The workup for bariatric surgery does not require a routine upper gastrointestinal series. *Obes Surg.* 1997;7:16-18.
9. Livhits M, Mercado C, Yermilov I, et al. Does weight loss immediately before bariatric surgery improve outcomes: a systematic review. *Surg Obes Relat Dis.* 2009;5:713-721.
10. Tarnoff M, Kaplan L, Shikora S. An evidence-based assessment of preoperative weight loss in bariatric surgery. *Obes Surg.* 2008;18:1059-1061.
11. Fris R. Preoperative low energy diet diminished liver size. *Obes Surg.* 2004;14:1165-1170.
12. Vargas MA, Fernandez NC, Serrano JO. Preoperative weight loss in patients with indication of bariatric surgery: which is the best method? *Nutr Hosp.* 2011;26:1227-1230.
13. Greenberg I, Sogg S, Perna MF. Behavioral and psychological care in weight loss surgery: best practice update. *Obesity.* 2009;17:880.
14. Tariq N, Chand B. Presurgical evaluation and postoperative care for the bariatric patient. *Gastrointest Endoscopy Clin N Am.* 2011;21:229-240.
15. Kinzi JF, Schrattenecker M, Traweger C. Psychosocial predictors of weight loss after bariatric surgery. *Obes Surg.* 2006;16(12):1609-1614.
16. Omalu BI, Cho P, Shakir AM. Suicides following bariatric surgery for the treatment of obesity. *Surg Obes Relat Dis.* 2005;1:447.
17. Katkhouda N, Mason RJ, Wu B, Takla FS, Keenan RM, Zehetner J. Evaluation and treatment of patients with cardiac disease undergoing bariatric surgery. *Surg Obes Relat Dis.* 2012;8:634-640.
18. Feringa HH, Bax JJ, Poldermans D. Perioperative medical management of ischemic heart disease in patients undergoing noncardiac surgery. *Curr Opin Anaesthesiol.* 2007;20:254-260.
19. Prophylactic measures to reduce the risk of venous thromboembolism in bariatric surgery patients. *Surg Obes Relat Dis.* 2007;3(5):494-495.
20. Gasa M, Salord N, Fortuna AM, et al. Optimizing screening of severe obstructive sleep apnea in patients undergoing bariatric surgery. *Surg Obes Relat Dis.* 2013;9(4):539-546.
21. Moretto M, Kupski C, Morrin CC. Hepatic steatosis in patients undergoing bariatric surgery and its relationship to body mass index and co-morbidities. *Obes Surg.* 2003;13:622-624.
22. Brody F, Vziri K, Garey C, et al. Preoperative liver reduction utilizing a novel nutritional supplement. *Journal of Laparoendoscopic and Advanced Surgical Techniques.* 2011;21(6):491-495.
23. Frangou C. *General Surgery News.* November 2012. Available at: http://www.generalsurgerynews.com/ViewArticle.aspx?d=In+the+News&d_id=69&i=October+2012&i_id=891&a_id=21954. Accessed November 2012.
24. Beymer C, Kowdley KV, Edmonson P. Prevalance and predictors of asymptomatic liver disease in patients undergoing gastric bypass surgery. *Arch Surg.* 2003;138:1240-1244.
25. Brolin RE, Gorman JH, Gorman RC. Prophlyactic iron supplementation after Roux-en-Y gastric byass: a prospective, double-blind randomized study. *Arch Surg.* 1998;133:740-744.

12

Anesthetic Issues in the Patient With Obesity Undergoing Surgery

Eugene Kim, MD and Stephanie B. Jones, MD

Patients undergoing bariatric procedures represent a subset of patients with a unique combination of comorbidities, some of which are discussed elsewhere in this book. The overall body habitus and body composition (relative proportion of fat and lean tissues) also have a role in determining anesthetic choices and management strategies. This combination of factors presents a variety of challenges for the anesthesiologist, which we will highlight in this chapter.

Preoperative Assessment

Preoperative assessment of morbidly obese patients may prove challenging. Clinical signs of organ dysfunction, such as hepatomegaly, or edema may be more difficult to discern on physical exam. Detection of cardiac murmurs or pulmonary abnormalities on auscultation may be problematic. Functional status of the patient may be limited, making cardiac or pulmonary dysfunction challenging to assess. The increased prevalence of significant cardiac, endocrine, and pulmonary comorbidity makes careful screening all the more critical.[1]

While it is important not to overuse diagnostic testing in the preoperative setting, patients with significant risk factors warrant additional evaluation. For that reason it is vital that preoperative anesthetic assessment occurs well ahead of the procedure. Sufficient time for advance preparation will help ensure proper preoperative assessment and optimization of comorbid conditions, which in turn will help avoid delays on the day of surgery and unnecessary risk to the patient.[2]

Intravenous Access

Difficulty in securing peripheral intravenous (IV) access in individuals with obesity relative to their nonobese counterparts has been noted in both adults and children.[3] The need to secure IV access prior to induction of anesthesia may result in case delays. While it is unnecessary to

Forse RA, Apovian CM, eds.
Bariatric Surgery: What Every Provider Needs to Know (pp 141-150).

preemptively secure central access on every patient with obesity, for those patients who have a history of difficulty with IV access it may be prudent to place a central line, peripherally inserted central catheter (PICC) line, or brachial midline prior to induction. If preoperative central access is not indicated, additional time should be allotted for peripheral access. Ultrasound visualization may facilitate IV placement.

Intraosseous (I/O) access has been used in emergent situations for individuals with obesity where IV access is difficult, but it is a less favorable solution for scheduled elective procedures or for prolonged access. However, it remains an important approach in the setting of crash resuscitation. I/O access is typically secured in the tibia or humerus. Flow rates of a 15-gauge I/O needle are similar to that of a 20-gauge peripheral IV. Medications that can be administered through an I/O catheter include all drugs of resuscitation, crystalloid and colloid solutions, as well as blood products.[4]

Physiologic Changes

Obesity is associated with numerous physiologic changes that can greatly affect management of the patient in the perioperative setting. Many of the changes are described in other chapters. We will discuss some that specifically impact anesthetic management.

Respiratory

Changes in static and dynamic lung volumes in obese vs nonobese individuals have been well studied. Individuals with obesity have been noted to have reduced expiratory reserve volume, as well as a rapid shallow breathing pattern.[5,6] Preoperative pulmonary function testing (PFT), typically done in the sitting position in an unsedated patient, can overestimate the functional respiratory status of a supine patient with obesity receiving anxiolytics, sedatives, or narcotics. While tests may show normal or near normal PFT values, there may be profound changes as the patient is placed supine, further exacerbated by Trendelenburg (head down) positioning.[7] Patient history should be elucidated as to sleeping habits and ability to breathe in the supine position.

Supine positioning of patients with obesity is accompanied by a decrease in an already compromised functional residual capacity (FRC). Preoxygenation, therefore, should be performed with the patient in 25 to 30 degrees reverse Trendelenburg (head up) position, with the addition of 10 cm H_2O continuous positive airway pressure (CPAP), if tolerated. This not only has the benefit of subjectively improving the patient's feeling of dyspnea during induction, but may also extend the time to desaturation during the apneic period prior to intubation by improving FRC and, by direct extension, oxygen reserve.[8-10]

Following anesthetic induction, increased difficulty in bag-mask ventilation may be observed. Patients with obesity have been noted to have decreased chest wall compliance and increased airway resistance due to an abundance of pretracheal soft tissue. In addition, high body mass increases the overall metabolic oxygen demand, thereby increasing the consumption of oxygen and decreasing time to desaturation.

Airway

The airway in the patient with obesity poses a potential challenge. While individual patients with obesity may or may not have an airway that is easy to manage, the incidence of the difficult airway is increased in obese vs lean patients.[11] Body mass index (BMI) or weight alone is not uniquely predictive of difficult intubation. Standard airway exams assist in planning for airway difficulty; parameters such as Mallampati classification, neck circumference, and thyromental distance all tend to be less favorable in this population but still have relatively poor positive predictive

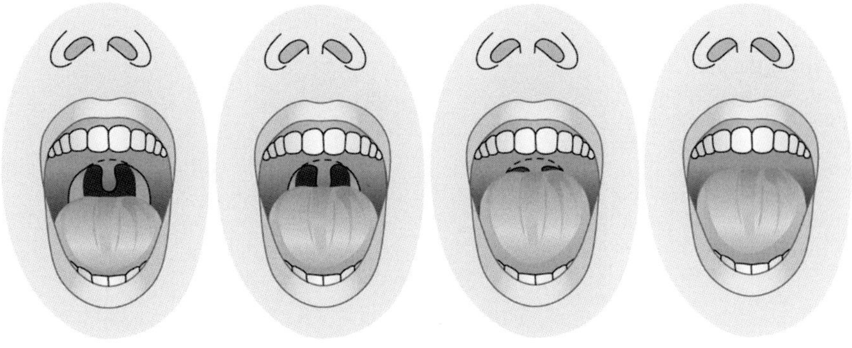

Figure 12-1. The Mallampati score is used to predict the potential difficulty of endotracheal intubation with direct laryngoscopy. It ranges from Class 1, where the soft palate, tonsillar pillars, and uvula are all visible, to Class 4, where only the hard palate is visible. Classes 3 and 4 predict difficult laryngoscopy.

value (Figure 12-1). Recent studies have suggested alternative measurements, such as the ratio of neck circumference to thyromental distance, that may be more reliably predictive.[12]

Of utmost importance in securing the airways of patients with obesity is proper positioning. Classic sniff position (ie, alignment of the ear to the sternal notch in a horizontal plane) is ideal for direct laryngoscopy as well as for bag-mask ventilation. However, in patients with increased central obesity, supine position on a flat surface (or even worse, on a soft surface) may place the ear far posterior, making direct visualization extremely difficult. Common practice in patients with obesity is to "ramp" the upper body to produce a more ideal position for laryngoscopy. Firm folded blankets or commercial foam or inflatable ramps are used to elevate the thorax to a more equal plane with the abdomen, and additional padding will align the ear with the sternal notch[13] (Figure 12-2). This simple act of repositioning can sometimes make easy intubations out of impossible ones.

Preparation for induction of anesthesia should include having additional personnel available for assistance, additional equipment for bag-mask ventilation, and special equipment for intubation. Adjuncts such as oral or nasal airways or even preemptive placement of a laryngeal mask airway (LMA) may help to maintain a patent airway in the setting of excessive oropharyngeal tissue and preserve oxygen saturation prior to endotracheal intubation.[14] Assistance should be sought without hesitation for 2-person bag-mask ventilation if necessary. Special airway equipment for endotracheal intubation may include intubating LMAs, video laryngoscopes, and fiber-optic bronchoscopes. Equipment for invasive techniques such as retrograde intubation and cricothyrotomy should be available, but such techniques are typically only used emergently, when other methods have failed.

In cases where suspicion of a markedly difficult airway is high, it is generally preferred to secure the airway awake or under light sedation, with the patient breathing spontaneously. This method has the benefit of ongoing ventilation during intubation attempts, as well as the option to abandon intubation with minimal risk to the patient should endotracheal intubation prove impossible. However, awake intubation requires a degree of patient understanding and cooperation. Typically the airway reflexes are blunted by topical, inhaled, and/or injected local anesthetic to prevent coughing and gagging during the procedure. An antisialagogue such as glycopyrrolate enhances the effectiveness of the inhaled local anesthetic by avoiding dilution with saliva. Decreasing the quantity of secretions present in the airway and oropharynx will also improve fiber-optic visualization. Bronchodilators may also be administered beforehand to help prevent bronchospasm during airway manipulation. Sedating agents such as benzodiazepines must be used with caution. Morbidly obese patients with coexisting obstructive sleep apnea may be very sensitive to the respiratory depressant effects of these drugs, defeating the purpose

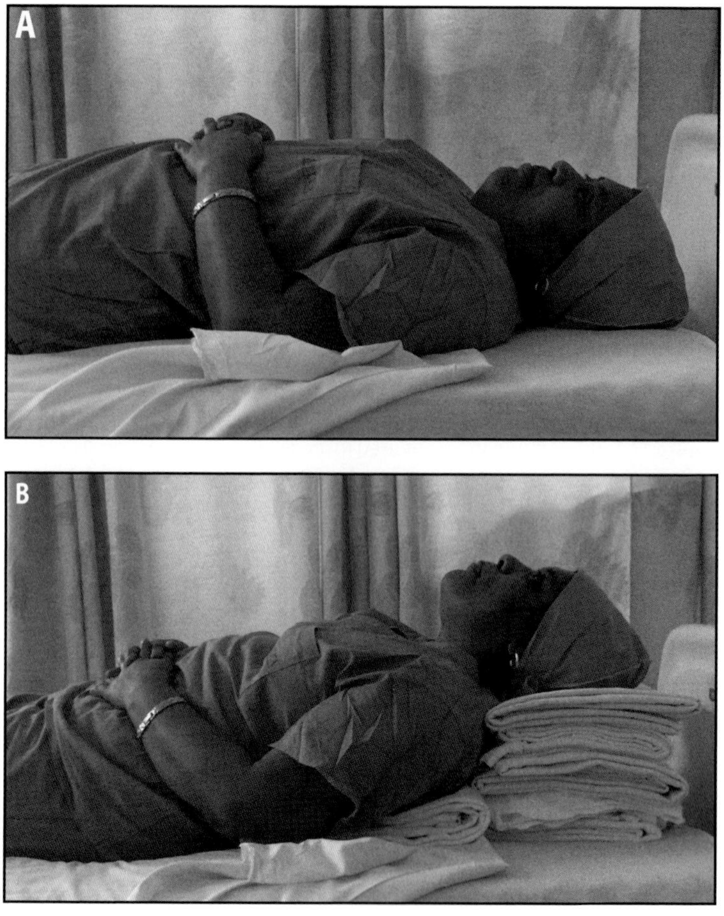

Figure 12-2. An example of "ramping" the upper body to produce a more ideal position for laryngoscopy. (A) Without ramping, the neck is minimally extended and both the chin and ear are well below chest level. (B) Once ramped, the patient's neck is better extended, the head is in the desired "sniff" position, and the ear is level with the sternal notch. This serves to better align the oral, tracheal, and laryngeal axes for direct laryngoscopy.

of choosing an awake technique. While many operators elect to secure the airway by fiber-optic bronchoscopy to minimize stimulation of the posterior oropharynx, the well-topicalized airway can be secured via either direct or video-assisted laryngoscopy as well.

Cardiac

Patients who present for bariatric surgery have a higher prevalence of cardiac comorbidity than their nonobese counterparts.[1] While some conditions may show improvement with presurgical weight loss and diet modification, others will persist.[15]

Total blood volume and cardiac output increase as a means to supply oxygen to the increased tissue mass. Concurrent obstructive sleep apnea may place additional stress on the heart, resulting in chronic pulmonary hypertension. Therefore, there may be strain on both left and right ventricles in the patient with obesity, despite a relatively asymptomatic presentation. Cardiac dysfunction may also be difficult to diagnose if patients live a sedentary lifestyle.

While the presence of morbid obesity alone should not be an indication for invasive cardiac testing, increased scrutiny is necessary during the preoperative assessment, with echocardiogram, stress testing, echocardiography, or angiography as indicated. Intraoperative monitoring may also be challenging. Often the upper arm may be poorly conducive to noninvasive blood pressure monitoring due to its conical shape. Alternatively, noninvasive blood pressure measurements may be obtained from the forearm with reasonable fidelity. Patients with large extremities may require intra-arterial blood pressure monitoring.

Obstructive Sleep Apnea

In the general population, 4% of middle-aged men and 2% of middle-aged women meet minimal diagnostic criteria for obstructive sleep apnea. However, prevalence of obstructive sleep apnea among bariatric surgery patients has been reported at greater than 70%.[6] While this statistic alone makes a compelling argument for weight loss surgery, it does present a unique set of perioperative concerns for the anesthesia provider.

Patency of the upper airway is determined by position, craniofacial and soft tissue structure, and muscle activity. During sleep, particularly pharmacologically induced sleep, upper airway muscles can relax, causing pharyngeal narrowing and decreased airway patency.[16]

Apart from higher incidences of hypertension, coronary artery disease, stroke, and atrial fibrillation present in patients with obstructive sleep apnea, obstructive sleep apnea has been associated with an increased incidence of postoperative adverse events and increased hospital length of stay. Most complications occur during the first day after surgery, but increased adverse events have been noted through postoperative day 5.[17,18] Observed complications include cardiac ischemia and respiratory failure. Speculation on anesthetic causes for complications included direct and indirect means; both direct sedative effects that increase the incidence of apneic episodes, and indirect effects of "REM (rapid eye movement) rebound." REM rebound is the phenomenon where loss of REM sleep in the immediate postoperative period leads to increased REM sleep in the subsequent days, a so-called rebound effect. As apneic episodes are more likely to occur during REM sleep, the rebound period can be a dangerous one in the days following major surgery.

Patients who present for bariatric surgery should be screened for obstructive sleep apnea and previous sleep study results reviewed. If the patient is not already on CPAP therapy, consideration should be given to fitting the patient for a device preoperatively. It has been suggested that postoperative compliance and perioperative risk reduction are more successful in patients previously experienced with CPAP therapy.[19] Risk factors for obstructive sleep apnea include increased BMI, increased neck circumference, and snoring, making its predominance in obese populations understandable. Other screening criteria include increased daytime somnolence, observed apnea, hypertension, male gender, and age greater than 50 years.[20] While preoperative weight loss may do a great deal to reduce the degree of obstructive sleep apnea, it is important to remain vigilant in patient management in the postoperative period.

Pain Management

Analgesia is of special concern as both intra- and postoperative opioid analgesics can contribute markedly to sedation and apneic events. While patient-controlled analgesia can be used to increase safety profiles and improve patient satisfaction, narcotic-only postoperative pain regimens may still be overly sedating and exacerbate issues with obstructive sleep apnea. Patients can often achieve better pain relief with less respiratory depression by using a multimodal approach to pain that utilizes non-narcotic medications as adjuvants.[21] At times, nonsteroidal anti-inflammatory agents will be given to provide analgesia without sedation; however, these concerns must be balanced against bleeding risks due to platelet effects. Medications such as dexmedetomidine and ketamine may be administered intraoperatively to provide adjunct analgesia; they may be associated with increased somnolence, although not necessarily increased respiratory depression. Acetaminophen, now available in IV form, can also be used with good effect in providing analgesia without respiratory depression.

Gabapentin is seeing increased utility in off-label usage as a perioperative medication in reducing postoperative pain as part of a multimodal approach to pain management. Meta-analysis of double-blind placebo-controlled trials have demonstrated efficacy in postoperative analgesia, including laparoscopic and open abdominal procedures. In open abdominal and thoracotomy procedures, perioperative use of gabapentin has been associated with improved respiratory mechanics postoperatively. However, its utility for bariatric surgery must be weighed against gabapentin's association with water retention and weight gain in chronic use.[22]

For open bariatric procedures or laparoscopic procedures with a high chance of conversion to an open incision, preoperative neuraxial analgesia may be the ideal method for pain control. Studies have shown epidural analgesia to be associated with earlier ambulation and shorter hospital stay, with improved gastrointestinal motility and respiratory function.[23] However, positioning of individuals with obesity for neuraxial anesthesia, as well as the placement itself, may be more difficult.[24] Longer needles and ultrasound localization of the epidural space and its distance from the skin may ease this process. Further, while rare, there is always the possibility of respiratory depression from neuraxial anesthesia by rostral spread of the local anesthetic, as well as delayed apnea from use of epidural or intrathecal narcotics. For these reasons, patients at high risk for postoperative apnea may be better served by narcotic-free epidural or intrathecal solutions.[8] Generally speaking, in patients undergoing laparoscopic procedures the level of associated surgical pain may not warrant neuraxial catheter placement.

Another regional technique that may be utilized is the transverse abdominus plane block. This can be done with ultrasound guidance in the pre- or postoperative period. The proper plane for injection can be more difficult to locate in individuals with obesity. Diazepam and other benzodiazepines have been used with great success as part of multimodal pain protocols, particularly for pain associated with abdominal surgical procedures. However, because of additive respiratory despression risk when combined with opioids they must be used with extreme caution.

Anesthetic Induction

Induction of patients begins with securing IV access, if it has not been done already. IV premedication for anxiolysis should be used with some caution, depending on the risk factors for obstructive sleep apnea. Fentanyl and midazolam are frequently selected for their quick onset and highly potent effects; however, when used together marked respiratory depression is often noted. Patients are preoxygenated with 100% oxygen in a head-up position (reverse Trendelenburg). The upper body should be placed in a ramped position to facilitate direct laryngoscopy, as previously described. The airway may be secured awake or asleep, depending on the level of anticipated difficulty with bag-mask ventilation and/or intubation. Immediately following intubation large sustained positive pressure breaths may be useful for lung volume recruitment. Significant atelectasis may occur during induction particularly if the patient was difficult to intubate, extending the apneic period, and if there was rapid absorption of the 100% oxygen in the alveoli.[25] Invasive monitors can be placed either preoperatively or post-intubation at the discretion of the anesthesiologist, depending upon patient acuity.

Drug Dosing

Anesthetic drug dosing of nonobese patients is typically by weight. However, in individuals with obesity, dosing may vary. Obesity is associated with a number of physiologic changes that can potentially affect the volume of distribution of medications and thus pharmacokinetics and pharmacodynamics. These include changes in plasma proteins, increased adipose tissue mass and lean body mass, decreased tissue perfusion (particularly in adipose tissue), increased splanchnic blood flow, and increased cardiac output.[26] The effects of higher cardiac output are particularly apparent in the more rapid redistribution of bolus medications, such as anesthetic induction agents. Medication characteristics, including lipid solubility, water solubility, time to onset, and half-life, must be taken into account as well.

For a few medications specific recommendations exist, but this is the exception rather than the rule as the Food and Drug Administration has not usually required inclusion of patients with obesity in drug-dosing studies. If specific information is unavailable, dosing based upon lean body weight (LBW) is typically a safe choice. LBW is defined as the difference between total body weight and fat mass and accounts for relevant changes in body composition due to obesity. It can be roughly calculated as 120% to 140% of ideal body weight. However, it must be kept in mind that while lean body mass increases as total body weight increases, it is not in direct proportion.[27] At more severe levels of obesity, adipose tissue continues to increase while the addition of lean tissue levels off. Ultimately what influences medication decisions and dosing are dependent on anesthesia provider preference, patient body habitus, and the clinical context of the patient.

Two notable exceptions to LBW-based dosing are succinylcholine and nondepolarizing neuromuscular-blocking drugs such as rocuronium and cisatracurium. The best intubating conditions are obtained following administration of succinylcholine calculated based upon total body weight. The need for the higher dose is felt to be due to increased pseudocholinesterase activity breaking down the drug before it reaches the neuromuscular junction and increased extracellular volume.[28] In contrast, rocuronium and cisatracurium should be dosed based upon ideal body weight, as larger doses prolong duration but do not improve intubating conditions.[29,30]

Maintenance of Anesthesia

Once induction is complete and the patient is asleep, agents used to maintain anesthesia for the patient can vary. In most general anesthetics in nonobese patients the maintenance agent of choice is an inhaled halogenated agent, such as sevoflurane, desflurane, or isoflurane. These agents are commonly used in individuals with obesity as well; however, some caution must be used in dosing. All 3 agents show remarkable fat solubility; therefore, emergence can be prolonged in individuals with obesity. This is likely more significant for procedures lasting more than 4 hours.[31] In addition, as patients may hypoventilate postoperatively, either from pain, oversedation, or obstructive sleep apnea, the potential exists for reaccumulation of agent and a need for reintubation. However, given ease of use, ability to titrate anesthetic effect, and the fact that drug levels can be continually measured by gas sampling during the procedure, they are often the agents of choice.

Nitrous oxide is an excellent adjuvant in the maintenance of anesthesia. It has the benefit of low lipid solubility and therefore fast elimination from the patient, and its use can reduce the amount of halogenated agents needed for anesthesia. Morbidly obese patients may not tolerate the decreased inhaled fraction of oxygen (FiO_2) associated with nitrous oxide administration. Nitrous oxide use is also discouraged during laparoscopic procedures as its solubility is significantly higher than oxygen or nitrogen, and thus may cause bowel distention during longer procedures. The same property increases the rate of expansion of pneumothorax, pneumoperitoneum, and subcutaneous emphysema, potentially worsening the severity of these conditions. As a result nitrous oxide is seldom used in laparoscopic bariatric procedures.

Other adjuvants may prove useful during the maintenance of anesthesia. Dexmedetomidine is an alpha-2 receptor agonist useful in its ability to provide sedation with minimal respiratory depression. While its time of onset and low level of amnestic properties preclude its use as a sole anesthetic, it provides excellent supplemental anesthesia and analgesia in patients with obesity. Remifentanil is a highly potent ultra-short-acting opioid. When run as an infusion it can contribute significantly to the anesthetic, decreasing the need for halogenated agents. It has the advantage of being quickly metabolized by nonspecific tissue and plasma esterases, and therefore is metabolized quickly when the infusion is terminated, allowing for prompt recovery. Studies, however, have associated its use with hyperalgesia, and therefore it does have the potential to increase pain medication requirements postoperatively.

Ventilation and Oxygenation

One frequently encountered issue during laparoscopic procedures in the morbidly obese patient is difficulty with ventilation.[32] Even in the absence of insufflation patients with obesity may be markedly difficult to ventilate with positive pressure ventilation. This varies from patient to patient, but is likely worse with central, compared to peripheral, obesity patterns. Increasing driving pressure in an attempt to improve ventilation can result in barotrauma and lung injury. As the peritoneum is insufflated ventilation can become more difficult, as the pressure in the abdomen elevates the diaphragm and transfers increased pressure in the thorax. In addition, the use of carbon dioxide as the insufflating agent will increase the amount of dissolved carbon dioxide in the blood. The excess carbon dioxide must be eliminated by increasing minute ventilation, creating a further challenge.

Oxygenation may also be impaired. General anesthesia and the supine position may decrease FRC and increase ventilation perfusion mismatch. During induction, patients are preoxygenated with 100% oxygen. During intubation, they are nearly always pharmacologically rendered apneic in order to create ideal intubating conditions. During that time significant atelectasis may occur as the freely permeable distal alveoli close during apneic oxygenation. After the endotracheal tube is secured, the patient should receive recruitment breaths to help open up these atelectatic portions of the lung.

A number of different ventilatory strategies can be used to improve oxygenation. Pressure-controlled delivery of breaths has the advantage over volume controlled as it decreases peak pressures for comparable tidal volumes. Positive end-expiratory pressure (PEEP) can be effective in maintaining patency of distal alveoli following recruitment maneuvers.[33] Morbidly obese patients may require fairly high levels of PEEP (10 to 12 mm Hg) to be effective. The respiratory benefits of PEEP must be weighed against the cardiovascular effects as excessive pressures may impair thoracic blood return and cardiac output. Increasing FiO_2 may help; however, running patients at 100% oxygen over the entire case may cause issues postoperatively with resorption atelectasis. Finally, placement of the patient in reverse Trendelenburg position, if compatible with the surgical procedure, can help with intrathoracic pressures, increasing FRC and decreasing the level of ventilation-perfusion mismatch.[34]

Emergence and Extubation

At the end of the procedure, a number of issues need to be considered for the successful and safe transition of the patient. Patients will typically be extubated in the operating room. This is generally preferred, because the anesthesia provider will be present to observe the patient in the immediate post-extubation period and intervene if necessary. There are well-established extubation criteria for perioperative extubation that assess whether the patient is awake, oxygenating and ventilating well, with no residual muscle relaxation, and is hemodynamically stable. Certain factors may result in preferentially keeping the patient intubated for a period of time following surgery. These include markedly difficult intubation, difficult or impossible bag-mask ventilation, large-volume resuscitation with possible airway edema, or history of severe obstructive sleep apnea. In such patients, it may be preferable to bring them to the post-anesthesia or intensive care unit, and have them emerge more slowly from their anesthetic, ideally in a head-up position to optimize FRC. The extubation criteria can then be reevaluated some time later when the patient's condition has been optimized.

Post Extubation Airway Management

Following extubation, patients with known or suspected obstructive sleep apnea may benefit from CPAP or BiPAP (bilevel positive airway pressure) treatment. This can aid in lung recruitment and prevention of hypoventilation. In the setting of early treatment of postoperative hypoxia, CPAP therapy has been shown to decrease the incidence of reintubation, pneumonia, and sepsis, as well as hospital length of stay.[35] At a minimum, it is important to have resources available so patients can readily be placed on CPAP if indicated. There have been concerns raised regarding the use of ongoing noninvasive positive-pressure ventilation in the absence of an endotracheal tube. Apart from issues of abdominal discomfort and increased reflux there are also worries that air insufflation may put new gastrointestinal anastomotic connections (eg, a Roux-en-Y gastric bypass) at risk for leak. Fortunately, there are studies that have shown these risks to be minimal[36]; however, the surgical team should be made aware of plans for CPAP.

Studies in obstructive sleep apnea patients see improvements in ventilation when patients sleep in the prone, lateral, or sitting positions, rather than supine. While the first two may not be practical in the postoperative period due to patient discomfort, placing the patient at an incline during recovery, up to and including a full sitting position, may help with ventilation and lung re-recruitment. Early use of incentive spirometry has also been demonstrated to decrease hospital length of stay, as marked atelectasis may occur over the patient's operative and postoperative course.[2]

Summary

The care of the morbidly obese patient can be complex due to a combination of anatomic and physiologic changes and associated comorbidities. Bariatric procedures are most commonly performed laparoscopically, adding the impact of pneumoperitoneum and positioning to the mix. While anesthesia in such patients does pose certain challenges, patients should receive assurance that their anesthesiologist has experience in dealing with these issues, and that careful adjustments in their management will be made to optimize safety and comfort.

References

1. Guh DP, Zhang W, Bansback N, et al. The incidence of co-morbidities related to obesity and overweight: a systematic review and meta-analysis. *BMC Public Health.* 2009;9:88.
2. Schumann R, Jones SB, Ortiz VE, et al. Best practice recommendations for anesthetic perioperative care and pain management in weight loss surgery. *Obes Res.* 2005;13:254-266.
3. Juvin P, Blarel A, Bruno F, Desmonts JM. Is peripheral line placement more difficult in obese than in lean patients? *Anesth Analg.* 2003;96:1218.
4. Voigt J, Waltzman M, Lottenberg L. Intraosseous vascular access for in-hospital emergency use: a systematic clinical review of the literature and analysis. *Ped Emerg Care.* 2012;28:185-199.
5. Pelosi P, Croci M, Ravagnan I, et al. The effects of body mass on lung volumes, respiratory mechanics and gas exchange during general anesthesia. *Anesth Analg.* 1998;87:654-660.
6. Isono S. Obstructive sleep apnea of obese adults: pathophysiology and perioperative airway management. *Anesthesiology.* 2009;110:908-921.
7. Paul DR, Hoyt JL, Boutros AR. Cardiovascular and respiratory changes in response to change of posture in the very obese. *Anesthesiology.* 1976;45:73-78.
8. Schumann R, Jones SB, Cooper B, et al. Update on best practice recommendations for anesthetic perioperative care and pain management in weight loss surgery 2004–2007. *Obes Res.* 2009;17:889-894.
9. Altermatt FR, Munoz HR, Delfino AE, Cortinez LI. Pre-oxygenation in the obese patient: effects of position on tolerance to apnoea. *Br J Anaesth.* 2005;95:706-709.
10. Gander A, Frascarolo P, Suter M, Spahn DR, Magnusson L. Positive end-expiratory pressure during induction of general anesthesia increases duration of nonhypoxic apnea in morbidly obese patients. *Anesth Analg.* 2005;100:580-584.

11. Juvin P, Lavaut E, Dupont H, et al. Difficult tracheal intubation is more common in obese than in lean patients. *Anesth Analg.* 2003;97:595-600.
12. Kim WH, Ahn HJ, Lee CJ, et al. Neck circumference to thyromental distance ratio: a new predictor of difficult intubation in obese patients. *Br J Anaesth.* 2011;106:743-748.
13. Brodsky JB, Lemmens HJ, Brock-Utne JG, Saidman LJ, Levitan R. Anesthetic considerations for bariatric surgery: proper positioning is important for laryngoscopy. *Anesth Analg.* 2003;96:1841-1842.
14. Abdi W, Dhonneur G, Amathieu R, et al. LMA supreme versus facemask ventilation performed by novices: a comparative study in morbidly obese patients showing difficult ventilation predictors. *Obes Surg.* 2009;19:1624-1630.
15. Alvarado R, Alami RS, Hsu G, et al. The impact of preoperative weight loss in patients undergoing laparscopic Roux-en-Y gastric bypass. *Obes Surg.* 2005;15:1282-1286.
16. Schwab RJ, Pasirstein M, Pierson R, et al. Identification of upper airway anatomic risk factors for obstructive sleep apnea with volumetric magnetic resonance imaging. *Am J Resp Crit Care Med.* 2003;168:522-530.
17. Gupta RM, Parvizi J, Hanssen AD, Gay PC. Postoperative complications in patients with obstructive sleep apnea syndrome undergoing hip or knee replacement: a case-control study. *Mayo Clin Proc.* 2001;76:897-905.
18. Kaw R, Pasupuleti V, Walker E, Ramaswamy A, Foldvary-Schafer N. Postoperative complications in patients with obstructive sleep apnea. *Chest.* 2012;141:436-441.
19. Rennotte MT, Baele P, Aubert G, Rodenstein DO. Nasal continuous positive airway pressure in the perioperative management of patients with obstructive sleep apnea submitted to surgery. *Chest.* 1995;107:367-374.
20. Chung F, Subramanyam R, Liao P, et al. High STOP-Bang score indicates a high probability of obstructive sleep apnoea. *Br J Anaesth.* 2012;108:768-775.
21. Schummann R, Shikora S, Weiss JM, et al. A comparison of multimodal perioperative analgesia to epidural pain management after gastric bypass surgery. *Anest Analg.* 2003;96:469-474.
22. Liu SS, Carpenter RL, Mackey DC, et al. Effects of perioperative analgesic technique on rate of recovery after colon surgery. *Anesthesiology.* 1995;83:757-765.
23. Kong VKF, Irwin MG. Gabapentin: a multimodal perioperative drug? *Br J Anaesth.* 2007;99:775-786.
24. Bamgbade, OA, Khalaf WM, Ajai O, et al. Obstetric anaesthesia outcome in obese and non-obese parturients undergoing caesarean delivery: an observational study. *Int J Obstet Anesth.* 2009;18:221-225.
25. Futier E, Constantin JM, Pelosi P, et al. Noninvastive ventilation and alveolar recruitement maneuver improve respiratory function during and after intubation of morbidly obese patients. *Anesthesiology.* 2011;114:1354-1363.
26. Jain R, Chung SM, Jain L, et al. Implications of obesity for drug therapy: limitations and challenges. *Clin Pharm Ther.* 2011;90:77-89.
27. Lemmens HJ, Ingrande J. Pharmacology and obesity. *Intl Anesth Clin.* 2013;51:52-66.
28. Lemmens HJ, Brodsky JB. The dose of succinylcholine in morbid obesity. *Anesth Analg.* 2006;102:438-442.
29. Leykin Y, Pellis T, Lucca M, et al. The effects of cisatracurium on morbidly obese women. *Anesth Analg.* 2004;99:1090-1094.
30. Leykin Y, Pellis T, Lucca M, et al. The pharmacodynamic effects of rocuronium when dosed according to real body weight or ideal body weight in morbidly obese patients. *Anesth Analg.* 2004;99:1086-1089.
31. Lemmens HJ, Saidman LJ, Eger EI 2nd, Laster MJ. Obesity modestly affects inhaled anesthetic kinetics in humans. *Anesth Analg.* 2008;107:1864-1870.
32. Pelosi P, Croci M, Ravagnan I, Vicardi P, Gattinoni L. Total respiratory system, lung, and chest wall mechanics in sedated-paralyzed postoperative morbidly obese patients. *Chest.* 1996;109:144-151.
33. Whalen FX, Gajic O, Thompson GB, et al. The effects of the alveolar recruitment maneuver and positive end-expiratory pressure on arterial oxygenation during laparoscopic bariatric surgery. *Anesth Analg.* 2006;102:298-305.
34. Perilli V, Sollazzi L, Bossa P, et al. The effects of the reverse Trendelenberg position on respiratory mechanics and blood gases in morbidly obese patients during bariatric surgery. *Anesth Analg.* 2000;91(6):1520-1525.
35. Squadrone V, Coha M, Cerutti E, et al. Continuous positive airway pressure for treatment of postoperative hipoxemia. A randomized controlled trial. *JAMA.* 2005;136:738-747.
36. Huerta S, DeShields S, Shpiner R, et al. Safety and efficacy of postoperative continuous positive airway pressure to prevent pulmonary complications after Roux-en-Y gastric bypass. *J Gastrointest Surg.* 2002;6:354-358.

13

Current Concepts in Perioperative Management of Adolescents Undergoing Bariatric Surgery

Kathleen B. Hrovat, MS, RD, LD; Linda Kollar, RN, MSN, CBN; and Thomas H. Inge, MD, PhD

The percentage of adolescents aged 12 to 19 years who are obese increased from 5% to 18% between 1980 and 2008,[1] and approximately 4% of youth meet criteria for severe obesity (body mass index [BMI] > 99th percentile).[2] Obesity in adolescents is accompanied by both immediate and long-term consequences to health and well-being; type 2 diabetes mellitus, nonalcoholic fatty liver disease, and obstructive sleep apnea are often seen in youth. Severely obese adolescents are more likely to have risk factors for cardiovascular disease and remain obese as adults.[3] In addition, severely obese adolescents and children experience psychological sequelae including depression and low self-esteem.[4] Conventional behavioral methods aiming to achieve weight loss are rarely effective in treating adolescents with obesity. Therefore, based on the success of bariatric surgery for reversing obesity, obesity-related comorbidities,[5] and obesity-related premature demise[6-8] in adults, weight loss surgery is increasingly considered an appropriate treatment avenue for adolescents who meet criteria.[9]

Surgical Options

The number of weight loss surgery procedures performed on adolescents has remained stable since 2003 at a rate of about 1000 procedures annually.[10] The laparoscopic Roux-en-Y gastric bypass (RYGB) is commonly performed in the adolescent age group. The laparoscopic sleeve gastrectomy (LSG) is gaining popularity, but lacks long-term information for the use in adolescent patients. The laparoscopic adjustable gastric band (LAGB) makes up about one-third of all procedures performed.[10] The LAGB has not been approved by the Food and Drug Administration for use in minors and is considered investigational. Procedures sometimes used in adults that result in significant malabsorption, such as the biliopancreatic diversion or duodenal switch, are not recommended for adolescents due to predictable long-term adverse effects on nutrition, especially if supplement adherence is suboptimal.[11,12]

Forse RA, Apovian CM, eds.
Bariatric Surgery: What Every Provider Needs to Know (pp 151-160).

Table 13-1

Surgical Weight Loss Outcomes in Adolescents

PROCEDURE	BMI REDUCTION AT 1 YEAR	DOCUMENTED COMORBIDITY IMPROVEMENT	COMPLICATIONS
Roux-en-Y gastric band	35% to 37%	Obstructive sleep apnea, type 2 diabetes, pseudotumor cerebri, dyslipidemia, insulin resistance, and psychosocial functioning	Anastomotic stricture, leak, wound infection, bowel obstruction, bleeding, ulceration, pneumonia, micronutrient deficiency, and other perioperative complications of general surgery
Laparoscopic sleeve gastrectomy	35%	Type 2 diabetes, dyslipidemia, insulin resistance	Staple line leak, gastroesophageal reflux, bleeding, micronutrient deficiency, and other perioperative complications of general surgery
Laparoscopic adjustable gastric band	28%	Hypertension, dyslipidemia, plasma insulin, gastroesophageal reflux, asthma, irregular menstruation	Reoperation for band complications, including high rates of band removal, and other perioperative complications of general surgery

There are limited but mounting data available to inform us about the outcomes of weight loss surgery in adolescents; at this time, there is not enough evidence available to determine which weight loss procedures are best for this age group. The results from surgical weight loss procedures in adolescents are comparable or better than those seen in adults in terms of safety, efficacy, and resolution of comorbidities (Table 13-1). A recent retrospective cross-sectional review of inpatient data found a low complication rate and no in-hospital deaths among adolescents undergoing weight loss surgery.[10] Weight loss surgery in adolescents has been found to far surpass conventional lifestyle modification in reducing BMI, improving comorbidities, and raising quality of life.[13] Additional outcome data are needed to understand the safety and efficacy of surgical weight loss in the adolescent population. Programs performing weight loss surgery in adolescents should participate in careful long-term data collection.

Patient Selection

Consideration for surgery in the adolescent should be driven by the presence of clinical comorbidities. Current recommendations suggest a BMI cut-off of ≥ 35 kg/m^2 with the presence of one or more serious comorbidities, such as type 2 diabetes mellitus, severe steatohepatitis, pseudotumor cerebri, or moderate to severe sleep apnea. Adolescents with less severe comorbidities are considered surgical candidates at a BMI ≥ 40.[12] In addition, timing of the referral for bariatric surgery is an important consideration to achieve optimal weight loss results. Our longitudinal results of adolescents undergoing RYGB in Cincinnati found that the decline in BMI at 1 year was 37% regardless of the BMI at time of surgery, thus late referral at a higher BMI may well preclude attainment of a BMI in the nonobese postoperatively.[14]

The psychological toll of severe obesity in the adolescent is high and often precedes the medical comorbidities. Adolescents with severe obesity have higher rates of depression, they are often socially isolated and have experienced victimization and bullying at school, and they have poor health-related quality of life.[15] Formal evaluation for psychological comorbidities must be conducted prior to weight loss surgery. The psychological evaluation includes interview and objective questionnaires to evaluate for psychopathology, eating disorders, family functioning, and adherence to medical regimens. Identified psychological comorbidities must be treated and controlled prior to surgery.

Additional considerations unique to the adolescent include evidence of completion of physical development. Typically, surgery is not recommended until Tanner stage IV or V has been reached, usually age 12 for females and age 14 for males. Radiographic assessment of bone age may assist with estimation of completion of linear growth, especially when considering weight loss surgery in younger adolescents.[12]

The more difficult assessment is related to cognitive development and the adolescent's ability to understand the long-term implications of the surgery. This includes ability to understand the lifelong dietary and exercise changes that will be required for optimal success, the need for daily nutritional supplements, and the importance of long-term follow-up. In addition, the adolescent should ideally show evidence of mature decision making with appropriate understanding of risks and benefits of surgery. This assessment is initiated with the psychological assessment and reassessed throughout the preoperative period as the adolescent and family demonstrate the ability to comply with treatment recommendations and attendance at appointments for weight management visits and other specialty care appointments as needed.

Adolescent Multidisciplinary Team

Adolescent bariatric procedures in the United States are most often performed in adult hospital units. Whatever the setting, the team caring for the adolescent patient must combine expertise in the medical and psychosocial care of pediatric and adolescent obesity with knowledge and skill in bariatric surgery. The multidisciplinary care team should include at a minimum an experienced bariatric surgeon, medical director with pediatric expertise, a clinical care coordinator, dietician, and a mental health professional.

The medical director should have pediatric expertise in order to provide appropriate evaluation and management of the unique health issues and syndromes that will be encountered in a pediatric referral population. The clinical care coordinator should be an advanced practice nurse or physician assistant with expertise in pediatrics or ideally adolescent health. This coordinator functions to provide close monitoring, acts as the adolescent and family advocate at each level of care, and assists with communication within the health care team. Ideally, this individual should seek subspecialty training in bariatric nursing care and be certified as a bariatric nurse.

A key piece of the assessment of the adolescent is provided by a psychologist or psychiatrist. Expertise in pediatric obesity, eating disorders, and adolescent mental health issues is essential to provide a comprehensive assessment of the adolescent and family. A social worker is a valuable member of the team to provide ongoing support and reassessment both before and after surgery.

The registered dietician must have pediatric weight management credentialing in order to provide a comprehensive nutritional assessment, address the nutritional needs, and monitor the adolescent's nutritional status after surgery. The registered dietician must have the flexibility and ability to communicate effectively with adolescents and families in order to provide the education for the necessary lifestyle changes after surgery.

An exercise physiologist or physical therapist with experience working with adolescents with severe obesity is a beneficial member of the team to assess conditioning, alignment, strength, and balance and encourage ongoing physical activity and fitness. At the very least, the team should know the community resources available for teens to promote regular and safe bouts of physical activity.

Developing a relationship with pediatric/adolescent consultation services will assist with timely referral and evaluation for the bariatric patients. These services include anesthesiology, pulmonary, cardiology, and endocrinology. A relationship with adolescent medicine or gynecology is beneficial to assist with menstrual disorders, reproductive health care concerns, and reliable contraception in the initial postoperative years.

Adolescent-Friendly Services

Clinicians working with young people require knowledge of adolescent development and the ability to respond to developmental, behavioral, and mental health concerns that are unique to the adolescent population. Establishing rapport and building a trusting relationship with teens takes time. Ideally, the adolescent will have at least one consistent member of the multidisciplinary team whom he or she sees at every visit. Each visit should begin with a description of what will take place that day, including whom the teen will meet with and approximately how long the visit will last. The parameters of the treatment plan process should be clearly explained to the adolescent and family to ensure understanding of the expectations before and after surgery.

Effective communication with adolescents requires an appreciation of the unique characteristics of adolescent cognitive development. Adolescents are egocentric, often consumed with thoughts of themselves. Recognition of this normal developmental process can be helpful when developing a treatment plan or understanding why adherence is a problem. For example, adolescents have a sense of always being "onstage," having a feeling that everyone is watching them. Therefore, it may be difficult to drink a protein shake for lunch at school or to exercise in a public setting. As with all patients, the adolescent must be involved in the development of the treatment plan in order to increase likelihood of adherence.

Balancing the needs of the adolescent and the parent requires special skills as well. Assisting teens with dietary and lifestyle changes requires a family approach that allows everyone time to be heard. The majority of the education should be conducted with the adolescent and parent together. However, there must be time for the adolescent to address his or her concerns with the provider alone. This provides an opportunity for the adolescent to speak for him- or herself and for the provider to explore risk-taking behaviors, such as smoking, sexuality, and diet/supplement adherence. It is essential to handle this separate visit time in a sensitive manner to maintain trust and rapport with the parent and adolescent. The concept should be introduced early and emphasized as an opportunity to foster growth and self-reliance. After the separate interview time, it is crucial to reunite with the parent to review the plan of care.

One size does not fit all when it comes to education materials for adolescent patients. Handouts designed for adults usually fail to address the issues relevant to the adolescent and parent. Materials should be tailored to the adolescent; when developing new materials, having a team of adolescents to review the handouts will help to make them most relevant. Information given to the patient/family should be offered in written, visual, and/or electronic form to accommodate varying learning styles. It is also important to identify the "family" as defined by the adolescent. All caregivers within the adolescent's network should be invited to attend pre- and postoperative visits.

Support groups provide adult patients who have undergone bariatric surgery with a sense of connection to peers and help them adhere to weight loss programs.[16] Professional organizations that credential bariatric specialty centers have promoted the need for bariatric programs to provide a support group to maintain certification. There is, however, a paucity of data regarding outcomes of support group attendance for adolescent patients undergoing bariatric surgery. In addition, there is a lack of data to guide the optimal structure of the support group for adolescents in bariatric surgery programs. We have appreciated the importance of professional facilitators in support groups, as they can reinforce counseling provided in the clinic setting and challenge misconceptions that may arise and be promulgated. Also, the addition of an adolescent peer education framework may be beneficial because the similarity of experience between young people facilitates communication and provides a positive model for behavior change.

Consent and Assent

Authorization (permission) for treatment must be obtained by the adult guardian for minors seeking weight loss surgery. However, ensuring the adolescent has provided informed assent for treatment is an equally important process. Obtaining legal permission and adolescent assent is a dynamic process that begins at the initial assessment and is completed with the signature on the surgical consent form. Ensuring psychosocial well-being and maturity is an important aspect of the consent process. The adolescent should participate to the degree possible with support for independent decision making. The assent should be obtained with the adolescent alone to ensure he or she has an opportunity to ask any questions he or she may have and respond without overt or subtle coercion from adults. The person obtaining assent should ascertain that the adolescent understands what will be required for his or her success, what will be done, basic purpose of the surgical intervention, the risks and benefits of the surgical and nonsurgical options, and future ramifications. Assessment of understanding can be completed through a written test or discussion with the adolescent and should be documented in the medical record. The actual signing of the consent document should be done with the adolescent and guardian together.

Preoperative Preparation

Adolescents and their families require a well-planned, developmentally appropriate pre- and postoperative program of education, preparation, and support. See Table 13-2 for patient education themes.

During the initial assessment, baseline anthropometric measurements are taken and laboratory assessment identifies potentially important nutritional deficiencies (Table 13-3). The registered dietician assesses previous weight management and weight loss attempts (and suspected reasons for failure), current eating habits, meal pattern, and fluid intake. This information will serve as the basis for developing the preoperative dietary plan specific to the patient. The preoperative weight management plan emphasizes adequate protein intake (1.0 to 1.5 g/protein/kg of ideal body weight), fruits, vegetables, whole grains, water, and sugar-free fluids to achieve weight stability or weight loss. The preoperative phase, 3 to 6 months in length, allows the patient to develop and practice the postoperative behaviors that will contribute to his or her weight loss success after surgery. Examples of the topics and behaviors addressed during this period include label reading for portion size and composition; measuring of foods and liquids with measuring cups, spoons, and liquid measure; journaling patient intake; and meal planning. At each of the preoperative treatment plan visits, the dietician sets nutrition goals with the patient. These goals should be measurable, attainable, and specific to the adolescent. An example would be: "I will drink water and sugar-free fluids equal to 64 ounces daily, and I will quantify this amount with my water bottle." It is important these goals are reviewed at subsequent visits.

Preoperative Liquid Diet

Many programs require a preoperative liquid diet 2 weeks prior to surgery. These meal plans typically recommend an intake of 1000 to 1200 kcal, 60 g protein distributed over 3 to 4 meals/day. A preoperative liquid diet introduces the adolescent to the postoperative dietary regimen and

Table 13-2
Patient Education Themes

- Risks/benefits of bariatric surgery
- Risks/benefits of medical treatment of obesity, including risks of persistent obesity
- Vitamin and mineral supplements and risks of deficiencies
- Basic nutrition information
- Mindful eating
- Assessing hunger and fullness
- Postoperative diet by stages
- Exercise and physical activity
- What to expect in the hospital
- Goal setting
- Getting back on track
- Pregnancy prevention

Table 13-3
Recommended Initial Laboratory Testing

- Complete blood count with differential
- Hepatic profile
- Lipid panel
- Fasting insulin
- Fasting glucose
- Hemoglobin A1c
- Thyroid-stimulating hormone
- Iron
- Ferritin

may well improve the safety of the surgical procedure by reduction of intra-abdominal fat stores and liver size.[17]

Postoperative Care

Routine supplementation with some form of multivitamins is recommended to begin upon discharge from the hospital. The American Society for Metabolic and Bariatric Surgery has published comprehensive nutritional guidelines, including suggested postoperative vitamin and mineral supplementation.[18] At this time, the recommendations are based on the surgery performed and not specific to the age of the patient.

Postoperative Dietary Progression

An upper gastrointestinal study is often done the first day after surgery to confirm that no leak or obstruction is present. If there are no contraindications to feeding, oral clear liquids are initiated. Patients who have had the LSG procedure advance to oral fluids on postoperative day 1. Adequate fluid intake is required for discharge.

The dietary progression postoperatively is patient driven based on his or her tolerance of foods at each of the stages (Table 13-4). Stage 2 typically begins at discharge from the hospital. The postoperative diet focuses on weight loss with preservation of lean body mass and consists of a diet high in protein, low in simple carbohydrates, free of added simple sugars, and with modest fat intake. The postoperative advancement of the dietary regimen for RYGB, LAGB, and LSG varies by the number of meals per day and consistency, texture, and the progression of the amount and type of food consumed at a meal. The use of food diaries or tracking forms should be encouraged to quantify intake.

In addition to ongoing management and evaluation of comorbidities after surgery, the team must remain attentive to adolescent risk-taking behavior. Risk taking is a normal part of adolescent development and may include no adherence to supplements, experimentation with substance use, and sexual activity. These behaviors need to be discussed at each visit with the adolescent as their risk taking may change over time. Assessment of risk behavior should be conducted privately with the assurance of confidentiality. A nonjudgmental approach to questioning within the context of associated health risks after weight loss surgery will allow for more open and honest communication between the adolescent and the provider.

There is no information available about the outcomes of pregnancy after bariatric surgery specific to adolescents. There is a potential increased risk associated with pregnancy prior to 18 months after weight loss surgery for women of all ages.[12] Counseling regarding appropriate methods for pregnancy prevention should be provided to all girls before and after surgery.

The frequency of follow-up visits proposed varies among programs. Frequent visits during the first year after weight loss surgery when rapid changes are occurring provide opportunities for monitoring, education, and support. These visits usually occur within 2 weeks after surgery, then every 3 to 6 months for the first 18 months. Annual follow-up visits should always be encouraged. The visits include weight assessment, nutritional status including micronutrient blood levels, comorbidities, risk behavior, and psychosocial status. In the event that annual visits cannot occur due to distance or other factors, a remote management (self-management) plan should be provided to ensure surveillance for the most commonly encountered long-term surgical and nutritional complications. These include, for example, cholelithiasis, partial/intermittent bowel obstruction, gastrointestinal ulceration, band erosions, micronutrient deficiencies, anemia, and bone health.

Adherence

Success after weight loss surgery requires ongoing adherence to the dietary, exercise, and supplementation recommendations. The health care team should anticipate and plan for adherence issues for all patients after surgery. The normal adolescent transition periods are high risk for adherence issues; preplanning with the teen and family prior to the life events can assist in preventing relapse and unwanted weight gain. Examples of transition periods include changing from the routines of the school year to summer vacation, transfer from junior high to high school, transfer from home school to traditional classroom, entering the work force, and entering college or moving out of parent's home.

Table 13-4

Postoperative Dietary Staging

	STAGE 1	STAGE 2	STAGE 3	STAGE 4	STAGE 5
	Ice chips, water, sugar-free clear liquids	Full liquids High protein	Smooth consistency foods and liquids	Soft foods	All textures Healthy foods
Roux-en-Y gastric bypass	1 oz/hour X 24-48 hrs then ad lib X 3-7 days	Weeks 2-4	Weeks 4-6	Weeks 7-9	Week 9 for life
Laparoscopic adjustable gastric band	1 oz/hour X 24-48 hrs	Weeks 0-2	Weeks 3-4	Weeks 5-6	Week 7 for life
Laparoscopic sleeve gastrectomy	1 oz/hour X 24-48 hrs then ad lib X 3-7 days	Weeks 1-5	Weeks 5-8	Weeks 9-12	Week 13 for life
Goals	48-64 ounces/day Acceptable sugar-free clear liquids include: Water, clear broth, sugar-free gelatin, sugar-free fruit-flavored drinks, sugar-free popsicles No carbonation, caffeine, or red dye	Calories: 500-600 kcal Protein: 50-60 g Fluid: 80-90 oz New foods: Skim or 1% milk, low-fat soy or Lactaid milk, high protein drinks, light plain or vanilla yogurt	Calories: 500-700 kcal Protein: 60 g Fluid: 80-90 oz New foods: Scrambled eggs, blenderized/minced turkey, chicken, flaked fish or mashed tofu, tuna, melted low-fat cheese, small curd low-fat cottage cheese, low-fat ricotta cheese Try new foods every 2-3 days	Calories: 700-800 kcal Protein: 60 g Fluid: 80-90 oz New foods: Shaved deli meats, low-fat cheese, lean pork, cooked beans, soft or canned fruit in own juice, no skin, soft cooked or canned vegetables, toast, low-sugar cereal, crackers, oatmeal, rice, pasta, mashed potatoes Choose whole grain foods	Calories: 800-900 kcal Protein: 60 g Fluids: 80-90 oz New foods: all healthy food choices
Meal pattern	Continuous sipping	3-6 meals/day Volume: ½ cup/meal	3-4 meals/day Volume: ½ cup solid or 5-6 oz protein drink/meal	3-6 meals/day Volume: ½-1 cup solid or 8 oz protein drink	3-6 meals/day Volume: ¾-1½ cup/meal

Adapted from Fullmer MA, Abrams SH, Hrovat K, et al. Nutritional strategy for adolescents undergoing bariatric surgery: report of a working group of the Nutrition Committee of NASPGHAN/NACHRI. *J Pediatr Gastroenterol Nutr.* 2011;54(1)125-135.

Transition to Adult Care

A thoughtful transition to an adult care model is an essential element of health care for adolescents. Ideally, as the adolescent becomes developmentally capable, he or she has begun to take more responsibility for the management of his or her health at home and in the medical office. If the surgical weight loss services are offered in a pediatric setting, the care will become more appropriate in an adult setting when the young adult reaches the early 20s. This transition should be coordinated with the primary care provider in partnership with the adolescent and family. If the young adult chooses to have follow-up through the primary care provider, a summary of supplement recommendations and laboratory follow-up should be reviewed with the young adult and forwarded to the primary care provider. Programs that provide surgical weight loss services to young people as well as adults still need to transition the young person to the adult model of care.

Summary

Bariatric surgery can be used safely to treat adolescent severe obesity. However, optimal patient care importantly involves consideration of choice of procedure, the contribution of a multidisciplinary team, unique consent issues, and certain aspects of pre- and postoperative care that differ from adult standards. The expectation is that increasingly outcome data will drive refinements in care paradigms for adolescents seeking surgical management of obesity.

References

1. Ogden CL, Carroll MD, Curtin LR, Lamb MM, Flegal KM. Prevalence of high body mass index in US children and adolescents, 2007-2008. *JAMA.* 2010;303(3):242-249.
2. Skelton JA, Cook SR, Auinger P, Klein JD, Barlow SE. Prevalence and trends of severe obesity among US children and adolescents. *Acad Pediatr.* 2009;9(5):322-329.
3. Freedman DS, Mei Z, Srinivasan SR, Berenson GS, Dietz WH. Cardiovascular risk factors and excess adiposity among overweight children and adolescents: the Bogalusa Heart Study. *J Pediatr.* 2007;150(1):12-17 e2.
4. Sjoberg RL, Nilsson KW, Leppert J. Obesity, shame, and depression in school-aged children: a population-based study. *Pediatrics.* 2005;116(3):e389-e392.
5. Buchwald H, Avidor Y, Braunwald E, et al. Bariatric surgery: a systematic review and meta-analysis. *JAMA.* 2004;292(14):1724-1737.
6. Sjostrom L, Narbro K, Sjostrom CD, et al. Effects of bariatric surgery on mortality in Swedish obese subjects. *N Engl J Med.* 2007;357(8):741-752.
7. Adams TD, Gress RE, Smith SC, et al. Long-term mortality after gastric bypass surgery. *N Engl J Med.* 2007;357(8):753-761.
8. Christou NV, Sampalis JS, Liberman M, et al. Surgery decreases long-term mortality, morbidity, and health care use in morbidly obese patients. *Ann Surg.* 2004;240(3):416-423; discussion 423-424.
9. Tsai WS, Inge TH, Burd RS. Bariatric surgery in adolescents: recent national trends in use and in-hospital outcome. *Arch Pediatr Adolesc Med.* 2007;161(3):217-221.
10. Kelleher DC, Merrill CT, Cottrell LT, Nadler EP, Burd RS. Recent national trends in the use of adolescent inpatient bariatric surgery: 2000 through 2009. *JAMA Pediatr.* 2013;167(2):126-132.
11. Michalsky M, Reichard K, Inge T, Pratt J, Lenders C. ASMBS pediatric committee best practice guidelines. *Surg Obes Relat Dis.* 2012;8(1):1-7.
12. Pratt JS, Lenders CM, Dionne EA, et al. Best practice updates for pediatric/adolescent weight loss surgery. *Obesity (Silver Spring).* 2009;17(5):901-910.
13. Bondada S, Jen HC, Deugarte DA. Outcomes of bariatric surgery in adolescents. *Curr Opin Pediatr.* 2011;23(5):552-556.
14. Inge TH, Jenkins TM, Zeller M, et al. Baseline BMI is a strong predictor of nadir BMI after adolescent gastric bypass. *J Pediatr.* 2010;156(1):103-108 e1.
15. Kolotkin RL, Zeller M, Modi AC, et al. Assessing weight-related quality of life in adolescents. *Obesity (Silver Spring).* 2006;14(3):448-457.

16. Glinski J, Wetzler S, Goodman E. The psychology of gastric bypass surgery. *Obes Surg.* 2001;11(5):581-588.
17. Edholm D, Kullberg J, Haenni A, et al. Preoperative 4-week low-calorie diet reduces liver volume and intrahepatic fat, and facilitates laparoscopic gastric bypass in morbidly obese. *Obes Surg.* 2011;21(3):345-350.
18. Aills L, Blankenship J, Buffington C, Furtado M, Parrott J. ASMBS allied health nutritional guidelines for the surgical weight loss patient. *Surg Obes Relat Dis.* 2008;4(5 Suppl):S73-S108.

14

Bariatric Surgery and the Elderly

Oliver A. Varban, MD, FACS

Measures and Prevalence of Obesity in the Elderly

It is unclear which measure of obesity best predicts the prevalence and impact of obesity on health in the elderly. Early studies revealed that for each pound gained after the age of 42 years, there was a 2% increase in mortality.[1] Furthermore, they noted that only 1 in 7 individuals with obesity will reach the US life expectancy of 76.9 years and that the life expectancy is reduced by 9 years in women and 12 years in men. When using body mass index (BMI) as a measure of obesity, a unique paradox occurs in that a higher BMI value predicts a lower relative mortality in older adults.[2,3] The relationship between BMI and disease risk in the elderly may be due to changes in both height and weight over time. For example, there is concomitant loss of height from vertebral compression and kyphosis along with increased omental and mesenteric fat and decreased muscle mass in the elderly. Thus, waist circumference, which correlates highly with total fat and intra-abdmoinal fat, may be a better predictor of adverse health effect of obesity in the elderly. This is evident from the Scottish Health Survey, which demonstrated a disproportionate increase in waist circumference along with ill health despite a smaller increase in BMI with age.[4] Other, confounding factors that contribute to the obesity paradox in the elderly include the presence of "resistant" survivors, unintentional weight loss from competing illnesses such as malignancy, and early death due to obesity-related comorbidities.[5] Nevertheless, the obesity paradox should not deter one from the harmful effects of obesity to the elderly. Moreover, as the life expectancy in the United States has risen, so has the prevalence of obesity among older age groups. In 2010, the predicted prevalence of obesity among Americans over 60 years old was 37%, and by the year 2030, it is predicted that 20% of the US population will be older than 65 years.[4,6]

Forse RA, Apovian CM, eds.
Bariatric Surgery: What Every Provider Needs to Know (pp 161-170).

Physiology of Obesity in the Elderly

Fat distribution changes significantly after the age of 70, as visceral fat mass increases and lean tissue decreases. This phenomenon results in a disproportionate increase in waist circumference despite a smaller increase in BMI.[4] Higher visceral fat is a main cause of impaired glucose tolerance in the elderly as increases in intramuscular and intrahepatic fat contribute to impaired insulin action through the release of fatty acids. Likewise, increased pancreatic fat decreases cell function, which also results in the progression of diabetes.[7]

Aging is associated with decreased energy expenditure as well as decreased fat oxidation. Loss of skeletal mass results in a decrease of basal metabolic rates up to 2% to 3% per decade after the age of 20 and 4% per decade after the age of 50. This corresponds to a decline of 150 kcal/day (630 kJ/d) or 30% between the age of 20 and 70 years.[8]

Visceral obesity and advanced age are associated with a proinflammatory state, resulting in reduced immune function, cognitive decline, and insulin resistance. Mediators of metabolic and insulin homeostasis are also affected with noted increases in levels of tumor necrosis factor (TNF), interleukin (IL)-6, and C-reactive protein. Moreover, TNF and IL-6 have catabolic effects on muscle mass resulting in sarcopenia.[9,10]

Endocrine changes related to obesity and aging included decreased growth hormone (GH), insulin-like growth factor-1 (IGF-1), and leptin as well as downregulation of ghrelin. Furthermore, these changes appear to be worsened in the presence of abdominal obesity and insulin resistance.[11]

Health Consequences of Obesity in the Elderly

The most significant health consequences of obesity in the elderly include glucose intolerance, hypertension, dyslipidemia, and cardiovascular disease, which is associated with metabolic syndrome.[12] These conditions peak at age 50 to 70 in men and age 60 to 80 in women, with an odds ratio (OR) of 5.8 in 65-year-old men and 4.9 in 65-year-old women compared to 20- to 34-year-old participants. Metabolic syndrome is also a risk factor for stroke and subclinical ischemic brain lesions. An increase in BMI is also associated with Alzheimer disease and vascular dementia.[13,14] Obesity doubles the risk of heart failure and is associated with a variety of comorbidities such as arthritis (with an OR of 4.8 for men and 4.0 for women), pulmonary dysfunction, obstructive sleep apnea, certain cancer types, decreased cognitive skills, sexual dysfunction, urinary incontinence, age-related macular degeneration, and cataracts.[4,15,16]

Finally, obesity results in many functional disabilities and impaired quality of life among the elderly. Along with decreased muscle mass and increased joint dysfunction, older people experience increased frailty, sarcopenia, chronic pain, and unintentional injuries.[4,17] Both elderly women and men exhibit an increased risk of functional decline with a BMI of 35 kg/m^2 or greater (OR of 2.61 and 3.32, respectively), which also results in an increase in the relative risk of nursing home admission by 31% for those aged 65 to 74 years.[10,18] The physiology and health consequences of obesity in the elderly are summarized in Table 14-1.

Management of Obesity in the Elderly

The benefits of weight loss in the elderly are many and include improvement or resolution diabetes, hyperlipidemia, hypertension, cardiopulmonary disease, and obstructive sleep apnea. In addition, weight loss improves functional capacity, mobility, and the ability to perform activities of daily living alone, which reduces the risk for unintentional injuries, disability, and depressive symptoms.[4,19] Treatment options for obesity in the elderly include lifestyle interventions (diet and

Table 14-1

Physiologic Changes and Consequences of Obesity in the Elderly

PHYSIOLOGIC CHANGES	HEALTH CONSEQUENCES
Increase in visceral fat mass and decrease in lean muscle tissue	Impaired glucose tolerance/diabetes Decreased cell function Proinflammatory state and decreased immune function
Decreased energy expenditure	Decrease metabolic rate (up to 4% per decade after the age of 50)
Decrease in GH and IGF-1, leptin and downregulation of ghrelin	Worsens in the presence of abdominal obesity and insulin resistance
Decrease in TNF, IL-6, CRP	Reduced immune function, sarcopenia, and insulin resistance
Decreased muscle mass and joint dysfunction	Increased risk of functional decline, unintentional injuries, and nursing home admission

CRP = C-reactive protein, GH = growth hormone, IGF-1 = insulin growth factor-1, IL-6 = interleukin-6, TNF-α = tumor necrosis factor-α.

exercise), pharmacotherapy, endoscopic treatments, and bariatric surgery. However, all treatments have inherent risks and limitations in the elderly.

Lifestyle Interventions

In a study that included men and women participants up to the age of 84 years, every kilogram of weight loss through diet and exercise reduced the incidence of diabetes type 2 by 16% over a period of 3.2 years.[20] However, changes in lifestyle among the elderly presents unique challenges. Diet-induced weight loss alone without the addition of exercise results in both a decrease in fat mass and fat-free mass, thus worsening sarcopenia and osteopenia, and can further impair physical function. Also, cognitive dysfunction, depression, isolation, dependency from others, institutionalization, chronic disability, and impairments in vision and hearing interfere with physical activity and exercise necessary for healthy weight loss.[21]

Pharmacological Management

Orlistat, a lipase inhibitor that blocks the digestion and absorption of fat, is currently approved for patients with a BMI $\geq$ 30 and in patients with a BMI of 27 to 29.9 in the presence of obesity-related comorbidities.[22] In a randomized study in the primary care setting, orlistat was just as effective adults aged 65 and older as in younger adults and gastrointestinal side effects were not different. However, the use of pharmacotherapy in the elderly is problematic as polypharmacy and drug interactions may result in complications. Moreover, most clinical trials that study the effects of new medications exclude older test participants.

Endoscopic Management

As with pharmacotherapy, endoscopic modalities, such as intragastric balloons, bypass devices, or plication mechanisms, have not been tested in the elderly since study participants are typically under the age of 50 years. Moreover, follow-up is short and comparative data with bariatric surgery are lacking. Although the technology is promising in a population of patients who are at higher risk for surgery, endoscopic treatments for elderly patients with obesity are unproven at this point.

Bariatric Surgery

Bariatric surgery results in sustained weight loss, reduction in comorbidities, and a marked survival advantage.[2,23-25] The most common bariatric procedures include gastric bypass, adjustable gastric banding (AGB), sleeve gastrectomy (SG), and biliopancreatic diversion with duodenal switch (BPD-DS).[23] Current guidelines from the National Institutes of Health state that bariatric surgery can be offered to patients with a BMI of > 40 or > 35 combined with weight-related comorbidities such as cardiorespiratory disease, diabetes, sleep apnea, and severe osteoarthritis.[26]

Performing bariatric surgery in the elderly is somewhat controversial. Data from more than 16,000 Medicare beneficiaries between 1997 and 2002 demonstrated a nearly 3-fold increase in the risk of early mortality (1.7% vs 4.8%).[27] However, more recent data from the Longitudinal Assessment of Bariatric Surgery Consortium (LABS) and the American College of Surgeon's National Surgical Quality Improvement Program (ACS NSQIP) did not identify advancing age as a perioperative risk factor for death.[28,29] In February 2006, the Centers for Medicare and Medicaid Services expanded national coverage for bariatric surgery procedures for Medicare beneficiaries. The procedures covered include laparoscopic and open gastric bypass, AGB, and BPD-DS. Procedures must be performed at high-volume centers (more than 125 procedures per year) that achieve a low mortality rate and are certified by the ACS or the American Society for Metabolic and Bariatric Surgery.

Surgical Risk Assessment

Risk estimation tools have been developed to predict mortality and serious complications after bariatric surgery. Thus far, all tools utilize age as a significant predictor for mortality.[30-32] Other risk factors that increase the probability of mortality and postoperative complications include BMI, preoperative dyspnea at rest, history of percutaneous intervention, history of peripheral vascular disease, history of venous thromboembolism, chronic corticosteroid use, type of bariatric surgery, serum albumin, functional status, smoking history, and male gender. Not surprisingly, the elderly suffer many of the same comorbidities that also increase their perioperative risk.

As a means of improving geriatric surgical care in an aging population, the ACS NSQIP and the American Geriatrics Society collaborated to create best practices guidelines around optimal perioperative care of the geriatric surgery patient.[33] The 21-member, multidisciplinary panel represented multiple specialties, including surgical oncology, gastrointestinal surgery, colorectal surgery, cardiothoracic surgery, endocrine surgery, advanced laparoscopic surgery, urology, anesthesiology, and geriatric medicine. Based on their consensus, optimal preoperative assessment of the geriatric surgical patient involves a multifaceted assessment of not only their baseline physiology but also of their cognitive ability, frailty, and functional status. A review of the guidelines has been summarized and revised for its application to bariatric surgery in Table 14-2. Given the number of comorbidities associated with the elderly bariatric patient, the guidelines provided by the expert panel assist in appropriate patient selection. Moreover, since bariatric surgery is entirely elective, the surgeon must advocate for the patient to receive all the appropriate preoperative evaluations and interventions so that the patient can make an informed decision with regard to perioperative risk.

Table 14-2

Preoperative Assessment of the Geriatric Surgical Patient

SCREENING EVALUATIONS	PREOPERATIVE LABORATORY TESTS	PREOPERATIVE IMAGING AND BODY FUNCTIONAL TESTS
• Cognitive impairment and dementia • Decision-making capacity • Depression • Postoperative delirium • Alcohol and substance abuse • Cardiac and pulmonary evaluation • Functional status • Mobility • Fall risk • Frailty • Nutritional status • Polypharmacy and medication dosing • Preoperative counseling on goals and expectations • Determine family and social support system • Designate a health care proxy or surrogate decision maker	• Hemoglobin, renal function, and albumin tests are indicated for all geriatric surgical patients • White blood cell count—for known or suspected infection, myeloproliferative disease or at risk for leukopenia • Platelet count—if at risk of thrombocytopenia or thrombocytosis • Coagulation tests—if at risk of bleeding disorders or medications affecting coagulation; on hemodialysis; or has malnutrition, malabsorption, or liver disease • Electrolytes—for baseline renal insufficiency; congestive heart failure; taking diuretics, digoxin, angiotensin-converting enzyme inhibitors, or other medications that increase likelihood of abnormal results • Serum glucose—known or suspected diabetes • Urinalysis—suspected urinary tract infection or diabetes	• Chest radiograph—cardiopulmonary disease (including smoking, asthma, and chronic obstructive pulmonary disease), > 70 years old with stable chronic cardiopulmonary disase without recent chest radiograph in the past 6 months • Electrocardiogram—known ischemic heart disease, previous myocardial infarction, cardiac arrhythmias, peripheral vascular disease, cerebrovascular disease, heart failure, diabetes, renal insufficiency, or respiratory disease • Pulmonary function test—poorly characterized dyspnea or exercise intolerance with diagnostic uncertainty between cardiac or pulmonary limitation vs simple deconditioning; obstructive lung disease with questionable preoperative optimization • Noninvasive stress testing—≥ 1 clinical risk factor and poor functional capacity

Outcomes After Bariatric Surgery in the Elderly

Bariatric surgery in the elderly is in evolution and data are conflicting at this point in time. Initial concerns regarding increased perioperative complications and poor results have led to a reluctance to offer such surgery to older patients. However, with the introduction of advanced laparoscopic techniques and optimization of perioperative care, bariatric surgery is safer and age alone is not an absolute contraindication. As evidence for this, a study utilizing the ACS NSQIP database noted that the proportion of bariatric procedures in the older population (>65 years) has risen significantly from 2.9% in 2005 to 4.8% in 2009, reflecting a 60% increase.[28] Furthermore, the type of bariatric procedures performed in the elderly has also changed over time. While the proportion of patients undergoing gastric bypass has decreased significantly, the proportion of patients undergoing AGB has increased significantly when compared to younger age groups.

Contemporary outcomes after bariatric surgery in the elderly are summarized in Table 14-3. In a comprehensive meta-analysis of 18 studies that included patients 55 years old undergoing laparoscopic gastric bypass and laparoscopic AGB only, clinically significant BMI reductions occurred for both procedures.[34] Patients experienced a mean excess weight loss (EWL) of 72.6% after gastric bypass and 39.1% after AGB. When compared to younger adults, older patients who have undergone bariatric surgery experience less weight loss and had a lower level of resolution of obesity-related conditions.[28,34-36] However, older patients also tended to have more comorbidities and required more medications prior to surgery. Despite these differences, the elderly experience successful weight loss after surgery and overall improvement of multiple comorbidities as well as a reduction in medication requirements. As with younger patients, comorbidity resolution was significantly higher after laparoscopic gastric bypass than with laparoscopic AGB.[34]

Laparoscopic SG has been proven to be a safe, effective, and durable procedure for morbid obesity even in high-risk patients, making it the ideal procedure in the elderly.[37,38] Although often considered safer than gastric bypass and more effective than AGB, there remains a paucity of data on the outcomes of laparoscopic SG in older populations. In a study consisting of 12 patients over the age of 59 years, Leivonen et al demonstrated that weight loss at 12 months in the elderly is comparable to younger patients after laparoscopic SG (median EWL of 48.4% and 48.5%, $p = .6$), as were resolution of comorbidities.[39] There was no operative mortality but early major complications were seen more often in the older age group (42% vs 9%, $p = .02$). Operative times and hospital length of stay were also longer in the older age group.

The oldest cohort of patients with reported outcomes after bariatric surgery are over 70 years.[40] Among this group of patients ($n = 42$), 52.4% had undergone laparoscopic AGB, 28.6% laparoscopic SG, and 19% laparoscopic gastric bypass with no reported mortality. The mean EWL percentage was 47.7% at 12 months, and postoperative use of medications for hypertension, hyperlipidemia, diabetes, and degenerative joint disease was reduced by 56%, 54%, 53%, and 66%, respectively. Complications included wound infections (9.5%), band removal (7.1%), anastomotic leak (2.3%), and megaesophagus (2.3%). All patients underwent medical screening with a detailed preoperative cardiac workup. Exclusion for any bariatric procedure included coagulopathy, meanwhile contraindications for gastric bypass included inflammatory bowel disease and severe bowel adhesions. Contraindications for SG included gastroesophageal reflux, Barrett's esophagus, and liver cirrhosis with severe portal hypertension.

Although early data on mortality rate were unfavorable in the elderly population, they also included many more open procedures. Advanced laparoscopic techniques have been shown to result in fewer intensive care unit admissions and shorter length of stay after bariatric surgery in the elderly.[41] As such, laparoscopy is likely a key reason why mortality rates after bariatric surgery have been improving over time. Contemporary reports of bariatric surgery in the elderly that include only laparoscopic techniques reveal a mortality rate of less than 0.6% (see Table 14-3). Of equal importance, elderly patients with obesity who undergo bariatric surgery and successfully lose weight benefit from significant improvements in weight-related comorbidities and have significantly increased survival rates when compared with a similar group of nonsurgical patients.[35]

Table 14-3

Contemporary Outcomes After Bariatric Surgery in the Elderly

REFERENCE (STUDY PERIOD)	PROCEDURE (N)	AGE (YEARS)	WEIGHT LOSS AT 1 YEAR	COMPLICATIONS	MORTALITY (30-DAY) %	LENGTH OF STAY (DAYS)
Wittgrove et al[42] (2002 to 2007)	LGB (120)	>60	NR	10.8% strictures, 2.5% bleeding, 1.7% wound infection, 1.7% reexploration (at 90 days)	0	NR
Ramirez et al[40] (2002 to 2008)	LAGB (22) LSG (12) LGB (8)	>70	32.8% EWL (LAGB) 39.4% EWL (LSG) 63.6% EWL (LGB)	7 complications after LAGB 3 complications after LSG 1 complication after LGB	0	4
Fazylov et al[43] (2003 to 2006)	LGB (33)	≥55	59.5% EWL	6% bleeding 3% anastomotic leak 6% intractable vomiting	0	3
Dorman et al[28] (2004 to 2009)	LGB LLGB OGB LAGB VBG BPD-DS (1994)	≥65	NR	4.3% in patients 65 to 69 years old 2.8% in patients ≥70 years old	0.4% (65 to 69 years old) 0.6% (≥70 years old)	NR
Willkomm et al[44] (2005 to 2008)	LGB (100)	>65	74.8% EWL	1.0% bleeding 3.0% pulmonary 2.0% cardiac 2.0% wound	0	1.97

(continued)

Table 14-3 (continued)

Contemporary Outcomes After Bariatric Surgery in the Elderly

REFERENCE (STUDY PERIOD)	PROCEDURE (N)	AGE (YEARS)	WEIGHT LOSS AT 1 YEAR	COMPLICATIONS	MORTALITY (30-DAY) %	LENGTH OF STAY (DAYS)
Leivonen et al[39] (2007 to 2011)	LSG (12)	> 59	45.6% EWL	42% complication rate overall	0	5.8
Busetto et al[45]	LAGB (216)	≥60	Mean postoperative BMI 38.6 kg/m^2	3.7% requiring reoperation	0.46	NR

BPD-DS = biliopancreatic diversion with duodenal switch, EWL = excess weight loss, LAGB = laparoscopic adjustable gastric band, LGB = laparoscopic gastric bypass; LLGB = long limb gastric bypass, LSG = laparoscopic sleeve gastrectomy, OGB = open gastric bypass, VBG = vertical banded gastroplasty.

Summary

With the advent of advanced laparoscopic techniques and centers optimizing bariatric care, bariatric surgery is safer and age alone should not be an absolute contraindication to surgery. No clear recommendations can be made as to a maximal age limit, and so each patient should undergo a comprehensive risk assessment, addressing factors that increase both perioperative mortality after bariatric surgery and also geriatric-specific factors that may contribute to prolonged hospitalization or disability. No recommendations can be made on the choice of procedure either, as each carries its own risk-benefit profile. gastric bypass offers the best weight loss, but it is also associated with more complications. Meanwhile, AGB has the safest operative profile, but underperforms with regard to weight loss. SG is often considered safer than gastric bypass while achieving superior weight loss when compared with AGB, however, data on its use in the elderly population are lacking at this time.

References

1. Hubert HB, Feinleib M, McNamara PM, Castelli WP. Obesity as an independent risk factor for cardiovascular disease: a 26-year follow-up of participants in the Framingham Heart Study. *Circulation.* 1983;67:968-977.
2. Janssen I, Mark AE. Elevated body mass index and mortality risk in the elderly. *Obes Rev.* 2007;8:41-59.
3. Kuk JL, Ardern CI. Influence of age on the association between various measures of obesity and all-cause mortality. *J Am Geriatr Soc.* 2009;57:2077-2084.
4. Han TS, Tajar A, Lean ME. Obesity and weight management in the elderly. *Br Med Bull.* 2011;97:169-196.
5. Osher E, Stern N. Obesity in elderly subjects: in sheep's clothing perhaps, but still a wolf! *Diabetes Care.* 2009;32(Suppl 2):S398-S402.
6. Arterburn DE, Crane PK, Sullivan SD. The coming epidemic of obesity in elderly Americans. *J Am Geriatr Soc.* 2004;52:1907-1912.
7. Lim EL, Hollingsworth KG, Aribisala BS, Chen MJ, Mathers JC, Taylor R. Reversal of type 2 diabetes: normalisation of beta cell function in association with decreased pancreas and liver triacylglycerol. *Diabetologia.* 2011;54:2506-2514.
8. Chau D, Cho LM, Jani P, St Jeor ST. Individualizing recommendations for weight management in the elderly. *Curr Opin Clin Nutr Metab Care.* 2008;11:27-31.
9. Florez H, Troen BR. Fat and inflammaging: a dual path to unfitness in elderly people? *J Am Geriatr Soc.* 2008;56:558-560.
10. Gutierrez-Fisac JL, Guallar-Castillon P, Leon-Munoz LM, Graciani A, Banegas JR, Rodriguez-Artalejo F. Prevalence of general and abdominal obesity in the adult population of Spain, 2008-2010: the ENRICA study. *Obes Rev.* 2012;13:388-392.
11. Kennedy RL, Chokkalingham K, Srinivasan R. Obesity in the elderly: who should we be treating, and why, and how? *Curr Opin Clin Nutr Metab Care.* 2004;7:3-9.
12. Goodpaster BH, Krishnaswami S, Harris TB, et al. Obesity, regional body fat distribution, and the metabolic syndrome in older men and women. *Arch Intern Med.* 2005;165:777-783.
13. Beydoun MA, Beydoun HA, Wang Y. Obesity and central obesity as risk factors for incident dementia and its subtypes: a systematic review and meta-analysis. *Obes Rev.* 2008;9:204-218.
14. Bokura H, Yamaguchi S, Iijima K, Nagai A, Oguro H. Metabolic syndrome is associated with silent ischemic brain lesions. *Stroke.* 2008;39:1607-1609.
15. Harrington J, Lee-Chiong T. Obesity and aging. *Clin Chest Med.* 2009;30:609-614, x.
16. McTigue KM, Hess R, Ziouras J. Obesity in older adults: a systematic review of the evidence for diagnosis and treatment. *Obesity (Silver Spring).* 2006;14:1485-1497.
17. McCarthy LH, Bigal ME, Katz M, Derby C, Lipton RB. Chronic pain and obesity in elderly people: results from the Einstein aging study. *J Am Geriatr Soc.* 2009;57:115-119.
18. Jensen GL. Obesity and functional decline: epidemiology and geriatric consequences. *Clin Geriatr Med.* 2005;21:677-687, v.
19. Mathus-Vliegen EM. Prevalence, pathophysiology, health consequences and treatment options of obesity in the elderly: a guideline. *Obes Facts.* 2012;5:460-483.
20. Crandall J, Schade D, Ma Y, et al. The influence of age on the effects of lifestyle modification and metformin in prevention of diabetes. *J Gerontol A Biol Sci Med Sci.* 2006;61:1075-1081.

21. Villareal DT, Apovian CM, Kushner RF, Klein S. Obesity in older adults: technical review and position statement of the American Society for Nutrition and NAASO, The Obesity Society. *Obes Res.* 2005;13:1849-1863.
22. Hauptman J, Lucas C, Boldrin MN, Collins H, Segal KR. Orlistat in the long-term treatment of obesity in primary care settings. *Arch Fam Med.* 2000;9:160.
23. Kissane NA, Pratt JS. Medical and surgical treatment of obesity. *Best Pract Res Clin Anaesthesiol.* 2011;25:11-25.
24. Lang IA, Llewellyn DJ, Alexander K, Melzer D. Obesity, physical function, and mortality in older adults. *J Am Geriatr Soc.* 2008;56:1474-1478.
25. Sjöström L, Lindroos AK, Peltonen M, et al. Lifestyle, diabetes, and cardiovascular risk factors 10 years after bariatric surgery. *N Engl J Med.* 2004;351:2683-2693.
26. National Institutes of Health. Clinical guidelines on the identification, evaluation, and treatment of overweight and obesity in adults: the evidence report. *Obes Res.* 1998;6(Suppl 2):51S-209S.
27. Flum DR, Salem L, Elrod JAB, Dellinger EP, Cheadle A, Chan L. Early mortality among Medicare beneficiaries undergoing bariatric surgical procedures. *JAMA.* 2005;294:1903-1908.
28. Dorman RB, Abraham AA, Al-Refaie WB, Parsons HM, Ikramuddin S, Habermann EB. Bariatric surgery outcomes in the elderly: an ACS NSQIP study. *J Gastrointest Surg.* 2012;16:35-44;discussion 44.
29. Flum DR, Belle SH, King WC, et al. Perioperative safety in the longitudinal assessment of bariatric surgery. *N Engl J Med.* 2009;361:445-454.
30. DeMaria EJ, Portenier D, Wolfe L. Obesity surgery mortality risk score: proposal for a clinically useful score to predict mortality risk in patients undergoing gastric bypass. *Surg Obes Relat Dis.* 2007;3:134-140.
31. Ramanan B, Gupta PK, Gupta H, Fang X, Forse RA. Development and validation of a bariatric surgery mortality risk calculator. *J Am Coll Surg.* 2012;214:892-900.
32. Turner PL, Saager L, Dalton J, et al. A nomogram for predicting surgical complications in bariatric surgery patients. *Obes Surg.* 2011;21:655-662.
33. Chow WB, Rosenthal RA, Merkow RP, Ko CY, Esnaola NF. Optimal preoperative assessment of the geriatric surgical patient: a best practices guideline from the American College of Surgeons National Surgical Quality Improvement Program and the American Geriatrics Society. *J Am Coll Surg.* 2012;215:453-466.
34. Lynch J, Belgaumkar A. Bariatric surgery is effective and safe in patients over 55: a systematic review and meta-analysis. *Obes Surg.* 2012;22:1507-1516.
35. Perry CD, Hutter MM, Smith DB, Newhouse JP, McNeil BJ. Survival and changes in comorbidities after bariatric surgery. *Ann Surg.* 2008;247:21-27.
36. Varela JE, Wilson SE, Nguyen NT. Outcomes of bariatric surgery in the elderly. *Am Surg.* 2006;72:865-869.
37. Fischer L, Hildebrandt C, Bruckner T, et al. Excessive weight loss after sleeve gastrectomy: a systematic review. *Obes Surg.* 2012;22:721-731.
38. Hamoui N, Anthone GJ, Kaufman HS, Crookes PF. Sleeve gastrectomy in the high-risk patient. *Obes Surg.* 2006;16:1445-1449.
39. Leivonen MK, Juuti A, Jaser N, Mustonen H. Laparoscopic sleeve gastrectomy in patients over 59 years: early recovery and 12-month follow-up. *Obes Surg.* 2011;21:1180-1187.
40. Ramirez A, Roy M, Hidalgo JE, Szomstein S, Rosenthal RJ. Outcomes of bariatric surgery in patients >70 years old. *Surg Obes Relat Dis.* 2012;8:458-462.
41. Gonzalez R, Lin E, Mattar SG, Venkatesh KR, Smith CD. Gastric bypass for morbid obesity in patients 50 years or older: is laparoscopic technique safer? *Am Surg.* 2003;69:547-553, discussion 553-534.
42. Wittgrove AC, Martinez T. Laparoscopic gastric bypass in patients 60 years and older: early postoperative morbidity and resolution of comorbidities. *Obes Surg.* 2009;19:1472-1476.
43. Fazylov R, Soto E, Merola S. Laparoscopic Roux-en-Y gastric bypass in morbidly obese patients > or =55 years old. *Obes Surg.* 2008;18:656-659.
44. Willkomm CM, Fisher TL, Barnes GS, Kennedy CI, Kuhn JA. Surgical weight loss >65 years old: is it worth the risk? *Surg Obes Relat Dis.* 2010;6:491-496.
45. Busetto L, Angrisani L, Basso N, Favretti F, Furbetta F, Lorenzo M. Safety and efficacy of laparoscopic adjustable gastric banding in the elderly. *Obesity (Silver Spring).* 2008;16:334-338.

15

Metabolic Surgery for Diabetes

Ashwin Soni, MD, BSc; Alpana Shukla, MD, MRCP(UK);
and Francesco Rubino, MD

Bariatric surgery (from the Greek "baros," which means weight) refers to surgery that is aimed primarily at weight loss, and has thus been referred to and is synonymous with "weight loss surgery." In recent years, it has been recognized that bariatric surgery confers benefits that extend beyond weight loss, and also that the mechanisms involved in amelioration of diabetes are in part weight independent.[1] While the benefits of bariatric surgery are now clearly established in the morbidly obese,[2-4] there is increasing evidence that less obese individuals (body mass index [BMI] < 35 kg/m^2) with type 2 diabetes mellitus may also benefit similarly. A group of multidisciplinary international experts convened at the Diabetes Surgery Summit in Rome in 2007,[5] and came to the consensus that gastrointestinal surgery should be considered in the treatment protocol of type 2 diabetes. The concept of metabolic surgery or "diabetes surgery" has thus evolved to define a surgical approach to correct hyperglycemia and other metabolic aberrations, and not simply excess weight.[6] Recently, the International Diabetes Federation (IDF) released a Position Statement that is intended to create awareness of the availability of other treatment options in type 2 diabetes. The IDF statement recommends that surgical options should be considered when existing therapies fail to achieve acceptable targets that are set to reduce complications and improve the quality of life.[7,8] Metabolic surgery introduces the possibility of eradicating type 2 diabetes or obtaining a long-term remission for diabetes.

Obesity and type 2 diabetes mellitus are worldwide epidemics. Obesity has an estimated worldwide prevalence of at least 400 million.[9] Type 2 diabetes mellitus had a worldwide prevalence among adults of at least 285 million in 2010, and this will increase to 439 million adults by 2030.[10] Nonsurgical treatment of severe obesity, including lifestyle intervention and approved pharmacotherapy, has not been demonstrated to provide adequate long-term results. The management of type 2 diabetes has conventionally been one of medical management combined with exercise and nutritional therapy. The progressive nature of type 2 diabetes requires escalating medical therapy, oral hypoglycemic agents, and insulin over time. Pharmacotherapy has advanced over the past few years; however, there are still limitations regarding the efficacy of drugs in achieving glycemic targets and prevention of cardiovascular disease. Conventional treatment of type 2 diabetes mellitus aims to control glycemia and not to induce remission of disease. Conversely, surgical treatment

Forse RA, Apovian CM, eds.
Bariatric Surgery: What Every Provider Needs to Know (pp 171-179).

has the potential to achieve disease remission and the prevention of cardiovascular disease and death.[4] In this chapter, we will review and discuss the outcomes of metabolic/bariatric surgery and indications for surgical treatment.

Overview of Metabolic Surgical Procedures

Conventional Surgical Procedures

Several gastrointestinal procedures are in use and have conventionally been used in bariatric surgery. These include laparoscopic adjustable gastric banding (LAGB), sleeve gastrectomy (SG), Roux-en-Y gastric bypass (RYGB), and biliopancreatic diversion (BPD). All procedures are currently performed primarily by a laparoscopic approach.

- LAGB is a restrictive procedure in which the upper part of the stomach is encircled with a saline-filled band to restrict the gastric volume and to produce early satiety during meals. The band is wrapped around the superior portion of the stomach, just distal to the gastroesophageal junction.[1]
- SG involves the removal of approximately 75% of the stomach along a line roughly parallel to the greater curvature, resulting in a thin, crescent-shaped stomach lacking the majority of its fundus.[1]
- RYGB is the most commonly performed bariatric procedure. A surgical stapler is used to create a small gastric pouch usually less than 30 cc in size, and a gastrojejunostomy is created between the small pouch and a portion of the jejunum. Bile and nutrients mix in the distal jejunum and can be absorbed through the remaining portion of the small bowel. Post-RYGB, ingested food bypasses approximately 95% of the stomach, the entire duodenum, and a short portion of the jejunum.[1]
- BPD is a malabsorptive procedure involving a gastric resection, usually leaving behind a 200- to 500-mL-sized stomach, in addition to a long intestinal bypass. Bile and nutrients mix in a short 50- to 100-cm "common limb" proximal to the ileocecal valve. The gastric resection can be horizontal as in the original Scopinaro procedure,[11] or vertical SG in its variant named biliopancreatic diversion with duodenal switch (BPD-DS).[12]

Novel Procedures

Novel surgical procedures specifically aimed at the control of diabetes without producing weight loss are currently the subject of translational and clinical research.[13] Recently, there has been an increasing interest in the development of potentially safer and reversible alternatives to conventional bariatric surgical procedures. Endoluminal and transgastric procedures are evolving concepts that combine the skills and techniques of flexible endoscopy with minimally invasive surgery.[14]

A vast array of endoscopic and less invasive methods is being investigated to address the issue of obesity and the associated metabolic derangements. These include endoscopic restrictive procedures, endoluminal sleeves, and intragastric balloons. The physiologic basis behind the use of endoluminal-duodenal sleeves is derived from the duodenal-jejunal bypass (DJB) developed by Rubino et al.[15,16] This operation was designed to investigate the mechanisms of action of gastric bypass surgery. The DJB is a gastric sparing variant of the RYGB, in which the stomach is left intact, and a short segment of the proximal intestine is bypassed, equivalent to the amount of intestine bypassed in a RYGB. This has demonstrated that duodenal exclusion can improve diabetes in rodent models and in humans with minimal or no weight loss.[17,18] Rubino et al developed an experimental model using an endoluminal sleeve to prevent contact between nutrients and duodenal mucosa in rats,[1] thereby producing a functional duodenal bypass without creating a rapid delivery of nutrients to the distal bowel. The endoluminal sleeve is essentially a flexible plastic sleeve that excludes the proximal intestine from ingested nutrients, thus mimicking the duodenal exclusion of the RYGB.[1,16] Rats undergoing the endoluminal sleeve showed dramatic improvement of glucose tolerance compared to matched controls in which the endoluminal sleeve had been fenestrated to allow nutrients to come into contact with the duodenal mucosa.[1] Consistent results regarding the antidiabetic effects of endoluminal sleeves were also reported by Aguirre et al[19] in a diet-induced rat model of insulin resistance. Recently, clinical trials have confirmed efficacy of the endoluminal sleeve approach also in humans.[20,21]

Glycemic Outcomes of Metabolic Surgery in Patients With Type 2 Diabetes Mellitus and a Body Mass Index > 35

The impact of metabolic surgery on diabetes in severely obese patients has been demonstrated consistently over the past few years. Type 2 diabetes mellitus has been shown to improve dramatically and very rapidly postoperatively after gastrointestinal surgery. The meta-analysis by Buchwald et al[22] including 22,094 patients with type 2 diabetes reported an overall 77% remission rate of type 2 diabetes (defined as persistent normoglycemia without diabetes medication after bariatric surgery). The mean procedure-specific resolution of type 2 diabetes mellitus was 48% for LAGB, 68% for vertical banded gastroplasty (VBG), 84% for RYGB, and 98% for BPD. The drawback of this study is that the majority of these studies included were retrospective and had a short follow-up duration of 1 to 3 years.

Mingrone et al conducted a randomized controlled trial[2] including 60 patients (BMI ≥ 35) and a glycated hemoglobin (HbA1c) level of 7.0% or more. These patients were randomly assigned to receive conventional medical therapy or surgical therapy including a gastric bypass or BPD. The primary endpoint was the remission of type 2 diabetes mellitus at 2 years (defined as a fasting glucose level of < 100 mg/dL and an HbA1c level of < 6.5% in the absence of pharmacologic therapy). At 2 years, diabetes remission had occurred in no patients in the medical therapy group vs 75% in the RYGB group and 95% in the BPD group. Age, sex, baseline BMI, duration of diabetes, and weight changes were not significant predictors of diabetes remission at 2 years or of improvement in glycemia at 1 and 3 months. At 2 years, the average baseline HbA1c level (8.65 ± 1.45%) had decreased in all groups, but patients in the 2 surgical groups had the greatest degree of improvement (average HbA1c levels, 7.69 ± 0.57% in the medical therapy group, 6.35 ± 1.42% in the RYGB group, and 4.95 ± 0.49% in the BPD group). This study thus demonstrated that in severely obese patients with type 2 diabetes, surgery resulted in more improved glycemic control than medical therapy alone did. Preoperative BMI and weight loss did not predict an improvement in hyperglycemia after these procedures.

Schauer et al conducted a randomized controlled trial[3] and evaluated the efficacy of intensive medical management vs medical therapy plus RYGB or SG in 150 obese patients (BMI 27 to 43) with uncontrolled type 2 diabetes mellitus. The primary endpoint was the proportion of patients with an HbA1c level of 6% or less, with or without glycemic medication, 12 months after randomization. The proportion of patients who reached the primary endpoint was 12% for the medical group, 42% in the RYGB group, and 37% in the SG group. Glycemic control was demonstrated to improve in all 3 groups with a mean HbA1c level of 7.5 ± 1.8% in the medical therapy group, 6.4 ± 0.9% in the gastric bypass group, and 6.6 ± 1.0% in the SG group. All patients in the RYGB group who achieved the primary endpoint did so without any glycemic medication, whereas 28%

in the SG group required the use of one or more glucose-lowering drugs. The improvement in glycemic endpoints was sustained over the 1 year with a reduction in glycemic medication. Patients in the medical therapy group had a more gradual improvement in glycemic control than the surgical group, and had an increase in the use of hypoglycemic medication.

In a recently published study by Adams et al,[23] 1156 severely obese patients (BMI ≥ 35) were prospectively followed for 6 years postoperatively. Diabetes remission rates 6 years after surgery were 62% in the RYGB group, 8% in control group 1 (sought to receive RYGB but did not have the surgery), and 6% in control group 2 (randomly selected from a population-based sample not seeking weight loss surgery). Among severely obese patients in this study, compared with nonsurgical control patients, the RYGB surgery group was associated with higher diabetes remission rates and a lower risk of cardiovascular and other health outcomes over 6 years.

Glycemic Outcomes of Metabolic Surgery in Patients With Type 2 Diabetes Mellitus and a Body Mass Index < 35

The effects and benefits of bariatric surgery in the morbidly obese (BMI > 35) population are well known. Recently, there has been an increasing amount of research in this field to look at the effects of metabolic surgery in those patients with a lower BMI (< 35). There is an abundance of data from both observational and retrospective studies; however, there are only a few prospective studies with regard to the lower BMI population. Several randomized controlled trials are ongoing, specifically looking at the effects of metabolic surgery on patients with a BMI < 35, comparing intensive medical vs surgical management.

Dixon et al published findings from their randomized controlled trial[24] comparing conventional medical management vs LAGB in 60 obese patients (BMI 30 to 40) with recently diagnosed type 2 diabetes mellitus (< 2 years). Two years post-surgery, 73% of the surgical group and 13% in the medical group achieved remission of diabetes (defined as fasting glucose level < 126 mg/dL and an HbA1c value < 6.2% while taking no glycemic therapy). This trial demonstrated that remission of diabetes was associated with weight loss (20.7% vs 1.7%) and lower baseline HbA1c levels.

Lee et al randomized 60 moderately obese patients (BMI 25 to 35) with poorly controlled type 2 diabetes mellitus (HbA1c > 7.5%) to either the RYGB or SG group.[25] The remission rate of diabetes (defined as fasting glucose < 126 mg/dL and an HbA1c value < 6.5% without glycemic therapy) was 93% for the RYGB group compared to 47% in the SG group.

Scopinaro et al have reported on the benefits of the BPD in 30 type 2 diabetic patients with a BMI 25 to 35.[26] One year after the BPD, mean HbA1c was 6.3% ± 0.8, with 83% of patients controlled (HbA1c ≤ 7%) without the use of hypoglycemic drugs, and the remaining showed improved glycemic control.

Shimizu et al conducted a review of the available 18 clinical studies and 477 patients, which described surgical treatment for type 2 diabetes mellitus with a mean BMI < 35.[27] Twelve studies were included in the mean estimation of fasting plasma glucose, which decreased from 203.5 to 112.5 mg/dL. Ten studies were included in the mean estimation of HbA1c, and it was found that it decreased from 9.0% to 6.3%. They also found that 86.8% of the patients were off antidiabetic medication after surgery. The main drawback is that the definition of remission or resolution of diabetes varies depending on the clinical study. Remission of diabetes was achieved in 66.0% of patients with a short history (8 years or less) of diabetes and 52.9% of those with a long history (more than 8 years). (Remission rate in this review was defined as the percentage of patients who had remission or resolution of type 2 diabetes mellitus according to the varied definition in the studies included.) From the review, it is clear that there are significant glycemic benefits after metabolic surgery, and that malabsorptive bariatric procedures (RYGB, BPD) have higher diabetes remission rates than restrictive ones (LAGB). Thus, metabolic surgery should be considered early in the diabetic stage before irreparable beta-cell damage occurs.

Cohen et al recently published their 6-year results from a prospective study investigating the effect of the RYGB on less obese patients (BMI of 30 to 35) with type 2 diabetes mellitus.[28] Their results show substantial and sustained improvement of diabetes in this population. Complete diabetes remission (defined as HbA1c < 6.5% without diabetes medication) was achieved in 88% of patients, with glycemic improvement in 11%. Interestingly, they found no association between the postoperative changes in body weight and the change in HbA1c at any postoperative time point from 6 months through to 6 years, thus suggesting weight-independent mechanisms of the RYGB. There was also no relationship between the change in weight and the magnitude of improvement in beta-cell sensitivity to glucose. The authors concluded that both the safety and efficacy of the RYGB to treat diabetes in less obese patients seemed as good, if not better, than is typically expected in patients with a BMI > 35. Therefore, the evidence suggests that a BMI cut-off of 35 is not an accurate parameter to predict the efficacy of metabolic surgery in this subset of patients.

The effects of ileal transposition associated with SG in less obese patients have also been reported, showing generally favorable results. The long-term efficacy and safety of these procedures, however, remain to be firmly established, and their use at present is recommended within experimental settings only.[29]

Extraglycemic Benefits of Gastrointestinal Surgery

Metabolic surgery results in a number of benefits beyond the reduction of glycemia, including the improvement of cardiovascular risk factors, dyslipidemia, hypertension, fertility in women with polycystic ovary syndrome (PCOS), as well as a beneficial effect on obstructive sleep apnea.

The meta-analysis by Buchwald et al[22] showed a significant reduction in total cholesterol, low-density lipoprotein cholesterol, and triglycerides after bariatric surgery. Hyperlipidemia improved in typically 70% of the patients, and the maximum improvements were shown after the RYGB and BPD or DS procedures. Hypertension was also demonstrated to resolve or improve in 78.5% of the patients.

Several studies have established that metabolic surgery improves cardiovascular risk factors such as type 2 diabetes mellitus, dyslipidemia, and hypertension. This reduction in cardiovascular risk factors may result in a reduced cardiovascular mortality.

Adams et al looked at long-term mortality by conducting a retrospective cohort study involving 7925 severely obese patients treated surgically with the RYGB, and 7925 similarly obese-matched controls.[30] After a mean follow-up of 8.4 years, surgery reduced overall mortality by 40%, cardiovascular mortality by 56%, cancer mortality by 60%, and diabetes-related mortality by 92%.

A recent study published by Romeo et al,[31] the prospective controlled intervention Swedish Obese Subjects study, aimed to specifically look at the effect of bariatric surgery on cardiovascular events on participants with type 2 diabetes, at a mean follow-up of 13.3 years. Bariatric surgery was shown to reduce myocardial infarction incidence (38 events among the 345 participants in the surgery group vs 43 events among the 262 participants in the control group). It was also noted that BMI was not related to the surgery outcome, which further supports the weight-independent effects of the surgery.

Cohen et al recently reported marked improvement in hypertension and dyslipidemia in their 6-year prospective follow-up of patients with a BMI of 30 to 35 after RYGB.[28] Hypertension resolved in 58%, hypercholesterolemia resolved in 64%, and hypertriglyceridemia resolved in 58%.

This resulted in 50% to 84% reductions in predicted 10-year cardiovascular disease risks of fatal and nonfatal coronary heart disease and stroke.

Obstructive sleep apnea has been shown to be associated with the metabolic syndrome in general, and specifically type 2 diabetes and insulin resistance. Obstructive sleep apnea is extremely prevalent in the obese population, but a relationship has been shown between obstructive sleep apnea and metabolic syndrome in patients of a lower mean BMI ranging between 29 and 36.7, demonstrating the relationship to be less weight dependent in these patients.[32] Obstructive sleep apnea syndrome is characterized by an apnea-hypopnea index (AHI) > 5 on polysomnography and excessive daytime sleepiness.

Metabolic surgery results in marked weight loss and very significant reductions in AHI allowing some patients to discontinue using continuous positive airway pressure (CPAP). However, in severely obese patients, even large reductions in AHI may still leave them with persistent obstructive sleep apnea that will continue to require ongoing treatment.[33] Greenburg et al performed a meta-analysis involving 342 patients, in which a mean reduction in BMI from 55.3 to 37.7 led to a combined 71% reduction in the AHI. Resolution of obstructive sleep apnea, defined as an AHI < 5, was seen in 38% of this patient population.[34] However, the effect on sleep apnea may vary with the type of surgical procedure. In fact, a recent study by Dixon et al[35] showed no statistically greater reduction in AHI in obese patients when comparing the LAGB to conventional weight loss therapy.

PCOS is also a very prevalent metabolic disorder and is closely associated with obesity, insulin resistance, and type 2 diabetes. Escobar-Morreale et al showed, in a case series of 17 patients,[36] that females who underwent either BPD or RYGB had almost complete resolution of PCOS, with serum androgen concentrations normalizing and an increase of sex hormone binding globulin. Hirsutism improved or normalized in all but one patient, and there was also an improvement of other metabolic parameters such as insulin sensitivity and dyslipidemia.

PCOS has been shown to be effectively managed by surgery, and the resolution of these problems occurs very soon postoperatively, thus improving fertility. However, further research is necessary in this field, especially focusing on the role of metabolic surgery in females with a lower BMI.

Metabolic Surgery for Type 2 Diabetes: Integration Into Clinical Guidelines

Several experimental and observational studies have been conducted, as well as the recent randomized controlled trials, prospectively analyzing the effects of metabolic surgery on type 2 diabetes. Cumulative data from both experimental and clinical studies indicate that a surgical approach may also be a viable treatment option in patients with BMI < 35 who fail medical therapy. It is envisaged that the collective evidence from the published and ongoing randomized controlled trials will help determine the optimal timing of surgery and selection of patients from the vast population of mild to moderately obese patients with diabetes. Long-term data from randomized controlled trials are required to assess the durability of these procedures and also the impact on micro- and macrovascular complications.

In keeping with current evidence, the IDF has included bariatric surgery in its treatment guidelines for type 2 diabetes mellitus and has called for its integration into other national and international treatment guidelines for diabetes. The IDF position statement recommends bariatric surgery as an accepted treatment option in people who have diabetes and BMI > 35, and that surgery should be considered as an alternative treatment option in patients with a BMI between 30 to 35 when diabetes cannot be adequately controlled by an optimal medical regimen, especially in the presence of other major cardiovascular risk factors. In Asians and some other ethnicities of increased risk, BMI action points may be reduced by 2.5.[7,8]

Physiological Mechanisms Behind the Metabolic Effects of Gastrointestinal Surgery

Gastrointestinal operations have been shown to improve insulin sensitivity and secretion. Insulin sensitivity improves after gastrointestinal surgery with a concomitant elevation in the levels of the insulin-sensitizing hormone adiponectin.[37] The concentration of insulin receptors and markers of insulin signaling increase and the lipid content within the muscle and liver also decreases after bariatric surgery.[37]

There has been growing evidence that the antidiabetes effect of gastrointestinal surgery is not just due to weight loss, but it is also caused by weight-independent effects. In lean diabetic Goto-Kakizaki rats, DJB rapidly and durably improves fasting glucose and post-prandial hyperglycemia, compared with sham-operated animals that have equivalent weight loss by food restriction.[15] Similar results for DJB have been reported by other groups.[38] Recently, Breen et al[18] reported that the effect of DJB on glycemia is weight and insulin independent owing to an enhancement of nutrient-sensing mechanisms in the gut.

Following the RYGB or BPD in humans, type 2 diabetes mellitus typically resolves within days to weeks, long before major weight loss has occurred. Schauer et al demonstrated that out of the patients who had preoperative diabetes treated with oral hypoglycemic medication and/or insulin, 30% had normalization of their plasma glucose levels and were discontinued from all diabetes medications at discharge post-RYGB.[39] In comparison, purely restrictive procedures, such as the LAGB, improve glycemia only after significant weight loss is achieved.[1] Growing evidence supports the fact that procedures (RYGB, BPD) involving rerouting of food may improve diabetes by enhancing insulin sensitivity and/or by improving beta-cell function, beyond what could be expected by weight loss alone.[27]

The exact physiological mechanisms behind the remission of type 2 diabetes mellitus still remain elusive. However, it is clear that these gastrointestinal surgeries induce a significant alteration of the gut hormonal milieu. Several gut hormones are altered postoperatively, and the ways in which they change depend largely on whether the procedure involves intestinal diversion or whether it is simply a restrictive procedure (LAGB). For instance, plasma levels of glucagon-like peptide-1, peptide YY, and ghrelin have all been shown to be altered after gastrointestinal surgery. The post-prandial glucagon-like peptide-1 and peptide YY response to oral glucose or a mixed test meal is consistently augmented following gastric bypass surgery or SG, while no change is observed after the LAGB.[12] Furthermore, ghrelin does not show the expected rise following weight loss after the RYGB.[12]

Other mechanisms behind the weight-independent effects of the RYGB that are currently being researched include bile acid perturbations, taste alterations,[40] and changes in intestinal nutrient-sensing mechanisms regulating insulin sensitivity.[18]

Summary

The newly emerging field of metabolic surgery aims to improve metabolic disease, including type 2 diabetes, which has become extremely prevalent in recent years. Despite the advancement in pharmacotherapy, many patients still fail to achieve adequate glycemic parameters and reduction of cardiometabolic risk. Metabolic surgery provides a suitable alternative for those who fail lifestyle interventions and medical therapy. Further research is required in this field to identify the long-term effects, and to better define the exact role of surgery among those patients who have a lower BMI. Ongoing research in this field also offers the potential to discover new therapeutic targets in order to improve and advance pharmacotherapy and the understanding of type 2 diabetes.

References

1. Rubino F, Schauer PR, Kaplan LM, et al. Metabolic surgery to treat type 2 diabetes: clinical outcomes and mechanisms of action. *Ann Rev Med.* 2010;61:393-411.
2. Mingrone G, Panunzi S, De Gaetano A, et al. Bariatric surgery versus conventional medical therapy for type 2 diabetes. *N Engl J Med.* 2012;366(17):1577-1585.
3. Schauer PR, Kashyap SR, Wolski K, et al. Bariatric surgery versus intensive medical therapy in obese patients with diabetes. *N Engl J Med.* 2012;366(17):1567-1576.
4. Carlsson LM, Peltonen M, Ahlin S, et al. Bariatric surgery and prevention of type 2 diabetes in Swedish obese subjects. *N Engl J Med.* 2012;367(8):695-704.
5. Rubino F, Kaplan LM, Schauer PR, et al. The Diabetes Surgery Summit consensus conference: recommendations for the evaluation and use of gastrointestinal surgery to treat type 2 diabetes mellitus. *Ann Surg.* 2010;251(3):399-405.
6. Rubino F, Shukla AP, Pomp A, et al. Bariatric, metabolic and diabetes surgery: what's in a name? *Ann Surg.* 2014;259(1):117-122.
7. Zimmet P, Alberti KG, Rubino F, et al. IDF's view of bariatric surgery in type 2 diabetes. *Lancet.* 2011;378(9786):108-110.
8. Dixon JB, Zimmet P, Alberti KG, et al. Bariatric surgery: an IDF statement for obese type 2 diabetes. *Diabet Med.* 2011;28(6):628-642.
9. Nguyen DM, El-Serag HB. The epidemiology of obesity. *Gastroenterol Clin North Am.* 2010;39(1):1-7.
10. Shaw JE, Sicree RA, Zimmet PZ. Global estimates of the prevalence of diabetes for 2010 and 2030. *Diabetes Res Clin Pract.* 2010;87(1):4-14.
11. Scopinaro N, Marinari GM, Camerini G. Laparoscopic standard biliopancreatic diversion: technique and preliminary results. *Obes Surg.* 2002;12(2):241-244.
12. Shukla AP, Ahn SM, Patel RT, et al. Surgical treatment of type 2 diabetes: the surgeon perspective. *Endocrine.* 2011;40(2):151-161.
13. Dixon JB, le Roux CW, Rubino F, et al. Bariatric surgery for type 2 diabetes. *Lancet.* 2012;379(9833):2300-2311.
14. Schauer P, Chand B, Brethauer S. New applications for endoscopy: the emerging field of endoluminal and transgastric bariatric surgery. *Surg Endosc.* 2007;21(3):347-356.
15. Rubino F, Marescaux J. Effect of duodenal-jejunal exclusion in a nonobese animal model of type 2 diabetes: a new perspective for an old disease. *Ann Surg.* 2004;239:1-11.
16. Soni A, Shukla AP, Rubino F. Interventional diabetology: the evolution of diabetes care in the XXI century. *Curr Atheroscler Rep.* 2012;14:631-636.
17. Rubino F, Forgione A, Cummings DE, et al. The mechanism of diabetes control after gastrointestinal bypass surgery reveals a role of the proximal small intestine in the pathophysiology of type 2 diabetes. *Ann Surg.* 2006;244(5):741-749.
18. Breen DM, Rasmussen BA, Kokorovic A, et al. Jejunal nutrient sensing is required for duodenal-jejunal bypass surgery to rapidly lower glucose concentrations in uncontrolled diabetes. *Nat Med.* 2012;18(6):950-955.
19. Aguirre V, Stylopoulos N, Grinbaum R, et al. An endoluminal sleeve induces substantial weight loss and normalizes glucose homeostasis in rats with diet-induced obesity. *Obesity.* 2008;16:2585-2592.
20. Tarnoff M, Rodriguez L, Escalona A, et al. Open label, prospective, randomized controlled trial of an endoscopic duodenal-jejunal bypass sleeve versus low calorie diet for pre-operative weight loss in bariatric surgery. *Surg Endosc.* 2009;23(3):650-665.
21. Espinet-Coll E, Nebreda-Durán J, Gómez-Valero JA, et al. Current endoscopic techniques in the treatment of obesity. *Rev Esp Enferm Dig.* 2012;104(2):72-87.
22. Buchwald H, Avidor Y, Braunwald E, et al. Bariatric surgery: a systematic review and meta-analysis. *JAMA.* 2004;292(14):1724-1737.
23. Adams TD, Davidson LE, Litwin SE, et al. Health benefits of gastric bypass surgery after 6 years. *JAMA.* 2012;308(11):1122-1131.
24. Dixon JB, O'Brien PE, Playfair J, et al. Adjustable gastric banding and conventional therapy for type 2 diabetes: a randomized controlled trial. *JAMA.* 2008;299(3):316-323.
25. Lee WJ, Chong K, Ser KH. Gastric bypass vs sleeve gastrectomy for type 2 diabetes mellitus. *Arch Surg.* 2011;146(2):143-148.

26. Scopinaro N, Adami GF, Papadia FS, et al. Effects of biliopancreatic diversion on type 2 diabetes with BMI 25 to 35. *Ann Surg.* 2011;253(4):699-703.
27. Shimizu H, Timratana, P, Schauer PR, et al. Review of metabolic surgery for type 2 diabetes in patients with a BMI < 35 kg/m^2. *J Obes.* 2012;2012:147256.
28. Cohen RV, Pinheiro JC, Schiavon CA, et al. Effects of gastric bypass surgery in patients with type 2 diabetes and only mild obesity. *Diabetes Care.* 2012;35(7):1420-1428.
29. DePaula AL, Stival AR, De Paula CCL, et al. Surgical treatment of type 2 diabetes in patients with BMI below 35: mid-term outcomes of the laparoscopic ileal interposition associated with a sleeve gastrectomy in 202 consecutive cases. *J Gastrointest Surg.* 2012;16(5):967-976.
30. Adams TD, Gress RE, Smith SC, et al. Long-term mortality after gastric bypass surgery. *N Engl J Med.* 2007;357(8):753-761.
31. Romeo S, Maglio C, Burza MA, et al. Cardiovascular events after bariatric surgery in obese subjects with type 2 diabetes. *Diabetes Care.* 2012;35(12):2613-2617.
32. Coughlin SR, Mawdsley L, Mugarza JA, et al. Obstructive sleep apnoea is independently associated with an increased prevalence of metabolic syndrome. *Eur Heart J.* 2004;25(9):735-741.
33. Lettieri CJ, Eliasson AH, Greenburg DL. Persistence of obstructive sleep apnea after surgical weight loss. *J Clin Sleep Med.* 2008;4(4):333-338.
34. Greenburg DL, Lettieri CJ, Eliasson AH. Effects of surgical weight loss on measures of obstructive sleep apnea: a meta-analysis. *Am J Med.* 2009;122(6):535-542.
35. Dixon JB, Schachter LM, O'Brien PE, et al. Surgical vs conventional therapy for weight loss treatment of obstructive sleep apnea: a randomized controlled trial. *JAMA.* 2012;308(11):1142-1149.
36. Escobar-Morreale HF, Botella-Carretero JI, Álvarez-Blasco F, et al. The polycystic ovary syndrome associated with morbid obesity may resolve after weight loss induced by bariatric surgery. *J Clin Endocrinol Metab.* 2005;90(12):6364-6369.
37. Thaler JP, Cummings DE. Minireview: hormonal and metabolic mechanisms of diabetes remission after gastrointestinal surgery. *Endocrinology.* 2009;150(6):2518-2525.
38. Liu S, Zhang G, Wang L, et al. The entire small intestine mediates the changes in glucose homeostasis after intestinal surgery in Goto-Kakizaki rats. *Ann Surg.* 2012;256:1049-1058.
39. Schauer PR, Burguera B, Ikramuddin S, et al. Effect of laparoscopic Roux-en Y gastric bypass on type 2 diabetes mellitus. *Ann Surg.* 2003;238(4):467-484.
40. Papamargaritis D, Panteliou E, Miras AD, et al. Mechanisms of weight loss, diabetes control and changes in food choice after gastrointestinal surgery. *Curr Atheroscler Rep.* 2012;14(6):616-623.

16

Immediate Postoperative Complications

Charles E. Thompson III, MD; Yaniv Cozacov, MD; Emanuele Lo Menzo, MD, PhD; and Raul J. Rosenthal, MD

For the past 20 years, the main bariatric procedures performed were the laparoscopic adjustable gastric band (LAGB) and the laparoscopic Roux-en-Y gastric bypass (RYGB). More recently, the laparoscopic sleeve gastrectomy (LSG) has been performed with increasing frequency.[1] These 3 procedures are currently the most common bariatric operations performed. The LSG seems to be positioned between the LAGB and RYGB in terms of its effectiveness in losing excess weight, treating comorbidities, and its morbidity and mortality profiles.[2] With patients often presenting to multiple emergency rooms postoperatively, it is essential that every general surgeon be aware of the possible early complications involved with these procedures.

Immediate complications are defined as those that happen within 30 days of surgery.

Laparoscopic Adjustable Banding

The placement of the LAGB is often thought of by the patient to be the least invasive of the 3 main bariatric procedures. The LAGB seems to be a safer procedure with frequent, but less severe, long-term complications.[3] While this may be true in the short term, it can still be associated with devastating postoperative complications.

Band Slippage

Band slippage is the most common postoperative complication after LAGB.[4] This complication can happen in the early or late postoperative period. Patients normally present with an abrupt onset of nausea and vomiting, followed by retching, after being completely asymptomatic. Any patient who presents with this constellation of symptoms and history of an LAGB placement should undergo prompt band deflation, in some selected patients nasogastric tube placement under radiographic visualization, followed by an upper gastrointestinal (UGI) series. The UGI will show a characteristic horizontal band configuration, as opposed to the normal obliquely situated band. Slippage occurs when gastric tissue slips through the band, severely decreasing or completely

Forse RA, Apovian CM, eds.
Bariatric Surgery: What Every Provider Needs to Know (pp 181-191).

closing the stoma. To prevent this from happening, most surgeons plicate gastric tissue around the band by suturing the gastric fundus proximal to the band to the fundus immediately distal to the band—in effect, holding the band in place. Others have added an additional stitch between the fundus and left crus of the diaphragm to further stabilize the stomach. Different types of slippage have been described: anterior, posterior, and total. Anterior slippage usually occurs when the anterior plicating suture is ineffective. Posterior slippage takes place when the lesser curve slips posteriorly into the lesser sac. Since the adoption of a different technique of band insertion, this complication has virtually disappeared. Total slippage occurs when the entire stomach, anterior and posterior, slips through the band, often completely closing the stoma. Once a band slippage has been diagnosed, all fluid in the band must be removed immediately. This, along with continuous nasogastric suction, should offer relief to most patients. If symptoms subside after band deflation, it is acceptable to electively schedule a patient for band reposition or possible removal. However, in cases where symptoms do not subside or patients have signs of possible infection, such as fever and leukocytosis, band slippage represents a surgical emergency where the band must be removed promptly.[4]

Gastric/Esophageal Perforation

Gastric or distal esophageal perforations present as a result of a variety of different mechanisms, most of them related to the dissection needed for placement of the band and sometimes with the advancement of nasogastric or calibrating tubes. Gastric perforations should be distinguished from gastric erosions where the band erodes into the gastric wall, often causing sepsis and critical illness (erosion is a late complication of gastric banding). In order to place the band in the proper position, the pars flaccida, angle of His, and left crus of the diaphragm are dissected, and a retroesophageal window is created. This manipulation exposes the stomach to potential iatrogenic perforation. Additionally, placing the band around the stomach is commonly done blindly, increasing the risk of gastric perforation.[5] In both cases, the band placement should be aborted; if the band is in place, it should be removed. The presence of a distal esophageal or gastric perforation along with a distal obstruction caused by the band will result in a nonhealing fistula and infection of the prosthesis.

Postoperative Obstruction

This complication is worth mentioning because of its relative frequency with which patients may complain of nausea and inability to tolerate even liquids immediately postoperatively. After placing the band, it is not uncommon for patients to have partially obstructive symptoms mainly due to an overadjusted band. Though the band is not filled until a later date, the mere presence of the band itself places mild restriction on the stomach, thus causing mild symptoms. The patient will eventually adjust to having the band in place, as postoperative swelling and edema subside. If the physician has extra concern about the patient's symptoms, a UGI with passage of contrast through the band will ease his or her concern. Occasionally an early endoscopy can facilitate resolution of the transient outlet obstruction. In a selected group of patients when symptoms do not resolve, or even get worse, the band has to be removed.

Port Flippage

Occasionally the subcutaneous port (used to adjust the band) may "flip" or rotate 180 degrees in its subcutaneous pocket. This usually happens because the port is not firmly stabilized to the fascia. Port flipping is important because it inhibits band adjustment, making it more difficult and causing tremendous patient anxiety. A skilled surgeon may be able to manipulate the port under fluoroscopy if only partially rotated. Occasionally, the patient may have to return to the operating room in order to stabilize the port in its subcutaneous pocket.

Sleeve Gastrectomy

In recent years, the enthusiasm for LSG as a definitive procedure for the treatment of morbid obesity has increased.[6] It has been associated with similar outcomes (resolution of comorbidities, postoperative complications, etc) as the gastric bypass[1] without the malabsorption and other long-term complications that can arise from the bypass procedure. Data reported by our center and many others place the LSG as one of the safest procedures when it comes to long-term morbidity. However, as with any surgical procedure, there are complications that may occur in the early postoperative period. LSG appears to be a simple but not easy procedure, with the longest staple line in surgery.

Staple Line Leaks and Abscesses

Staple line leaks are the most dreaded early postoperative surgical complication after a sleeve gastrectomy and are the most common cause of major morbidity and mortality after LSG.[7] These leaks are usually detected postoperatively when a routine UGI series is performed to detect this complication. Most of these leaks occur at or near the gastroesophageal junction. According to the law of Laplace, as the radius of a hollow, tubular object decreases, the intraluminal pressure increases, creating increased tension on the wall of the object. With a competent lower esophageal sphincter and pylorus, the intraluminal pressure inside the remaining stomach (sleeve) increases. This might cause an increased intragastric pressure on the staple line in the region of the gastroesophageal junction. Other potential reasons for this complication are ischemia, staple line hematoma, and use of nonabsorbable sutures for staple line reinforcement. Despite this rise in intraluminal pressure in all sleeve gastrectomies, the incidence of staple line leak is very low.[1,8-10] When using a stapler to create the sleeve, it is important to stay lateral to the fat pad at the angle of His that lies immediately to the left of the gastroesophageal junction. Using a stapler device or even dissecting too close to this region exposes the patient to an increased risk of leak in that region. While it is imperative to mobilize the fundus so as not to include it in the sleeve, going lateral to the gastroesophageal junction fat pad often leaves a "dog ear" of stomach that is seen on a postoperative UGI.

Management options for sleeve-related staple line leaks are numerous and are debated in the metabolic surgery community. Invasive techniques include immediate reoperation with an attempt at suture reinforcement of the leak site, laparoscopic or open exploration with drainage, and placement of a drain, creating a controlled fistula. Conversion to a Roux-en-Y esophagojejunostomy bypass procedure should be considered as a contraindication in the immediate postoperative period. In emergencies, surgeons should always choose the smallest procedure and RYGB should be a treatment option not before 12 weeks after the leak was diagnosed and provided the patient is not showing signs of infection and malnutrition. Exploration with an attempt at suture repair is generally not advised. When the leak is discovered, the area of the leak is often inflamed and friable, making suture reinforcement difficult. It is likely that the suture repair will not hold, and the leak will manifest again. Laparoscopic exploration with irrigation, debridement, and placement of a drain is the more conservative management option. This is a temporizing procedure that is used as a bridge to a more definitive operation in the future. Doing so, however, will require the patient to be placed on long-term total parental nutrition (TPN) and nothing-by-mouth status until the concomitant inflammation/infection cools down. After this period of recovery, conversion to a Roux-en-Y esophagojejunostomy with proximal gastrectomy should be performed in experienced hands.

Less invasive techniques have been described and reported in small series. Those include radiology-guided percutaneous drainage of the resultant left upper quadrant abscess cavity with placement of draining catheter, endoscopic placement of an esophageal stent to cover the leak and decrease the relative distal obstruction of the pylorus, and endoscopic plication maneuvers to "pinch" the tissue around the leak in an effort to promote closure. Radiology-placed drainage catheters are as appropriate as laparoscopically placed drains. However, depending on the clinical status of the patient, laparoscopic or open placement may be preferred because it offers the ability for debridement and irrigation should the patient present critically ill. Self-expanding esophageal stenting is another, less invasive option in treating these leaks, particularly near the gastroesophageal junction. Stenting seems to be better suited for massive leaks to control systemic symptoms.[4] Several studies have reported esophageal stenting as having acceptable success rates without requiring another operation for LSG leaks near the gastroesophageal junction.[11,12]

Postoperative Bleeding

During the postoperative period, hemorrhage should be suspected by observing a drop in the hematocrit, persistent tachycardia despite the administration of fluid boluses, a decreased pulse pressure, or hypotension. There are 3 areas in which bleeding may occur: intra-abdominal, intraluminal, and from the trocar sites.[4] The overall incidence of postoperative bleeding is low and rarely requiring operative intervention. When the hematocrit has dropped unacceptably low, transfusion of blood products usually corrects vital signs and improves physiologic conditions. On occasion invasive measures must be undertaken to treat postoperative hemorrhaging.

Intra-abdominal bleeding after a sleeve gastrectomy normally takes place in the following locations: the gastrocolic ligament, the left upper quadrant, at the site of dissection of the fundus and ligation of the short gastric vessels takes place, and on the staple line created during the gastrectomy. In preparing the stomach for a gastrectomy, the greater omentum must be separated from the greater curve of the stomach. In doing so, the gastroepiploic artery and vein are at risk for being damaged. Usually this is seen and managed intraoperatively. Smaller vessels branching off the gastroepiploic artery and vein may bleed, and not be seen as readily, and could become the cause of a delayed presentation of hemorrhaging. The way to prevent this complication is to stay close to the greater curve of the stomach, leaving no more than a few millimeters of tissue between the greater curve and path of dissection. After the greater omentum has been removed, the short gastric arteries at the fundus must be ligated to allow full mobilization of the stomach. Often, this requires meticulous dissection in the left upper quadrant between the spleen and stomach, the gastrosplenic ligament. Without careful attention to detail, hemorrhaging in this area can be significant. Lastly, intra-abdominal bleeding can occur along the staple line when the stomach is transected. This can be treated with clip appliers or imbricating sutures, both of which readily control the bleeding. Some surgeons choose to imbricate the entire suture line routinely.

Intraluminal bleeding occurs during the deployment of the stapler along the greater curve. Just as the stapling device has the ability to cause extraluminal bleeding (intra-abdominally), it can also cause intraluminal bleeding. Unless intraoperative endoscopy is performed (usually not necessary), there is no way to know if intraluminal bleeding has occurred. If it indeed occurred, it is rarely of significance. After the operation, the patient may feel mildly nauseous, a symptom that is ubiquitous in the postoperative patient. Bleeding from a trocar site is usually seen at the conclusion of the operation when the trocars are removed. With the laparoscope, it is important to visualize the trocars being removed so that trocar site bleeding can be observed and managed.

Kinking/Stenosis/Obstruction

Though there are no surgical anastomoses in the sleeve gastrectomy, there are several points where partial obstruction or kinking can occur in the newly made sleeve. One of the most common sites of obstruction is at the incisura angularis. This is the area on the lesser curve of the stomach where the corpus transitions to the antrum, creating an almost 90-degree angle. Without proper attention to stapling techniques while forming the sleeve, this area can become a narrowing where food has difficulty passing through. Should the patient experience persistent nausea and vomiting, a conversion to an RYGB may be necessary.

The size of bougies in creating the sleeve also has an effect on the obstructive nature of the sleeve. In our experience, bougie sizes less than 38 Fr. seem to be associated with increased symptoms of nausea and vomiting without having the benefit of increased weight loss.

Roux-en-Y Gastric Bypass

The RYGB has until recently been the gold standard procedure in bariatric surgery. For the past 30 years it has been the most common procedure performed for the purpose of weight loss. Different than the previously mentioned procedures, it is both a restrictive and malabsorptive procedure, resulting in the most amount of weight loss and greater resolution of comorbidities. However, with the RYGB comes a host of complications, many nonsurgical. Below we will discuss immediate postoperative surgical complications from the RYGB.

Anastomotic/Staple Line Leak

As with the sleeve gastrectomy, an anastomotic or staple line leak is considered to be one of the most devastating postoperative complications in the gastric bypass procedure. An anastomotic leak can be defined as an area of inadequate tissue healing allowing for exit of gastrointestinal material through the staple/suture line.[13] The incidence of anastomotic leaks is between 0 to 5.6% in large series.[14] Though thought to occur in the first 5 to 7 days postoperatively as a result of ischemia, 95% occur within the first 48 hours due to technical error.[14] There are 5 potential areas for anastomotic leak: (1) the pouch staple line, (2) the remnant staple line, (3) the gastrojejunostomy, (4) the Roux limb staple line, and (5) the jejunojejunostomy. Most leaks occur at the gastrojejunostomy; however, leaks are more devastating at the jejunojejunostomy because of the increase in biliary/pancreatic fluid passing through and lowered sensitivity/specificity of diagnostic tests in this region of the abdomen.[13]

Several studies have outlined risk factors associated with higher incidence for anastomotic leaks. Ischemia has been touted as the number one risk factor in the etiology of leaks.[13] Those that are at highest risk are superobese, male patients with multiple comorbidities.[15] Several technical factors may also affect the rate of anastomotic leaks in patients. The use of sealants or fibrin glues, buttressing materials on the staple line, suture reinforcement, appropriate staple sizing, bowel size matching (for the jejunojejunostomy), and the presence of tension-free anastomosis can affect the likelihood of leak postoperatively. On occasion, the surgeon may secure the Roux limb to the distal remnant stomach to prevent extra tension being placed on the gastrojejunal anastomosis. Most surgeons use some type of reinforcement of the staple lines/anastomoses. There have not been any definitive prospective randomized studies to determine the effectiveness of one form of reinforcement over the other. In making the gastrojejunal anastomosis, one can either use suture to close or use a circular stapler device. Again, no large studies have shown a significant difference in the rate of anastomotic leaks between these 2 techniques. Intraoperatively, a leak test is routinely performed to ensure the surgeon that no leak is present. This is typically done by 2 methods: (1) submerging the gastrojejunostomy in saline and forcing air from a nasogastric tube or endoscope placed distal to the anastomosis or (2) instilling methylene blue into the nasogastric tube to visualize leakage from the staple lines or suture lines.

An important piece to detecting leaks is having a high suspicion for this devastating complication. A patient who is persistently tachycardic and tachypneic postoperatively should be suspected of having a leak. A UGI is routinely obtained on postoperative day 1 on all patients to further ensure no leak is present, although the utility of this test has been challenged by some authors. Some surgeons leave drains in place after sleeve gastrectomies and gastric bypasses. If this is done, having the patient drink methylene blue and observing its presence in the drainage bulbs will confirm the presence of a leak. If neither of these techniques shows evidence of a leak but clinical suspicion remains high, a computed tomography (CT) scan of the abdomen and pelvis without contrast can aid in the diagnosis by detecting free air in the peritoneal cavity, diffuse fluid throughout the abdomen, abscess/fluid collections in the left upper quadrant, or residual contrast from the earlier UGI.[4] Normally, the UGI will show a leak, but if not, and the patient remains tachycardic with a declining clinical picture, then diagnostic laparoscopy should be performed emergently. When considering all diagnostic tests, these tests have been negative in 40% of all documented leaks.[13]

Management options vary, depending on the patient's clinical picture, surgeon experience, and judgment. All hemodynamically unstable patients require immediate surgical exploration. Operative management of gastrojejunal leaks includes copious irrigation and washing out of the abdomen with wide drainage. Placement of a gastrostomy tube through the remnant stomach is a necessity that will facilitate enteral nutrition, instead of the chronic use of TPN. Depending on the severity of inflammation and infection, primarily suturing the leak could be difficult. The tissue in the area of the leak may be too friable to hold sutures, making suture repair useless. However, if the leak is caught early, suture repair may work and would certainly decrease the time of convalescence for the patient. Though, even with healthy tissue and suture repair, drains and a feeding tube should still be placed. All the early and clinically significant jejunojejunostomy leaks should be managed operatively. The leaks, as stated before, are more devastating because of their usually delayed diagnosis and leakage contents.

In some instances, there has been a trend toward the nonoperative management of anastomotic leaks. If the patient is hemodynamically stable and a drain is left in place after the operation, a reasonable management option is to watch the patient clinically. If the patient's clinical status remains the same or improves, then the drain is serving its purpose. Experience has shown that these leaks normally close in 1 week and less than 10% of patients require reoperative intervention.[13] If the surgeon chose not to leave a drain in place, then a small leak with visible collection may be drained percutaneously (leaving the drain in place).

Postoperative Hemorrhage

Bleeding may occur either in the early or the late postoperative periods as a result of different etiologies. Early postoperative bleeding usually is a result of staple line bleeding; late postoperative bleeding usually occurs as a result of marginal ulceration or peptic ulcer disease. The incidence of postoperative hemorrhage overall is 1.1% to 4%.[13] Studies have shown that there is a slight increase in bleeding incidence in the laparoscopic technique when compared to open bypass procedures.[14] The reason behind this is thought to be the decreased tendency to buttress or reinforce the staple line in the laparoscopic technique as compared to the open. Most of these patients will stop bleeding spontaneously without the need for further intervention. On occasion, endoscopic, radiologic, or reoperative interventions are necessary.

Clinical manifestations of early gastrointestinal bleeding can vary depending on the location and timing of presentation. Signs of immediate postoperative bleeding usually manifest within the first 6 hours: tachycardia, low urine output, hypotension, and decreased pulse pressure. Hematemesis can rarely manifest as a result of intraluminal bleeding. At the same time, immediate postoperative hemorrhaging can occur in the absence of these signs, only detectable by a precipitous fall in the hematocrit. In those patients who have had drains placed, the continuous collection of frank blood in the drain can confirm the presence of active bleeding. However, the absence of the latter does not automatically rule out the presence of bleeding. Postoperative bleeding can manifest later in the early postoperative period. This bleeding is usually a result of slow oozing manifesting as melena or hematochezia. Finally, intraluminal bleeding can cause functional obstruction, especially at the level of the jejunojejunostomy. There have been risk factors associated with postoperative hemorrhaging. Chronic use of anticoagulants, antiplatelet drugs, and deep venous thrombosis prophylaxis can contribute to the incidence of postoperative bleeding.

If postoperative bleeding is diagnosed or highly suspected, judgment is used to determine the best course of treatment. A patient with tachycardia, hypotension, decreasing urine output, and a falling hematocrit immediately postoperatively (in the first 6 hours) certainly requires operative intervention. A patient who presents 5 days or more after a gastric bypass may respond to transfusion of blood products, and careful observation in the intensive care unit would be a prudent choice. The site of hemorrhaging presents a dilemma as well. If the bleeding occurs on the staple line, a laparoscopic approach would seem logical. If the bleeding is intraluminal, an endoscopic approach would seem appropriate. Without the presence of an intra-abdominal drain, nasogastric tube, or the presence of hematemesis, it is difficult to ascertain the location of bleeding. A patient with intraluminal bleeding presenting later in the postoperative period may not have melena because the intraluminal clots may produce an ileus, making the passage of blood-containing stool difficult.

The initial management of postoperative bleeding after gastric bypass is the same as with any other surgery—intravenous fluid resuscitation, insertion of foley catheter to monitor urine output, complete blood count, coagulation profile, and type and screen are mainstays. If the patient does not respond to these conservative measures, administration of blood products is required. If symptoms fail to improve despite these interventions, a more invasive approach is indicated. Usually the bleeding is intra-abdominal, thus a diagnostic laparoscopy is indicated. However, one must keep in mind the possibility of intraluminal bleeding, particularly in the patient 6 hours from surgery. In this case endoscopic management would be indicated. If bleeding arises in the gastric remnant intraluminally, laparoscopic or open approaches are the only valid options. Evacuation of blood clots and control of intraluminal bleeding inside the remnant can be controlled via transgastric enteroscopy.

Endoscopic management of active bleeding includes the injection of epinephrine solution, clipping of bleeding sites, and thermal coagulation. A UGI should be performed after any endoscopic procedure to test for leaks because of the newly fashioned anastomosis. Operative management is reserved for those with hemodynamic instability and those unresponsive to transfusion of blood products. Laparoscopic exploration is contraindicated in the unstable patient. Oversewing of all bleeding sites and evacuating intraluminal clot is the goal, especially in the gastric remnant. Postoperative observation of these patients in the intensive care unit for 24 hours is advisable.

Since postoperative bleeding remains a serious complication, prevention is key in avoiding this problem. Several innovative methods have been devised to prevent staple line bleeding. Using appropriate staple height is essential. The white staple cartridge is 2.5 mm and should be used for creation of the jejunojejunostomy because it provides for more tissue compression for the relatively thin-walled jejunum. The blue stapler cartridge (3.5 mm) or green (4.8 mm) provides appropriate tissue compression for the stomach (thicker tissue). The use of buttressing material on the staple line can be used to help decrease the incidence of bleeding. Peri-Strips Dry (Synovis) are strips of biological tissue derived from bovine pericardium applied to the linear stapler and act as buttressing material. Seamguard (WL Gore & Associates, Inc) is a bioabsorbable staple line reinforcement product that works in a similar fashion. Lastly, some surgeons oversew the staple lines, slightly imbricating and burying the staples.

Internal Herniation and Small Bowel Obstruction

Internal herniation (IH) and small bowel obstruction (SBO) are complications of the gastric bypass procedure that can have devastating consequences. In particular, IH often presents abruptly and requires immediate operative intervention, since it determines, in most cases, a closed-loop obstruction. The clinician should be aware of the numerous etiologies to both of these problems, as operative management is sometimes emergent.

IH is defined as a protrusion of intestine through a defect within the peritoneal cavity, as opposed to an external or incisional hernia through an abdominal wall defect.[13] Three sites of potential IH are created by the retrocolic gastric bypass, while 2 areas are created in the antecolic gastric bypass: (1) behind the jejunojenunostomy, (2) behind the Roux limb, known as Peterson's defect, and (3) through the mesocolic defect (retrocolic bypass only). There is a slightly higher incidence of IH in laparoscopic gastric bypass procedures,[13] thought to be secondary to decreased adhesion formation in these cases when compared to open procedures. Timing of presentation for IH varies widely, occurring within 1 week of the original operation up to 6 to 24 months postoperatively, but the risk persists for life. The patient will usually present with an abrupt onset of severe abdominal pain, vomiting, and retching. With this constellation of symptoms, the clinician should be highly suspicious of IH.

SBO could be the result of IH or a myriad of other causes. In order for having better ways of communicating, studying, and analyzing SBO, a simplified classification system has been devised.[16] The first part relates to the site of obstruction: at the level of the alimentary limb (type A), the biliopancreatic limb (type B), or at the level of the common channel (type C). The second part of the classification pertains to the time of onset: acute early (30 days or less), acute late (more then 30 days, less then 12 months), or chronic (more then 12 months).

Obstruction at the jejunojejunostomy usually occurs when the anastomosis is closed using a stapler. Hemobezoars develop as a result of bleeding in the gastric remnant and can cause obstruction in the biliopancreatic limb, leading to the dreaded complication of closed-loop obstruction. Intussusception often occurs at or in the vicinity of the jejunojejunostomy, while adhesions can form at any site along the gastrointestinal tract. Patients with SBO present with symptoms similar to that of IH, but the severity of their symptoms can range from mild to severe.

When patients present with symptoms of SBO, a diagnostic evaluation is warranted. However, with unstable vital signs and high clinical suspicion, resuscitation and immediate exploration should be performed without diagnostic tests. In the stable patient, appropriate labs (though rarely helpful in this case), including amylase and lipase, should be drawn. Abnormal liver function tests indicate type B SBO. The most sensitive radiologic exam in the case of SBO is a CT scan with oral contrast.[4] Even a small amount of contrast (patients usually cannot tolerate much) is useful and provides a shorter delay to the CT scanner. Though it is the most sensitive test, the CT scan may be normal in 20% of SBO cases.[4] Indications of SBO on CT scan include dilated small bowel, air-fluid levels or a dilated remnant stomach, free fluid in the peritoneal cavity, mesenteric vascular congestion, the "swirl" sign indicating IH, or the target sign of an intussusception. Less efficacious studies include UGI with small bowel follow-through, abdominal ultrasound, and flat and upright abdominal series. They should only be performed in the clinically stable patient if the CT scan is unrevealing. If enough clinical suspicion exists, a diagnostic exploration is warranted even in the face of normal radiographic evaluations.

The often unrevealing CT scan and persistent nonspecific signs and symptoms can lead the surgeon to operative exploration using an open or laparoscopic approach. An operation should be performed in a systematic approach, inspecting all areas of the abdomen regardless the cause of obstruction. Starting at the gastrojejunostomy, the entire bowel should be ran looking for distended bowel segments, stenosis or strictures, adhesive bands, internal hernias, or kinking of the bowel. Adhesions should be taken down with sharp dissection with careful attention not to create serosal defects. Stenoses and strictures often require bowel resection with reanastomosis, making sure the anastomosis is widely patent. If an IH is found, and no signs of ischemia are present, or if they quickly resolve, simple reduction and closure of the defect with nonabsorbable suture is sufficient. When evidence of permanent vascular compromise is present, appropriate resection is necessary.

When initially described, the gastric bypass was performed with the Roux limb passing through the transverse colon mesentery, a retrocolic approach. Some have since described the lowered incidence of IH with an antecolic approach, eliminating a potential space for herniation.[13] Closing other areas of mesenteric defects to prevent IH is also a subject of debate. There are those who advocate routine closure of defects, citing higher rates of IH in patients whose mesenteric defects were left open.[13] To date, there are no randomized controlled trials indicating whether routine closure of mesenteric defects leads to decreased IH incidence.

Incorrect Roux Limb Constructions

The so-called Roux-en-O bypass is a rare entity, but deserves mention because of its devastating consequences and the relative ease for which it can be avoided. The Roux-en-O bypass happens when the proximal biliopancreatic limb is inadvertently anastomosed to the gastric pouch, being mistaken for the Roux limb (distal jejunum). This complication is precipitated when one of the ends of the transected jejunum, in preparation for anastomosis to the gastric pouch, is not marked with a clip or suture. In our practice, we routinely place a small clip on the biliopancreatic limb immediately after transecting the jejunum. Additionally, we rerun the biliopancreatic limb back toward the ligament of Treitz to ensure we have properly identified each limb. Many of the diagnostic tests fail to identify this complication (CT, x-ray, ultrasound). Interestingly, a hepatobiliary scan has been shown[4] to detect this serious complication by revealing contrast entering the duodenum and promptly travelling in a cephalad direction to fill the esophagus. A Roux-en-O configuration can also be formed by anastomosing the distal end of the transected jejunum to itself. This happens when the jejunojejunostomy is created before the gastrojejunostomy. Prevention of these rare complications is achieved by using a systematic approach to the entire procedure, paying meticulous attention to identifying each limb appropriately.

Nonsurgical Early Postoperative Complications

Due to the frequent presence of comorbid conditions, bariatric surgery patients are considered at high risk for a number of complications, the most serious being myocardial infarction and pulmonary embolism. Often, the patient's own comorbidities (morbid obesity, diabetes, hypertension, hyperlipidemia, cardiovascular disease, arrhythmias) predispose him or her to these sometimes catastrophic outcomes. The clinician should have a low threshold in obtaining cardiac enzymes, 12-lead echocardiograms, arterial blood gas analysis, and a spiral CT scan of the chest with intravenous contrast. On occasion, the patient may not be able to tolerate intravenous contrast or obtain a CT scan (allergy, unstable), in which case, if a pulmonary embolism is clinically suspected, therapeutic administration of anticoagulation medication should be initiated, along with a pulmonary medicine consult. Signs and symptoms that may lead one to suspect myocardial infarction or pulmonary embolism are tachypnea, tachycardia resistant to fluid boluses, diaphoresis, desaturation on room air, chest pain, shoulder pain, and pain on inspiration.

A report from the American College of Surgeons Bariatric Surgery Center Network in 2011 revealed an incidence of myocardial infarction in 0%, 0.02%, and 0.06% for LSG, LAGB, and LGB out of a total of 28,616 patients within the 30-day postoperative period, respectively.[1] This same paper reported an incidence of pulmonary embolism in 0.32%, 0.02%, and 0.12% for LSG, LAGB, and LGB, respectively. Interestingly, the rate of pulmonary embolism in LSG is higher than in the LGB group, despite the decreased dissection and bowel manipulation in the LSG procedure. Depending on the patient's risk factor, some surgeons would insert a caval interruption device (inferior vena cava filter) preoperatively to decrease the risk of pulmonary embolism. Surgical judgment in combination with the patient's comorbidities and risk factors should determine whether a filter should be placed preoperatively. The filter can be placed immediately before the operation, under the same anesthesia. Caval filters should be considered in all patients with a history of deep vein thrombosis and pulmonary embolisms who present preoperatively on long-term or life-long anticoagulation.[12]

Postoperative deep venous thrombosis occurs with varying frequency in this population, most studies quoting between 0.14% to 3.8%. Age, male gender, prior venous thromboembolism, pulmonary disease, cardiac disease, and smoking have all been associated with risk of morbidity after bariatric surgery.[17] These deep vein thromboses can lead to fatal pulmonary embolisms, and so prophylaxis against deep vein thrombosis formation is an important part of perioperative management. The administration of preoperative subcutaneous unfractionated or fractionated heparin as well as intraoperative stockings and sequential compression devices are essential. Postoperatively, most surgeons have a standard protocol for which the administration of prophylactic doses of anticoagulation is given.

Summary

With the epidemic of obesity, it stands to reason that the numbers of bariatric procedures will only increase throughout the near future. The majority of bariatric operations are being performed at bariatric Centers of Excellence (COE), of which not every hospital is a member. As more patients undergo these procedures and arrive in the emergency room of non-COE hospitals, it is imperative that clinicians, especially surgeons, be mindful of the immediate postoperative complications of bariatric procedures and the correct course of action in treating these patients.

References

1. Jackson TD, Hutter MM. Morbidity and effectiveness of laparoscopic sleeve gastrectomy, adjustable band, and gastric bypass for morbid obesity. *Adv Surg.* 2012;46:255-268.
2. Hutter MM, Schirmer BD, Jones DB, et al. First report from the American College of Surgeons Bariatric Surgery Center Network: laparoscopic sleeve gastrectomy has morbidity and effectiveness positioned between the band and the bypass. *Ann Surg.* 2011;254(3):410-420.
3. Franco JV, Ruiz PA, Palermo M, Gagner M. A review of studies comparing three laparoscopic procedures in bariatric surgery: sleeve gastrectomy, Roux-en-Y gastric bypass and adjustable gastric banding. *Obes Surg.* 2011;21(9):1458-1468.
4. Deitel M, Gagner M, Dixon JB, Himpens J, Madan Atul. *Handbook of Obesity Surgery.* Toronto, Canada: FD Communications; 2010.
5. Snow JM, Steverson PA. Complications of adjustable gastric banding. *Surg Clin North Am.* 2011;91:1249-1264, ix.
6. Nadler EV, Barefoot LC, Qureshi FG. Early results after laparoscopic sleeve gastrectomy in adolescents with morbid obesity. *Surgery.* 2012;152(2):212-217.
7. Lalor PF, Tucker ON, Szomstein S, Rosenthal RJ. Complications after laparoscopic sleeve gastrectomy. *Surg Obes Relat Dis.* 2008;4(1):33-38.
8. Deitel M, Gagner M, Erickson AL, Crosby RD. Third International Summit: current status of sleeve gastrectomy. *Surg Obes Relat Dis.* 2011;7:749-759.
9. Aurora AR, Khaitan L, Saber AA. Sleeve gastrectomy and the risk of leak: a systematic analysis of 4,888 patients. *Surg Endosc.* 2012;26(6):1509-1515.
10. Serra C, Baltasar A, Andreo L, et al. Treatment of gastric leaks with coated self-expanding stents after sleeve gastrectomy. *Obes Surg.* 2007;17:866-872.
11. Nguyen NT, Nguyen XM, Dholakia C. The use of endoscopic stent management of leaks after sleeve gastrectomy. *Obes Surg.* 2010;20:1289-1292.
12. Rosenthal RJ, Jones DB. *Weight Loss Surgery: A Multidisciplinary Approach.* Edgemont, PA: Matrix Medical Communications; 2008.
13. Al Harakeh AB. Complications of laparoscopic Roux-en-Y gastric bypass. *Surg Clin North Am.* 2011;91:1225-1237, viii.
14. Fernandez AZ Jr, DeMaria EJ, Tichansky DS, et al. Experience with over 3,000 open and laparoscopic bariatric procedures: multivariate analysis of factors related to leak and resultant mortality. *Surg Endosc.* 2004;18(2):193-197.
15. Finks JF, English WJ, Carlin AM, et al. Predicting risk for venous thromboembolism with bariatric surgery: results from the Michigan Bariatric Surgery Collaborative. *Ann Surg.* 2012;255:1100-1104.

16. Tucker ON, Escalante-Tattersfield T, Szomstein S, Rosenthal RJ. The ABC system: a simplified classification system for small bowel obstruction after laparoscopic Roux-en-Y gastric bypass. *Obes Surg.* 2007;17(12):1549-1554.
17. Rosenthal RJ, International Sleeve Gastrectomy Expert Panel, et al. International Sleeve Gastrectomy Expert Panel Consensus Statement: best practice guidelines based on experience of >12,000 cases. *Surg Obes Relat Dis.* 2012;8(1):8-19.

17

Long-Term Complications of Bariatric Surgery

Judy Y. R. Chen, MD, FACS and Scott A. Shikora, MD, FACS

Bariatric surgery, also referred to as weight loss surgery, has never been safer or more efficacious. It usually results in 40% to 70% excess weight loss and the resolution of many of the severe comorbidities associated with obesity. As currently performed, bariatric surgery has an extremely favorable risk to benefit ratio. Perioperative mortality is generally less than 1%. Additionally as the result of these procedures, there is a decreased risk of death related to coronary artery disease, diabetes, and cancer.[1] Despite the many benefits associated with bariatric surgery, there are still potential complications and consequences that may occur, even many years later. A general knowledge of these possible adverse events will minimize the likelihood of these events developing, and early recognition of these events may minimize their severity when they do occur. This chapter will discuss the complications associated with the most popular bariatric procedures: the laparoscopic Roux-en-Y gastric bypass (RYGB), laparoscopic adjustable gastric band (LAGB), and laparoscopic sleeve gastrectomy (LSG). As the early complications will be discussed elsewhere in this book, we will focus on the long term complications.

The Growing Epidemic of Obesity

Obesity is an incurable, chronic disorder that is well known to be associated with multiple metabolic and debilitating illnesses. The prevalence of obesity is increasing in the United States and worldwide. Currently, more than 67% of adults in the United States are overweight or obese and almost 16 million are morbidly obese. Even more astounding, it has been estimated that 1.8 billion humans are overweight, a prevalence that for the first time in human history equals the number of malnourished individuals.[2] Obesity is not just a cosmetic problem or benign condition. It is recognized as a serious disease with devastating consequences. While many laypeople have come to recognize that individuals with obesity are at higher risk for contracting type 2 diabetes mellitus, hypertension, and sleep apnea, obesity adversely influences nearly every organ system in the body and results in premature death. It has been estimated that obesity represents the second leading cause of preventable death behind smoking. Additionally, it adversely affects quality of life

Forse RA, Apovian CM, eds.
Bariatric Surgery: What Every Provider Needs to Know (pp 193-209).

for those individuals afflicted with it and is predicted to increase treatment costs for preventable obesity-related diseases estimated to be between $147 billion to $210 billion by 2030.[3]

The Growth of Bariatric Surgery

Long considered a fringe discipline that suffered from poor long-term results, high perioperative morbidity, and weak science, bariatric surgery has evolved into a highly respected field of surgery. The rapid adoption of minimally invasive surgery to the field and the introduction of a dramatically safer operative procedure, the laparoscopic gastric bypass, has led to a greater acceptance of the field. The increased number of procedures performed further demonstrated the improving safety and metabolic benefits. Ultimately, even nonsurgeon physicians were more accepting of bariatric surgery. More than 103,000 procedures were performed in the United States in 2003.[4] This represented a 644% increase in the decade, making bariatric surgery the fastest growing field in surgery. Today, approximately 150,000 to 200,000 procedures are performed in the United States annually.

Current Conventional Bariatric Surgical Procedures

Understanding the different procedures currently being performed and their mechanisms of weight loss are important in order to appreciate the potential long-term consequences of bariatric surgery. Bariatric surgical procedures were traditionally classified into 3 categories of weight loss: restrictive, malabsorptive, and a combination of these. Today, we appreciate that these descriptions are overly simplistic and that neurohormonal factors may have significant roles in the resulting weight loss and metabolic benefits.

LAGB is an inflatable device that encircles the proximal portion of the stomach to create a small pouch. This slows and limits the amount of food that is eaten, provides early satiety, and overall reduces caloric intake. The reduction in appetite and slow progression of food through the band provides restrictive weight loss. The tightness of the band is modified by injecting saline into a palpable subcutaneous port system to increase restriction over time.

LSG is an operative procedure in which 75% to 85% of the stomach is removed to create a tube or sleeve that both eliminates the gastric hormones that stimulate hunger and provides a reduced stomach capacity that limits food intake. The combination of neurohormonal inhibition and decreased capacity of the stomach size can lead to 50% to 70% excess body weight loss.

RYGB is an operation that divides the stomach to create a small pouch that holds approximately 30 cc and restricts the volume of food intake. The small gastric pouch is anastomosed to the small intestine so that the ingested nutrients travel directly into the intestine from the gastric pouch, bypassing the most of the stomach, the duodenum, and the proximal jejunum. The gastric bypass is thought to have several mechanisms of action beyond the long-held concepts of nutrient restriction by the small pouch capacity and mild malabsorption by the small bowel rerouting. Bypassing the upper foregut seems to have profound hormonal effects that reduce appetite (inhibit the appetite hormone ghrelin) and improve blood sugar homeostasis in patients with type 2 diabetes mellitus (incretins).

Biliopancreatic diversion (BPD) is an operation that removes most of the distal stomach and connects a moderately large gastric pouch to the ileum. The BPD with duodenal switch ([BDP-DS] or just duodenal switch [DS]) is a modified version of the BPD where the greater curvature of the stomach is removed similar to a sleeve gastrectomy with the pylorus intact and the duodenum anastomosed to the ileum. Both of these operations create a "controlled malabsorption" that results in significant weight loss and beneficial effects for patients with metabolic disease such as type 2 diabetes mellitus and hyperlipidemia.

Immediate Postoperative Period

Although the foci of this chapter are the long-term complications that may been seen after bariatric surgery, to put them in the proper perspective, it is beneficial to briefly discuss the immediate and early postoperative complications. Bariatric patients can suffer from the same postoperative complications as any other patient undergoing gastrointestinal surgery. These universal complications include wound infections, hemorrhage, incisional hernias, deep venous thrombosis, gastrointestinal leakage, pneumonia, atelectasis, organ injury, intestinal obstruction, and pulmonary embolism. As with other gastrointestinal surgeries (and in many cases, maybe to a greater degree), bariatric surgeons take the usual precautions to reduce the likelihood of sustaining these complications. These include meticulous surgical technique, experienced anesthesia support, prophylactic antibiotics, thromboprophylaxis, early ambulation, and pulmonary toilet. Surgeons should always be on alert for these serious complications. Even subtle signs or concerns warrant attention. The universal nature of these complications places them, however, outside the scope of this chapter. As such, they will not be discussed further. There are other complications more specifically related to bariatric surgery that must be recognized as well during the immediate postoperative period.

Perioperative Period

In the perioperative period after any bariatric surgery, dehydration is the most likely reason for readmission. Dehydration occurs when patients fail to achieve their fluid requirements. Factors that contribute to dehydration include the altered gastrointestinal anatomy, greater fluid requirements for the obese than the nonobese, nausea and vomiting, and even warm weather. Additionally, patients who have had a malabsorptive procedure may be more prone to dehydration from watery stools. Dehydration often exacerbates further symptoms of nausea, headache, dizziness, fatigue, weakness, and overall poor well-being. Generally speaking, patients are encouraged to take in 64 ounces or 8 cups of fluid a day. On occasion, intravenous hydration may be necessary to restore the fluid deficit in patients unable to consume adequate fluid by mouth.[5]

Protein intake is also very important after surgery. High-protein, low-carbohydrate liquid supplements are very helpful for the patient's needs after bariatric surgery. Protein-calorie malnutrition is a risk for several reasons. Many patients do not tolerate red meat, so they avoid these high-protein foods. The unpleasant sensation of restriction and nausea felt by many patients places them at risk for not ingesting enough protein in their diet. Small meals may not provide adequate protein. High-protein foods and even the use of supplemental protein shakes are essential to patient well-being. Protein-calorie malnutrition, if not corrected, may lead to poor wound healing, fatigue, edema, skin changes, muscle wasting, cachexia, and, in the extreme, infection and death. Most bariatric programs recommend that patients have a daily intake of 60 to 80 g of protein. In extreme cases, parenteral or enteral tube feeding may be required.

Long-Term Complications and Consequences

As more and more patients undergo bariatric surgery, the long-term complications of these procedures will be seen in an ever-increasing frequency. While bariatric surgeons will manage the lion's share of perioperative complications, other clinicians, such as primary care physicians, may be the ones managing the long-term complications. It is critical for all clinicians to be able to recognize and manage these problems. While there is considerable overlap, most of the long-term problems associated with bariatric surgery can be categorized into nutritional and anatomic categories.

Once the patient has recovered from the operation, it is important to emphasize to the patient that he or she requires close follow-up and routine surveillance. These visits include evaluation of the overall health of the patient and titration of his or her medications during the rapid weight loss. As patients lose weight, there will be changes in other health issues. Discussions with the patients regarding activity level, dietary habits, bowel function, and hydration status are important. Along with the adequacy of caloric restriction to induce weight loss, a practitioner also must evaluate the patient for the risk of nutrient malabsorption due to the alterations created by the weight loss surgery. Annual bloodwork to evaluate nutrient and micronutrient status is mandatory.

Nutritional Issues

Dysfunctional eating habits are probably the most common causes of nausea and emesis. Proper eating after most bariatric surgery procedures requires behavioral modification. Patients are trained to eat slowly, chew well, limit portion size, and not to drink fluid during the meal. However, many patients either cannot or do not successfully adapt their eating habits. Overeating can result in epigastric pain, discomfort, and heartburn, as well as nausea and vomiting. Drinking during the meals can "wash" the food out of the stomach pouch, thereby offsetting the desired early satiety and restriction resulting in insufficient weight loss or weight regain. Patients are generally counseled to drink 30 minutes before eating their meal or wait until 30 minutes after the meal to drink. Patients are also encouraged to eat slowly, take small bites, and chew food to a liquid consistency. Patients who complain of abdominal pain, nausea, and vomiting should be thoroughly evaluated to focus on time of inset, location, severity, pattern, and quality, to differentiate whether the etiology is dysfunctional eating or other causes, such as strictures, ulcers, etc.

Vitamin and mineral abnormalities are common after all bariatric surgeries. The etiologies are multifactorial. Patients eat dramatically less food and therefore ingest less nutrients and micronutrients. In addition, many develop food intolerances and may eat less nutrient-rich foods such as meats. Lastly, all of the operative procedures except for the band result in some degree of nutrient and micronutrient malabsorption. The mechanisms of micronutrient absorption may be altered to different degrees based on the operation performed and the patient's dietary habits. In addition, certain digestive processes and/or hormones secreted by the gastrointestinal system may be altered after bariatric surgery and may also impact nutrient absorption. For example, the achlorhydria that occurs when the stomach is either removed or diverted is associated with reduced levels of intrinsic factor, which negatively impact vitamin B_{12} absorption.

Severe nutritional deficiencies, if not recognized, can lead to devastating and permanent consequences. Any practitioner caring for a bariatric patient must be able to identify and correctly treat any deficiencies that develop. Table 17-1 lists symptoms associated with common long-term deficiencies seen in bariatric patients. Typically, nutritional abnormalities are insidious and usually occur over months to years. Also, some complications are multifactorial, thus careful history with particular attention to the patient's diet, serum vitamin levels, and physical exam can assist with the diagnosis. All patients should have yearly surveillance and life-long supplementation. Although there is a consensus for the recommendation of life-long supplementation, there is no consensus as to how to supplement. The American Society for Metabolic and Bariatric Surgery recommendations are based on best practice and the current literature, not on any specific scientific data.[6]

To best understand the risk for nutrient deficiencies with the different bariatric operations, clinicians must first be familiar with where the nutrients or minerals are normally absorbed in the gastrointestinal tract. See Table 17-2 for normal absorption levels of vitamins and minerals.

TABLE 17-1
SYMPTOMS ASSOCIATED WITH NUTRITIONAL DEFICIENCIES

DEFICIENCIES	EFFECT
Iron	Microcytic anemia, brittle nails, macroglossia, constipation, fatigue
Zinc	Hair loss, poor wound healing, rash, amnesia, lethargy, depression
Calcium	Bone disease
Thiamine	Wernicke's encephalopathy, cardiomyopathy, peripheral neuropathy
Cyanocobalamin	Megaloblastic anemia, peripheral neuropathy, beefy tongue
Protein	Poor wound healing
Vitamin A	Night blindness
Folate	Megaloblastic anemia, glossitis

TABLE 17-2
ABSORPTION OF VITAMINS AND MINERALS IN THE GASTROINTESTINAL TRACT

	STOMACH	DUODENUM	JEJUNUM	ILEUM
Iron		+++		
Zinc		++	+++	+
Calcium		+++		
Thiamine (B_1)		+++		
Cyanocobalamin (B_{12})				+++ (requires intrinsic factor)
Protein		++	++	++
Vitamin A				+
Folate		+	+++	

Iron Deficiency

Iron deficiency is multifactorial and most problematic in menstruating women. During a gastric bypass procedure, the duodenum and proximal jejunum, where iron is normally absorbed, are excluded. Additionally, the small gastric pouches produce dramatically less acid than normal-sized stomachs. Stomach acid is important for the normal absorption of iron. Iron deficiency can also be dietary related. In many of these patients, overall intake of dietary iron can be inadequate. Food volume is reduced and many patients find iron-rich food to be difficult to digest.[7] The total body reserve of iron is only is 3.5 to 4 g, and deficiencies can develop quickly. Patients with iron deficiency may present with brittle nails, macroglossia, constipation, headaches, fatigue, and depression. Microcytic anemia is normally seen in laboratory values. Once iron deficiency is identified, patients should start oral iron supplementation of 325 mg 1 to 3 times a day. Iron infusions may be necessary if oral iron is not tolerated or not effective.

Zinc Deficiency

Symptoms most often seen with zinc deficiency are skin related, such as eczema, acne, hair loss, and white spots seen on the nails. Other complaints include amnesia, lethargy, and depression. On the molecular level, zinc is important for the immune system, protein synthesis, wound healing, cell reproduction, smell, and taste. The total body reserve of zinc is 3 g. Red meat, shellfish, liver, and integral grains are the richest source of readily available zinc, and only 35% is absorbed in healthy patients. Zinc deficiency is frequently underestimated in the bariatric population both before and after surgery. In a study by Salle et al, 42.5% patients had evidence of zinc deficiency after gastric bypass, 18% of patients after sleeve gastrectomy, and 91% for patients after BPD.[8]

It is also important to note that zinc requirements are especially high during pregnancy. Zinc deficiency has also been associated with other nutrient malabsorption, diarrhea, and anorexia. Zinc levels can also be low due to vitamin A and D deficiency. The normal daily recommendation for zinc is 12 to 15 mg daily, and if zinc levels are found to be low, then administering 1 to 3 mg/kg is recommended. Follow-up zinc and copper levels are recommended after supplementation.

Calcium Deficiency

Calcium is mostly absorbed in the proximal small bowel and, like iron, is at risk for deficiency with the bypass procedures. In addition, it also requires an acidic environment for absorption. Calcium deficiencies can contribute to bone and dental disease. It also is important in muscle contraction, relaxation, nerve conduction, hormonal function, blood pressure, and cardiac regulation. Calcium must be ingested daily and absorbed effective to maintain optimal health. In the bariatric patient, the supplemental calcium needs to be given in a more absorbable form, such as calcium citrate (not sulfate) with vitamin D. Recommendations are 1200 to 1500 mg of a chewable calcium supplement daily, but limit the dose to 600 mg at one time. The maximum a body can absorb at one time is 600 mg. The doses should be separated by at least 4 hours. Also, it is important to not prescribe supplements that contain both iron and calcium, since they may interfere with each other's absorption. Evaluation of calcium deficiency will show laboratory values with decreased calcium and vitamin D. An elevated serum parathyroid hormone is consistent with reduced bone calcium. Vitamin D levels should be optimally greater than 30 ng/L.

Vitamin D and calcium deficiencies are seen in 50% to 80% of patients even by the first year after bariatric surgery. This range depends on multiple factors such as the amount of exposure to daylight, sequestration of vitamin D in fat, and the negative feedback in the 25 OH vitamin D cycle.[9] Overall, osteoporosis and bone disease due to calcium and vitamin D deficiency is a potential long-term consequence of bariatric surgery, but may be prevented with supplementation and close surveillance of all bariatric surgical patients.

Thiamine Deficiency

Thiamine (vitamin B_1) deficiency should be suspected in patients with intractable vomiting and dehydration. Thiamine in its active form functions as a coenzyme for the metabolism of carbohydrates as well as axonal conduction of nerves. It is normally absorbed in the duodenum and proximal jejunum by either active or passive receptors, depending on the intraluminal concentration. Normally the body can only store a limited amount of thiamine and cannot produce it if storage is low. Since the half-life of thiamine is only 9 to 18 days, it only takes a month for stores to become insufficient. If thiamine deficiency is associated with neurologic symptoms, it is known as beriberi. Bariatric patients are susceptible to beriberi, especially if they are not eating thiamine-rich foods such as pork, fish, pine nuts, and pistachios. Symptoms of a thiamine deficiency include peripheral neuropathy of the distal limbs as well as weakness. Rehydration with a glucose-based intravenous fluid without supplementation of thiamine can result in Wernicke-Korsakoff syndrome, a terrible neurologic condition due to demyelination of nerves. Initially Wernicke is characterized by the development of confusion, ocular nystagmus, and ataxia. Wernicke-Korsakoff syndrome is the diagnosis when the patient also exhibits amnesic confusion. Development of these symptoms is a medical emergency and only partly reversible with supplementation. Patients will require hospitalization and further workup for cardiac failure, as well as other deficiencies that can be associated with Wernicke-Korsakoff syndrome. Only half will recover all the neurologic deficits. Therefore, for all patients at risk for a thiamine deficiency, 100 mg of intravenous thiamine should be given prior to administering any glucose-containing fluid.

Vitamin B_{12} Deficiency

Cyanocobalamin (vitamin B_{12}) deficiency is a common cause of macrocytic anemia in the surgical bariatric population. Pernicious anemia occurs not due to the lack of intrinsic factor but rather to the inability to liberate cyanocobalamin from food in the gastric pouch. Vitamin B_{12} usually is found in animal protein and requires an acidic gastric environment to help cleave it for absorption. As stated previously, the gastric pouch produces only a small amount of acid. In the proximal foregut, further pancreatic enzymes break down and free the cobalamin, which then binds to intrinsic factor. Intrinsic factor transports the cobalamin into the distal ileum where it is normally absorbed. However, without the proper binding to intrinsic factor, less than 1% of vitamin B_{12} is absorbed. However, oral administration of pure cobalamin is generally well absorbed. The recommended daily intake of vitamin B_{12} is 2 mcg a day, and it is normally stored in the liver. Vitamin B_{12} is essential for the conversion of the inactive methyltetrahydrofolic acid to the active tetrahydrofolic acid, thus hematologic abnormalities are seen, such as megaloblastosis of the bone marrow. Symptoms of a B_{12} deficiency include weakness, ataxia, peripheral neuropathy, and a sore, beefy tongue. Neurologic complications of vitamin B_{12} include myeloneuropathy, encephalopathy, peripheral or optic neuropathy, and even behavior problems. When a deficiency is identified supplementation is required. Multiple studies have shown that 300 to 500 mcg administered daily is sufficient. One thousand to 3000 mcg vitamin B_{12} can be administered sublingually and intramuscularly every month to every 6 months as well, especially if deficiency is profound.[10]

Folate Deficiency

Folic acid deficiency can also occur after bariatric surgery. Like a B_{12} deficiency, it can result in a macrocytic anemia. Patients may also be found to have a leukopenia and thrombocytopenia. Other symptoms include glossitis. In one study, 19% of patients after gastric bypass surgery were found to have folic acid deficiency.[10] Close surveillance is especially important in women of child-bearing age due to the neural tube defects that can be associated with low levels of folic acid. Recommended supplementation is 1 mg folic acid orally or intravenously per day.

Vitamin A Deficiency

Vitamin A is normally absorbed as a fat-soluble vitamin in micelles across the brush border of the terminal ileum. Vitamin A deficiency is rarely seen after banding, short limb bypasses, or sleeves, but can occur after BPD due to malabsorption. Although uncommon after short limb gastric bypass, it was reported to occur in 11% of patients at 1 year after RYGB and 8% after 2 years.[11] Vitamin A is important for immune function, skin health, and antioxidant activity. Vitamin A is also essential for vision, and severe deficiency leads to night blindness. Early symptoms may include fatigue, dry hair, dry skin, pruritis, fragile fingernails, as well as an increased risk of developing respiratory and diarrheal-associated infections. Vitamin A is stored in the liver for up to 1 year but is also affected by multiple other factors, such as liver function, infections, and nutritional status of zinc and iron. The recommended daily allowance is 800 to 1000 mcg daily, and treatment of vitamin A deficiency is 3000 mcg daily. Many of the multivitamins that are over the counter contain 3500 IU of vitamin A, which is about 70% of daily intake. Vitamin A-rich foods include liver, fortified dairy products, fish, dark-colored fruits, and leafy vegetables. If severe deficiency is identified, it is recommended to administer 50,000 to 100,000 IU intramuscularly per day for 3 days, then 50,000 IU intramuscularly for 2 weeks or until clinical improvement is seen.[6,12]

Cholelithiasis

Cholelithiasis can be seen with the rapid weight loss associated with bariatric surgery. Historically, cholecystectomies were performed at the same time as the weight loss surgery to reduce the potential risks associated with gallstones. This was particularly true prior to the laparoscopic era. Open cholecystectomy was morbid and the common bile duct was endoscopically inaccessible; therefore, most bariatric surgeons removed most gallbladders (even normal gallbladders) at the time of the bariatric procedure. However, it is reported in the literature that biliary disease can also be managed expectantly. In a prospective study by Portenier, 19% of patients who had an RYGB had preoperative biliary findings such as sludge, stones, or polyps, yet only 8.1% became symptomatic and required a delayed cholecystectomy.[13] Currently, most bariatric surgeons only remove diseased gallbladders because performing a laparoscopic cholecystectomy at some point after the bariatric procedure (particularly after weight loss) is rarely morbid. Recent advancements in laparoscopic and endoscopic interventions also can treat common duct stones. For patients interested in reducing their risk of developing gallstones, the administration of ursodiol 300 mg twice a day for 6 months has been shown to decrease gallstone formation.[14]

Weight Loss Failure

Despite the best patient selection and properly conducted surgical procedures, approximately to 25% to 30% of patients will either lose insufficient weight or regain significant weight back by 2 to 5 years after surgery. While most bariatric surgery failures are due to poor eating habits or maladaptive behaviors, failure may also be due to anatomic derangements. A thorough evaluation is always indicated when confronted with a patient who has failed his or her procedure. The evaluation should include a comprehensive history, dietary and behavioral assessment, endoscopy, and radiographic studies. Anatomic etiologies for weight loss failure include dilated gastric pouches and/or stoma, gastrogastric fistulas, dilated gastric sleeves, and band prolapses. Revisional surgery for failed bariatric patients is discussed elsewhere in this book.

Incisional Hernias

Incisional and trocar hernias can occur at any time. While the risk of incisional hernias from open bariatric surgery was as common as 20% to 30% of patients, trocar hernias after laparoscopic surgery occur much less frequently. The symptoms range from just an enlarging bulge with mild discomfort to peritonitis from a strangulated hernia. Hernias that present shortly after surgery are more likely to present as a partial small bowel obstruction from a Richter's hernia where part of the intestinal wall is incarcerated in the abdominal wall defect from an incision. Ultimately, it is up to the clinician to determine the severity of the hernia and how urgent it is to offer a repair. Since many bariatric patients are still overweight when they present for evaluation, physical exam can be inadequate. Computed tomography (CT) scanning is very helpful in identifying if a hernia exists and whether there is bowel at risk. There is no uniform consensus regarding trocar closure. Some surgeons close all trocar wounds, while other chose to not close them. Still others selectively close the larger trocar wounds (12 mm or greater) or those in specific locations (midline or lower abdominal).

Internal Hernias and Bowel Obstructions

Internal hernias can occur from several tissue defects created during gastric bypass surgery. These spaces or defects are not created during band or sleeve procedures. Unlike ventral hernias, internal hernias are spaces within mesenteries that can trap bowel resulting in bowel obstruction, volvulus, and even strangulation if not promptly recognized and corrected. The location of these spaces is fairly consistent. If the Roux limb was brought up in an antecolic/antegastric orientation (anterior and over the transverse colon and gastric remnant), 2 such spaces are created. These are the intermesenteric space between the leaves of the mesenteries at the jejunojejunostomy and the Peterson's defect that can be found under the Roux limb mesentery just below the transverse colon. If the Roux limb is brought retrocolic/retrogastric (under the transverse colon through an

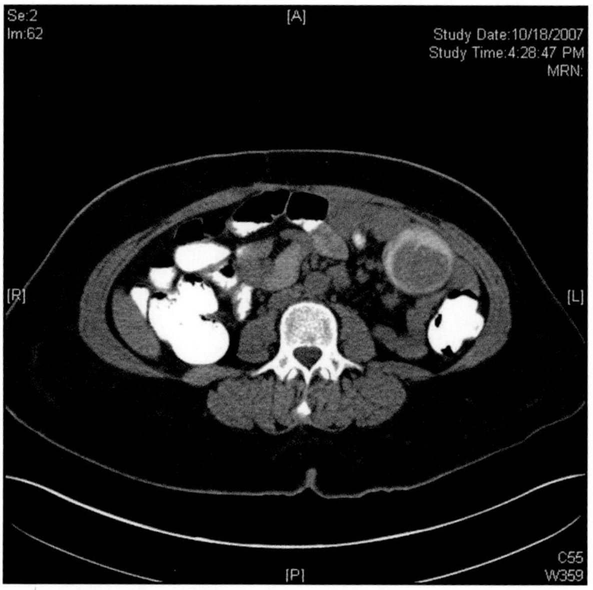

Figure 17-1. CT scan appearance of an intussusception. See the "target sign" on the left.

opening created in the transverse mesocolon), a third space is created alongside the Roux limb in the mesocolonic tunnel. This creates a hernia into the lesser sac under the gastric remnant. An internal hernia should always be suspected in any patient who presents to the clinic complaining of severe episodic pain, retching, or vomiting. Additionally, it should always be considered for all patients who present emergently with signs of intestinal obstruction, especially if there is bilious emesis. Due to the length of the Roux limb, bile should not be normally seen in emesis, unless there is an obstruction below the jejunojenunostomy that allows for the bilious contents from the biliopancreatic limb to be backed up into the Roux limb. If the biliopancreatic limb is obstructed, there is no mechanism for decompression resulting in a massively distended gastric fundus. This would result in upper abdominal pain, retching, dyspnea, and chest pain. Emergent percutaneous or operative decompression may be necessary. In addition to internal hernias, patients may also develop small bowel obstructions from adhesions or even ventral hernias, so these diagnoses must also be considered. Intussusception is also seen in gastric bypass patients where the intestine can telescope upon itself either in the antegrade or retrograde fashion. If obstructing, the patient should be taken to surgery and the intussusception reduced. The viability of the bowel will dictate if a bowel resection is necessary. If it is the first episode of intussusception, pexy is not necessary since recurrences may still occur despite pexy. If multiple episodes of intussusception occur, revision of the jejunal-jejunal anastomosis may be necessary. CT scan can be helpful for identifying the source. Treatment is usually operative repair (Figure 17-1).

Marginal Ulcers (Figure 17-2)

Marginal ulcers occur after gastric bypass surgery with an incidence of 0.6% to 16%. Symptoms include burning, midepigastric pain (63%), bleeding (24%), nausea, and emesis.[15] Ulcers are usually located at the anastomosis on the jejunal side. Risk factors that may contribute to the formation of ulcers are tobacco, alcohol, or nonsteroidal anti-inflammatory drug (NSAID) use; ischemia; diabetes; gastric pouch length; and gastrogastric fistulas. Although the pathogenesis may not always be specifically known, intractable ulcers may be due to ischemia at the anastomosis and should be suspected especially after difficult procedures such as revisional surgeries. While most marginal ulcers related to acid production will respond to nonoperative means, about 9% of marginal ulceration will require surgical resection.[15] Typically, the small gastric pouch produces a minimal amount of acid. However, even a small amount of acid production may be enough to result in ulceration. While gastric mucosa is resistant to ulceration, the small intestinal mucosa has no

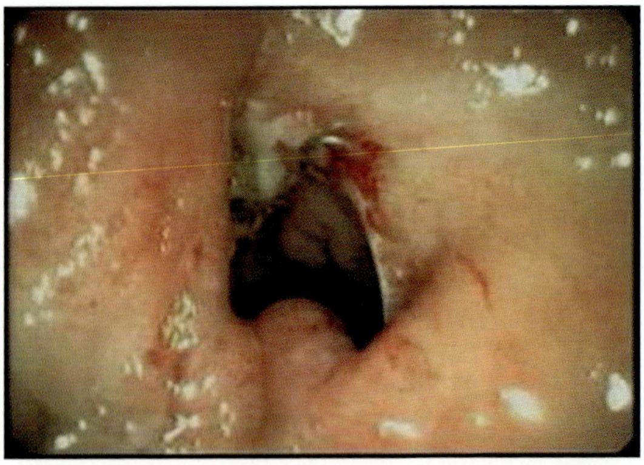

Figure 17-2. A marginal ulcer (see the white plaque near the staple) visualized on an endoscopy.

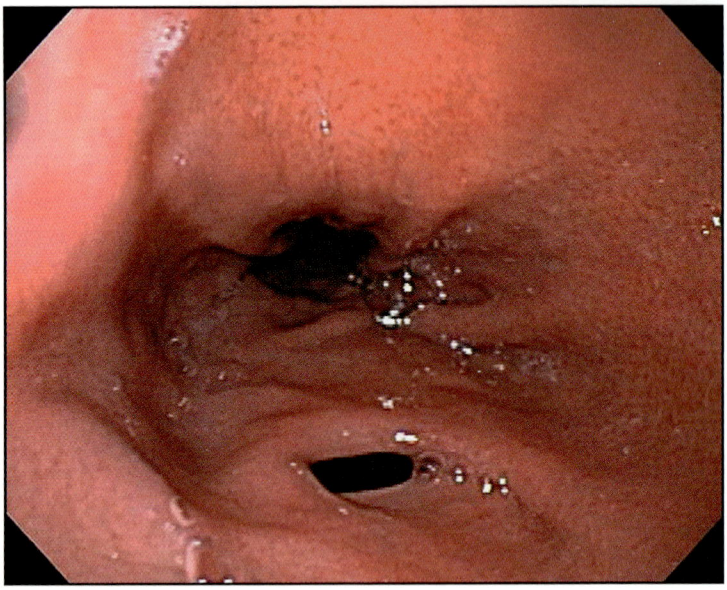

Figure 17-3. A gastrogastric fistula (seen at 6 o'clock) visualized on an endoscopy.

inherent natural protection to acid injury and may be susceptible. If not recognized and addressed early, marginal ulcers can result in potentially devastating consequences, such as hemorrhage and perforation. Like perforated peptic ulcers in nonbariatric patients, perforated marginal ulcers usually require immediate attention, most often surgical exploration and repair.

Gastrogastric Fistulas (Figure 17-3)

Gastrogastric fistulas, while uncommon with divided staple lines, have a reported incidence from 1.5% and up to 49% in nondivided staple lines.[16] They are a common cause for intractable ulceration. With gastrogastric fistula, acid from the "excluded" fundus can enter the pouch across the fistula ulcerating the jejunum. Medical management is rarely successful, and the treatment of choice is to resect the fistula and upper fundus.[16] The diagnosis can be made by endoscopy or upper fluoroscopy.

The usual treatment for marginal ulcers is similar to the medical therapy of peptic ulcers. As previously stated, marginal ulcers not associated with ischemia or gastrogastric fistula usually respond to sucralfate, a high dose of proton pump inhibitors, and the cessation of contributing factors such as tobacco, alcohol, and NSAIDs. On occasion, patients with marginal ulcers have significant oral intake intolerance and benefit from a short course of parenteral or enteral nutrition until the ulcer and its inherent inflammation resolve.

There has been some suggestion that like peptic ulcers there may be an association of marginal ulcers with *Helicobacter pylori*.[17] Many programs screen all patients preoperatively and eradicate *H pylori* when a patient screens positively for the bacteria. Currently, there is no consensus among bariatric surgeons.

Anastomotic and Staple Line Leaks

Anastomotic or staple line leaks are the most deadly complications of gastric bypass surgery and can occur early in the postoperative period. The incidence is reported to be 1% to 3%. This complication is unique to the gastric bypass because the sleeve and band do not require an anastomosis; however, the presentation, treatment, and outcome would be similar to a perforation of the gastric pouch above a band or a staple line leak after a sleeve. Leakage most commonly occurs at the gastrojejunostomy but can occur at the jejunojejunostomy or any of the staple lines. The typical signs and symptoms of a leak include fever, tachycardia (typically a sustained heart rate greater than 120 beats/min), severe abdominal pain, hypotension, tachypnea, anxiety, or the "feeling of doom." Unrecognized leaks may lead to peritonitis, shock, organ failure, and ultimately death or long-term morbidity. Treatment usually requires early surgical intervention either laparoscopic or open. The goal of treatment is to control the sepsis, and this is accomplished by irrigation, wide drainage, antibiotics, and nutritional support. Debridement and oversewing of the perforation with or without omental patching are options for surgical repair that may be tried but are rarely successful. Recently, there has been growing success with percutaneous drainage, endoscopic stenting, nutritional support, and antibiotics.

The timing of leaks can be divided into different categories, such as early, intermediate, or late leaks, as described by Csendes in his prospective study.[18] Late leaks usually are seen more than 10 days after surgery but can be seen anytime in patients with inadequately treated ulcers. Patients are managed depending on the clinical presentation, evidence of systemic instability, and the location and severity of the leak. Late leaks tend to be less deadly than early leaks and can be managed by a number of options. Intra-abdominal collections can often be addressed by percutaneous guided drain placement, broad-spectrum antibiotics, enteral or parenteral nutritional support, and close clinical observation. Other options may include endoscopic therapies such as stents and fibrin glue.

Upper Gastrointestinal Bleeding

Upper gastrointestinal bleeding can be seen in 0.5% to 2% of cases and in the early postoperative period is most often due to bleeding at a staple line. Heneghan found that 71% of gastrointestinal bleeding occurred in less than 30 days postoperatively and late gastrointestinal bleeding was likely from a marginal ulcer. Of those who had late bleeding, only 33.3% required surgical intervention.[19] Late bleeding can be occult and discovered during the workup for unexplained anemia or present with acute hemorrhage (hematemesis and/or bright red blood per rectum). Acute hemorrhage can usually be addressed with therapeutic endoscopy and cauterizing or clipping of any source of bleeding. However, if indicated, surgery and oversewing of the bleeder need to be performed. All gastrointestinal bleeding needs to be watched carefully and blood transfusions administered if anemia is profound. Nonoperative management can be feasible in a patient who is hemodynamically stable. Proton pump inhibitors and carafate are an adjunct as they are helpful for ulcer healing.

Peptic Ulcers

Peptic ulcers are uncommon after gastric bypass but may present with occult gastrointestinal bleeding or acute bleeding. Hematemesis is unlikely but patients may present with bright red blood per rectum and or melena and symptomatic anemia. The diagnosis is often made by exclusion. However, if the diagnosis is uncertain, the duodenum can often be accessed endoscopically and if unsuccessful by laparoscopic-assisted endoscopy.

Stomal Stricture

Stomal stricture is another known complication associated with RYGB and is seen in 3% to 27% of cases.[20-22] A stricture at the gastrojejunal anastomosis causes dysphagia and intolerance to solid food. Strictures can occur any time after surgery but generally present within the first 2 months. Strictures can occur thereafter often in association with marginal ulceration, and the associated inflammation and swelling. The etiology is often multifactorial. Additional factors include the blood supply to the pouch, method of surgery such as laparoscopic vs open, primary vs revisional procedure, and the size and surgical technique for constructing the gastrojejunal anastomosis.[23] It has also been proposed that chronic inflammation may also increase the likelihood of stricture formation as the result of scar tissue depositing into the anastomotic ring. Strictures are best diagnosed by endoscopy. Since the gastrojejunostomy is intentionally constructed to be narrow (1 to 1.5 cm), an anastomosis is only considered to be strictured if the endoscope cannot traverse it. Most strictures are successfully corrected by endoscopic dilation. Sequential placement of balloon catheters through the stricture can be used to safely dilate the stricture. Smaller balloons are attempted first; progressively larger balloons are used up to about 20 mm. Most symptoms resolve after the first dilation, but in one-third of patients a second dilation (or even more) may be required. Balloon dilation can result in perforation. Therefore, it is up to the judgment of the endoscopist to determine balloon size, how large to increase it in one session, and how many sessions are required. If dilation is not successful, revisional surgery is warranted to resolve the patient's dysphagia.

Gastric Remnant Distension

Gastric remnant distension is an uncommon complication that occurs with a less than 1% incidence. Patients will complain of bloating, hiccups, and, in extreme circumstances, peritonitis from perforation. Most often the distension is due to a distal intestinal obstruction whether it be from adhesions, internal herniation, intussusception, or other causes. The gastric remnant cannot be decompressed by vomiting or nasogastric tube suction, so the condition requires early attention. The treatment of choice is surgical correction of the intestinal obstruction. Sometimes, percutaneous gastric decompression may be indicated to temporize the situation prior to proceeding with surgery. However, delay in management can lead to profound distension that may result in fundic ischemia and even necrosis and perforation. For the above reasons, any intestinal obstruction after gastric bypass should be managed by early surgical intervention.

Nephrolithiasis

Nephrolithiasis is due to changes in calcium and oxalate absorption. There are multiple mechanisms proposed for the absorption of oxalate and calcium. Stone formation depends on the absolute concentration of intraluminal oxalate that creates hyperoxaluria. The pathophysiology is related to increased absorption due to excess bile salts and fatty acids creating increased permeability of oxalate in the colon. The initial treatment of nephrolithiasis is aggressive hydration. Large fluid intake with a goal of 3 L/day is the most effective therapy to minimize nephric intratubular oxalate deposition and stone formation. Additionally, the avoidance of oxalate-rich foods like tea, chocolate, spinach, or rhubarb is recommended. Furthermore, medications such as pyridoxine (5 mg/kg a day) can convert glyoxylate to glycine instead of oxalate. Medications that inhibit calcium oxalate precipitation include orthophosphate, potassium citrate, and magnesium oxide.[24-27] If symptoms are severe and persistent, revisional surgery may be considered.

Dumping Syndrome

Dumping syndrome is a condition where food, particularly simple sugars, pass too quickly through the gastrojejunal anastomosis and create an osmotic load in the small intestine. The symptom complex is caused by 2 mechanisms. Early dumping that occurs shortly after eating is due to the hyperosmolar ingested food entering into the small intestine causing a shift of fluid from the intravascular space to the intestinal lumen. This leads to vasomotor symptoms of flushing, sweating, dizziness, and palpitations. Late dumping is due to reactive hypoglycemia. Symptoms include early satiety, cramping, and explosive diarrhea. The constellation of dizziness, nausea, and sweating after a carbohydrate-heavy diet can be seen in up to 75% of gastric bypass patients but rarely with bands and sleeves. The episodes last approximately from 1 to 2 hours and may be alleviated by ingesting simple sugars or by lying down. In order to minimize the risk, patients are often advised to avoid calorie-dense foods and select those supplements with approximately 13 g of carbohydrates (or less) per serving. Patients who suffer from dumping syndrome are also encouraged to eat multiple small high-protein meals. Medications such as acarbose or octreotide may also be helpful. On rare occasions, patients may opt for reversal of their gastric bypass. Although there is limited information in the literature, at our institution, patients have presented with severe, intractable neurogylopenia and required reversal.

Bacterial Overgrowth

Bacterial overgrowth is a syndrome that is thought to be due to a change of the bacteria strains in the upper digestive system as a result of the surgical alteration of the gastrointestinal tract. Normally there are a low number of bacteria in the stomach, duodenum, jejunum, and ileum, but with either removing the body of the stomach or diverting it from the small bowel there are changes to the body's normal digestion and immunity. The foregut typically has 1×10^5 bacteria compared to the 1×10^{11} in the colon. In normal anatomy, gastric acid, bile, and digestive enzymes help to destroy bacteria and prevent overgrowth. After a gastric bypass, digested food no longer is exposed to an acidic environment of the stomach. Furthermore, the lack of bile in the Roux limb may also contribute to abnormal bacterial growth. Other factors include intestinal stasis and changes in the luminal digestive enzyme levels. The symptoms of bacterial overgrowth include abdominal cramping, bloating, discomfort, and diarrhea. The mechanism may be multifactorial and is not fully understood. The diagnosis is often one of exclusion. The workup includes a gastrointestinal fluoroscopic evaluation of the intestinal tract to rule out other possible causes, such as strictures, stasis, and dysmotility of the bowel. Hydrogen, bile, and xylose breath tests may also be helpful but the diagnosis is best made by endoscopy with biopsies and culturing of the intestinal fluids. The treatment of bacterial overgrowth syndrome includes correction of primary underlying disease, if any, antibiotic therapy, and even the use of probiotics.

Sleeve Gastrectomy

Sleeve Stricture

Sleeve stricture most commonly occurs at the incisura. The incidence is reported from 1% to 3.5%. The etiology is likely multifactorial but may depend on bougie size used.[23-29] The symptoms are similar to those seen with a gastric bypass anastomotic stricture, namely dysphagia and solid food intolerance. Endoscopic dilation is the first-line treatment and often effective for treating the stricture. If endoscopic dilation fails, surgical conversion of the sleeve to a gastric bypass may be indicated.[23]

Sleeve Leak

Sleeve leak occurs approximately in 0.5% to 3% of cases. It is most commonly seen at the angle of His just below the esophagogastric junction but can occur anywhere along the staple line. A sleeve leak presents very much like a leak after a gastric bypass, and treatment is also similar. When identified, surgical exploration is important to control the contamination of gastric fluid in the peritoneum. While debridement and repair may be attempted, wide drainage is the optimal intervention. Once the leak is controlled, endoscopic stenting may provide exclusion of the fistula in hopes to allow further healing. Unlike the gastric bypass leak, sleeve leaks are more resistant to conservative management and more likely to persist as a gastric fistula. This may be due to the higher intraluminal pressure in the sleeve than the gastric bypass pouch. If the fistula persists despite stenting, further endoscopic interventions, such as fibrin glue or clipping, may promote closure of the fistula. Should that fail, surgical repair or, depending on the location of the leak, conversion to a gastric bypass or esophagojejunostomy might be required.

Gastroesophageal Reflux

Gastroesophageal reflux is commonly associated with obesity and can resolve with weight loss. While gastric bypass and even the band improve severe reflux, the sleeve may actually worsen it. Reflux is caused by the backflow of acid or alkaline intragastric contents into the esophagus. The gastric sleeve is a high-pressure system that may facilitate the movement of gastric fluid into the esophagus. Should a patient fail medical management, surgery might be indicated. If a hiatal hernia is found at the time of surgery, it should be repaired, which may reduce the likelihood of reflux. Should a hiatal hernia be discovered in a patient with intractable reflux symptoms after the sleeve procedure, reoperation for hiatal hernia repair may be effective. Severe, intractable reflux may require conversion of the sleeve to a gastric bypass. Since the sleeve may worsen reflux symptoms, patients with severe reflux preoperatively should be counseled as such and may be better served by a gastric bypass.

Gastric Banding

Band Slippage (Figure 17-4)

Band slippage or prolapse occurs in approximately 2% to 13.2% of cases.[30] It is the result of the fundus distal to the band herniating through the band, resulting in a large, baggy gastric pouch. Some patients may be asymptomatic and the prolapse found incidentally. For those patients who present with symptoms, they will vary from new onset reflux to post-prandial pain and vomiting. In extreme cases, prolapse may be associated with outlet obstruction of the stomach and potentially ischemia and necrosis. Upper gastrointestinal fluoroscopy is the diagnostic study of choice. The first treatment for prolapse is deflating the band. Many patients will experience instant relief, and small prolapses may spontaneously resolve over time. For patients without improvement after band deflation or signs and symptoms of peritonitis, early surgical intervention may be mandated. Operative options include reduction of the prolapse and band repositioning or band removal. The appropriate choice will depend on patient wishes and the appearance of the stomach at surgery.

Band Erosion (Figure 17-5)

Band erosion or migration occurs in 1.5% to 2%[30] of cases and represents the migration of the band (that was placed on the outside of the stomach) through the wall of the stomach and the penetration into the lumen. The etiology of this complication is likely multifactorial. Possible causes include injury to the wall of the stomach at band placement, overtightening of the band, and chronic overeating. Like prolapse, patients may be asymptomatic and the erosion found incidentally or patients may complain of pain, reflux, vomiting, or the sensation that the band is no longer in place. Additionally, a late port infection may be due to a band erosion. Band erosion does not usually lead to free perforation. It is a slowly developing process, and the surrounding tissues seal off the erosion, minimizing the likelihood of free perforation. Endoscopy is the best modality to diagnose a band erosion as x-ray studies are rarely helpful. Often, an erosion will be seen on endoscopy for the workup of the patient's dysphagia. Once identified, the band must be surgically removed and erosion repaired. In some cases, the band can even be removed endoscopically.

Stomal Obstruction

Stomal obstruction is most frequently caused by impacted food and is due to poor dietary compliance, where patients do not chew their food adequately. Food gets lodged in the outlet. Patients will present with vomiting and describe the vomitus as "foam" as it is predominantly swallowed saliva. Many patients will vomit up the food and require no further treatment. For those patients

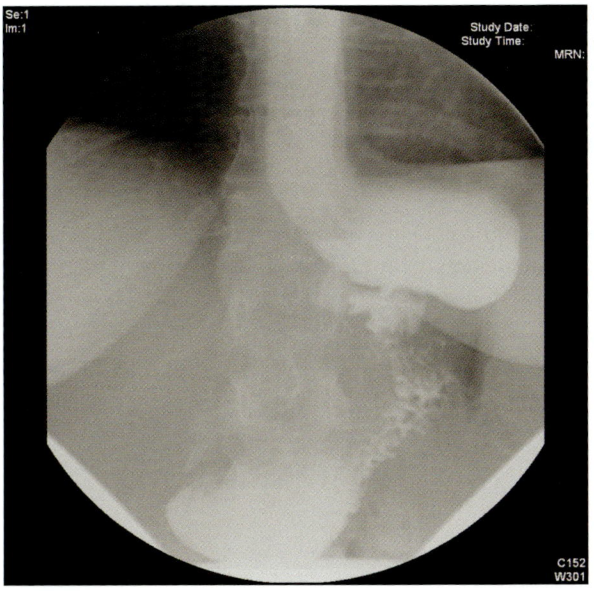

Figure 17-4. A gastric band prolapse demonstrated on upper GI series.

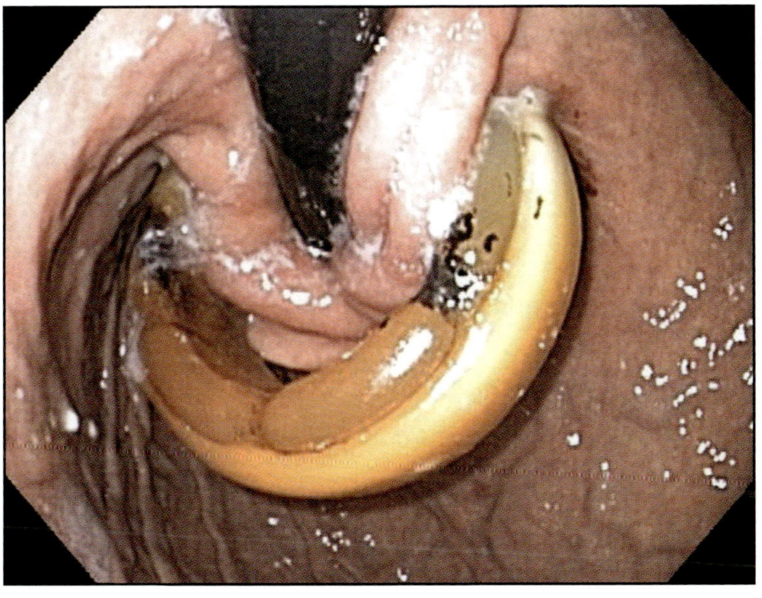

Figure 17-5. A gastric band erosion found on endoscopy. Most of the band is located inside the lumen of the stomach.

who present with foamy vomiting secondary to a food impaction, deflation of the band will usually solve the problem. If deflation of the band and a liquid diet for 48 hours does not relieve the obstruction, endoscopic removal of obstruction can be an option.

Port Problems

Port problems include infection, inversion, leak, or dislodgement. Superficial infections can initially be treated with antibiotics, but for the majority of cases, the port must be removed. Like all foreign bodies, the band port once contaminated will not clear infection with antibiotics. Only superficial skin infections at the port site where the port is not exposed to the bacteria will respond to conservative therapy. After port removal, a new port should generally not be attempted for several months to allow for maximal clearance of the infection. As stated previously, if there is a persistent or late port infection, further investigation should occur to rule out band erosion.

Inversion occurs if the fixation stitches dislodge and the port flips over, thereby it can no longer be accessed. A minor surgical procedure is needed to resecure it. A tube leak is suspected when after a band fill the restriction is quickly lost or when the volume of fluid recovered from the port will be less than the recorded volume inserted. Injecting contrast into the port under fluoroscopy may demonstrate the site of the leakage. The band and port system should then be revised.

Esophageal Dilation

Esophageal dilation occurs as a result of an acquired esophageal dysmotility secondary to a tight band. The incidence is thought to be 1% of patients, although the incidence may be higher as many patients are asymptomatic until the dilation and dysmotility are severe. Thus, yearly fluoroscopic surveillance is recommended. The first-line treatment for a mild dilation is deflation of the band. If resolution of the dilation does not occur after deflation of the band, then surgical explantation of the band is recommended.

Summary

Despite the success of weight loss and resolution of comorbidities, a bariatric patient who has undergone surgery is always considered as a bariatric patient for life and requires long-term follow-up. The currently performed operative procedures each have unique mechanisms of action to promote weight loss and potential long-term consequences. Therefore, to best manage these patients, an understanding of the anatomy and physiology of each procedure is important. The risk of micronutrient depletion is life-long and needs to be evaluated. Supplementation is critical to prevent adverse health conditions. Particular attention must also be given to bariatric surgical patients who present with concerns or symptoms. A life-long partnership between knowledgeable clinicians and bariatric patients is important to get the most benefits from the procedures and to minimize the risks.

References

1. Adams TD, Gress RE, Smith SC, et al. Long-term mortality after gastric bypass surgery. *N Engl J Med.* 2007;357(8):753-761.
2. Flegal KM, Carroll MD, Ogden CL, Johnson CL. Prevalence and trends in obesity among US adults, 1999-2000. *JAMA.* 2002;288(14):1723-1727.
3. Voelker R. Escalating obesity rates pose health, budget threats. *JAMA.* 2012;308(15):1514.
4. Steinbrook R. Surgery for severe obesity. *N Engl J Med.* 2004;350(11):1075.
5. Hong B, Stanley E, Reinhardt S, et al. Factors associated with readmission after laparoscopic gastric bypass surgery. *Surg Obes Relat Dis.* 2012;8:691-695.
6. Allied Health Sciences Section Ad Hoc Nutrition Committee, Aills L, Blankenship J, Buffington C, Furtado M, Parrott J. ASMBS allied health nutritional guidelines for the surgical weight loss patient. *Surg Obes Relat Dis.* 2008;4(5 Suppl):S73-S108.
7. Avinoah E, Ben-Yehuda A, Ovnat A, Pilpel D, Charuzi I. Long-term weight changes after Roux-en-Y gastric bypass for morbid obesity. *Harefuah.* 1993;124(4):185-187.
8. Salle A, Demarsy D, Poirier AL, et al. Zinc deficiency: a frequent and underestimated complication after bariatric surgery. *Obes Surg.* 2010;20:1660-1670.
9. Flores L, Osaba MJ, Andreu A, Moizé V, Rodríguez L, Vidal J. Calcium and vitamin D supplementation after gastric bypass should be individualized to improve or avoid hyperparathyroidism. *Obes Surg.* 2010;20:738-743.
10. Aarts EO, van Wageningen B, Janssen IM, Berends FJ. Prevalence of anemia and related deficiencies in the first year following laparoscopic gastric bypass for morbid obesity. *J Obes.* 2012;2012:193705.
11. Clements RH, Katasani VG, Palepu R, et al. Incidence of vitamin deficiency after laparoscopic Roux-en-Y gastric bypass in a university hospital setting. *Am J Surg.* 2006;(72):1196-1204.
12. Eckert MJ, Perry JT, Sohn VY, et al. Incidence of low vitamin A levels and ocular symptoms after Roux-en-Y gastric bypass. *Surg Obes Relat Dis.* 2010;(6):653-657.

13. Portenier DD, Grant JP, Blackwood HS, Pryor A, McMahon RL, DeMaria E. Expectant management of asymptomatic gallbladder at Roux-en-Y gastric bypass. *Surg Obes Relat Dis.* 2007;3(4):476-479.
14. Sugerman HJ, Brewer WH, Shiffman ML, et al. A multicenter, placebo-controlled, randomized, double-blind prospective trial of prophylactic ursodiol for the prevention of gallstone formation following gastric-bypass-induced rapid weight loss. *Am J Surg.* 1995;169:91-96.
15. Azagury DE, Abu Dayyeh BK, Greenwalt IT, Thompson CC. Marginal ulceration after Roux-en-Y gastric bypass surgery: characteristics, risk factors, treatment and outcomes. *Endoscopy.* 2011;43:950-954.
16. Salimath J, Rosenthal RJ, Szomstein S. Laparoscopic remnant gastrectomy as novel approach for treatment of gastrogastric fistula. *Surg Endosc.* 2009;23:2591-2595.
17. Schirmer BD, Meyers WC, Hanks JB, Kortz WJ, Jones RS, Postlethwait RW. Marginal ulcer. A difficult surgical problem. *Ann Surg.* 1982;195:653-661.
18. Csendes A, Burgos AM, Braghetto I. Classification and management of leaks after gastric bypass for patients with morbid obesity: a prospective study of 60 patients. *Obes Surg.* 2012;22:855-862.
19. Heneghan HM, Meron-Eldar S, Yenumula P, Rogula T, Brethauer SA, Schauer PR. Incidence and management of bleeding complications after gastric bypass surgery in the morbidly obese. *Surg Obes Relat Dis.* 2012;8:729-735.
20. Sugerman et al. Stomal complications of gastric bypass: incidence and outcome of therapy. *Am J Gastroenterol.* 1992;(9):1165-1169.
21. Espinel J, Pinedo E. Stenosis in gastric bypass: endoscopic management. *World J Gastrointest Endosc.* 2012;4:290-295.
22. Matthews BD, Sing RF, DeLegge MH, Ponsky JL, Heniford BT. Initial results with a staples gastrojejunostomy for the laparoscopic isolated Roux-en-Y gastric bypass. *Am J Surg.* 2000;179:476-481.
23. Abdel-Galil E, Sabry AA. Laparoscopic Roux-en-Y gastric bypass—evaluation of three different techniques. *Obes Surg.* 2002;(5):639-642.
24. Asplin JR, Coe FL. Hyperoxaluria in kidney stone formers treated with modern bariatric surgery. *J Urol.* 2007;177(2):565-569.
25. Whitson JM, Stackhouse GB, Stoller ML. Hyperoxaluria after modern bariatric surgery: case series and literature review. *Int Urol Nephrol.* 2010;42(2):369-374.
26. Cochat P, Hulton SA, Acquaviva C, et al. Primary hyperoxaluria type 1: indications for screening and guidance for diagnosis and treatment. *Nephrol Dial Transplant.* 2012;27:1729-1736.
27. Milliner DS, Eickholt JT, Bergstralh EJ, Wilson DM, Smith LH. Results of long-term treatment with orthophosphate and pyridoxine in patients with primary hyperoxaluria. *N Engl J Med.* 1994;331:1553-1558.
28. Parikh A, Alley JB, Peterson RM, et al. Management options for symptomatic stenosis after laparoscopic vertical sleeve gastrectomy in the morbidly obese. *Surg Endosc.* 2012;(3):738-746.
29. Gagner M, Deitel M, Kalberer TL, Erickson AL, Crosby RD. The second international consensus summit for sleeve gastrectomy, March 19-21, 2009. *Surg Obes Relat Dis.* 2009;(4):476-485.
30. Owers C, Ackroyd R. A study examining the complications associated with gastric banding. *Obes Surg.* 2013;23:56-59.

III

Medical Issues Post Bariatric Surgery

18

Nutritional Consequences Following Bariatric Surgery

Ashley Cuellar, MD; Pradeep K. Pallati, MBBS, FACS; and Amanda Powell, MD

The nutritional consequences of bariatric surgery are broad and require long-term oversight. Preexisting nutritional deficiencies may become exacerbated by bariatric surgery, and de novo deficiencies may occur as a result of reduced food intake, changes in digestion or absorption, or nonadherence to recommended supplementation.[1] The postoperative nutrition and metabolic evaluation of the bariatric patient should be guided by the specific procedure performed. Bariatric surgery may be purely restrictive, purely malabsorptive (these are rarely, if at all, offered), or a combination of restrictive and malabsorptive techniques. Purely restrictive procedures are not associated with alterations in intestinal continuity; therefore, nutritional deficiencies may be less frequent. Alternatively, nutritional deficiencies occur often following operations involving malabsorptive techniques due to the significant alterations in gastrointestinal anatomy. Any preoperative nutritional disturbances, which are common in patients with obesity, should be optimized prior to any surgery to minimize postoperative ramifications. The postoperative period should include systematic laboratory evaluation as well as a multidisciplinary team approach to detect and manage potential nutritional complications. It is also imperative patients seeking a bariatric procedure understand the life-long commitment to vitamin and nutritional supplementation, as well as to frequent metabolic and nutritional monitoring.

Restrictive Procedures

Laparoscopic Adjustable Gastric Band

The laparoscopic adjustable gastric band (LAGB) achieves weight loss by reducing available gastric volume and inducing satiety with a small amount of food.[2] This is a purely restrictive procedure with no element of malabsorption. A hollow, flexible silicone band is placed around the upper stomach, which reduces stomach capacity and causes rapid feelings of satiety. The band is tightened by injecting saline via a subcutaneous port located just inferior to the sternum or lateral to the

Forse RA, Apovian CM, eds.
Bariatric Surgery: What Every Provider Needs to Know (pp 213-227).

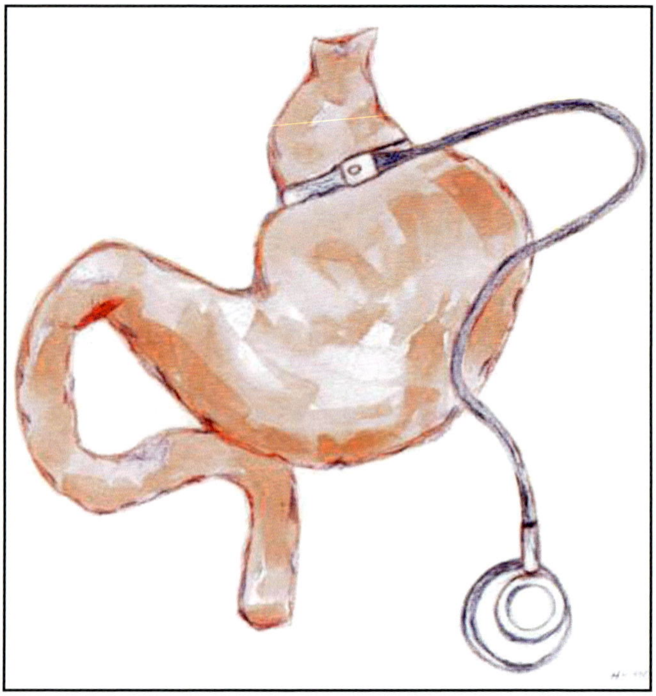

Figure 18-1. Laparoscopic adjustable gastric band. (Illustration by Kyisook Hong.)

umbilicus. The gastric pouch above the band usually restricts the volume of intake to around 15 to 30 mL. In the first 1 to 2 years following surgery, energy intake averages approximately 1000 to 1400 kcal daily, significantly reduced from presurgery intake.[2] The nutritional consequences of this procedure are a result of decreased intake of calories and subsequently nutrients (Figure 18-1).

Sleeve Gastrectomy

The sleeve gastrectomy involves resection of a significant portion of the stomach body and the fundus, leaving a long tubular stomach. This results in smaller available gastric volume, usually between 75 to 120 mL, and hormone changes, which induce early satiety and subsequent weight loss.[3] Compared to adjustable gastric banding, these patients are able to tolerate larger quantities of food. Unlike the gastric band, however, the sleeve gastrectomy does not allow for volume adjustments. Because there is no alteration in the small bowel anatomy, absorption is not affected. The nutritional consequences of this procedure are a result of restricted calorie intake similar to adjustable gastric banding (Figure 18-2).

Combination Restrictive and Malabsorptive Procedures

Roux-en-Y Gastric Bypass

Roux-en-Y gastric bypass (RYGB) acts to both restrict gastric volume and induce malabsorption. A small pouch, 15 to 30 mL, is created from the proximal portion of the stomach. The jejunum is subsequently divided a distance away from the ligament of Treitz. The distal jejunal segment is anastomosed to the gastric pouch creating the Roux or alimentary limb. A jejunojejunostomy is

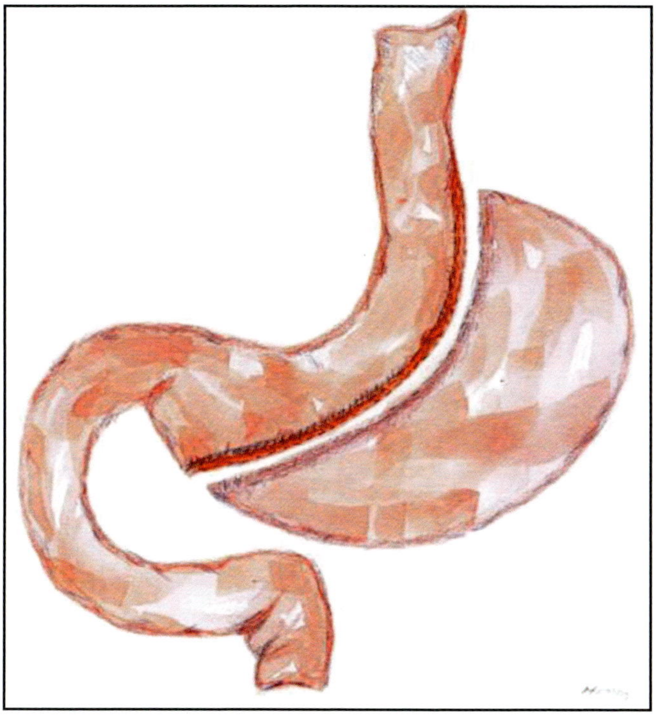

Figure 18-2. Sleeve gastrectomy. (Illustration by Kyisook Hong.)

then created by anastomosis of the proximal portion of the jejunum or the biliopancreatic limb to the side of the Roux limb. This procedure leads to food restriction, as a result of the small pouch, as well as malabsorption, as the majority of the stomach, the entire duodenum, and the proximal jejunum are bypassed (Figure 18-3).

Biliopancreatic Diversion With Duodenal Switch

Biliopancreatic diversion with duodenal switch (BPD-DS), also a restrictive and malabsorptive procedure, is a variant of the BPD procedure. The BPD procedure with and without gastrectomy proved wrought with post-surgical complications. The DS, originally described as a therapy for bile acid reflux, alleviated some of the complications seen with BPD alone.

The restrictive component of this procedure is achieved with a pylorus-sparing partial gastrectomy, often a sleeve gastrectomy, which leaves a gastric volume of approximately 100 mL.[4] The duodenum is transected, leaving only a small portion associated with the stomach. This duodenal stump is anastomosed to transected ileum, which allows for bypass of the remaining duodenum and jejunum. The length of this alimentary limb is approximately 40% of the original length of the small bowel.[4] An anastomosis between the biliopancreatic limb and alimentary limb is constructed to form a short common channel, approximately 50 to 100 cm from the ileocecal valve.[4] This surgery is the most malabsorptive of the procedures discussed here. The remaining stomach produces gastric acid and pepsinogen, which initiate protein digestion. The absorption of peptides and carbohydrates is somewhat preserved along the length of the alimentary limb because of the presence of brush border enzymes. Absorption of dietary fat, however, depends on emulsification by bile salts and can only take place in the short common channel. Protein-calorie malnutrition and vitamin and mineral deficiencies may occur with this method. Additionally, fat malabsorption and the excretion of bile acids may predispose patients to deficiencies of fat-soluble vitamins (Figure 18-4).

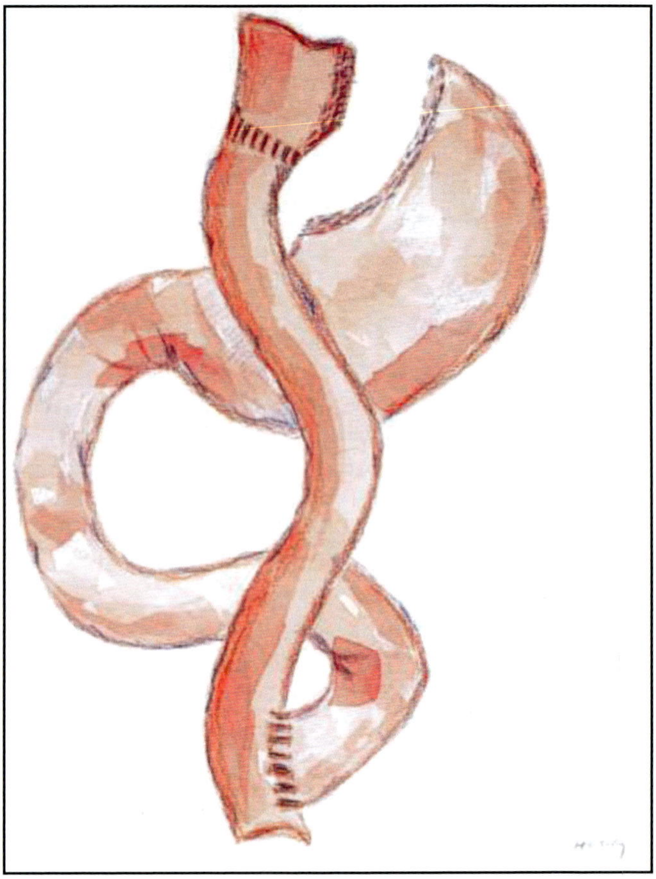

Figure 18-3. Roux-en-Y gastric bypass. (Illustration by Kyisook Hong.)

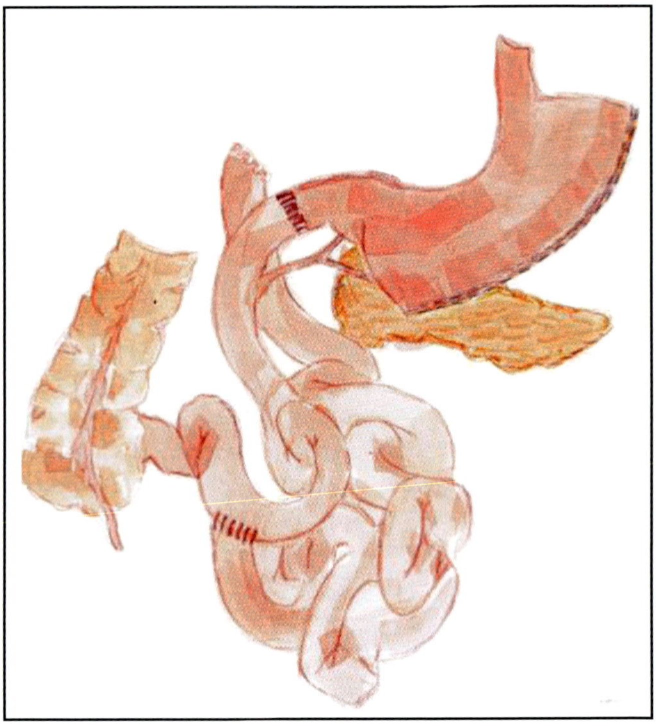

Figure 18-4. Biliopancreatic diversion with duodenal switch. (Illustration by Kyisook Hong.)

Energy and Macronutrient Needs

Energy

Total caloric intake usually begins with approximately 400 kcal per day during the first 4 weeks following bariatric surgery and increases slowly over the subsequent months to 800 to 1000 kcal per day, divided into multiple small meals and snacks.[5] The optimal long-term macronutrient combination for a post-surgical bariatric patient is not well defined. Despite initial weight loss, indelible changes and weight loss maintenance is difficult.[6] Observational studies have shown patients undergoing restrictive surgeries typically follow a dietary composition similar to his or her presurgical diet in the 12 months following surgery, regardless of recommendations.[7] In order to achieve sustained weight loss, ensure proper nutrition, and minimize deficiencies, an individualized long-term diet plan should be guided by a trained dietician and monitored by the multidisciplinary team.

Protein

Adequate protein intake is encouraged postoperatively for improved healing, to decrease lean body mass loss, and increase satiety. Protein calorie malnutrition is rare following the LAGB and LSG. It is more common after RYGB due to intolerance of protein-rich foods and in BPD ± DS as the ingested protein may be poorly absorbed and lost in the stool.[8] Protein malnutrition is the most common and severe macronutrient complication associated with malabsorptive procedures.[9] Importantly, however, protein malnutrition can occur in any patient due to inadequate protein intake.

Current medical guidelines for the nutritional support of the bariatric surgery patient recommend an average daily protein intake of 60 g daily at a minimum and up to 1.5 g/kg of ideal body weight.[10] Additional protein intake may require adjustment by a trained professional. It is imperative to properly educate all patients on how to achieve an adequate amount of protein per day. If a patient is unable to tolerate solid food proteins, alternative sources must be offered, such as liquid protein shakes. Despite these recommendations a large proportion of bariatric patients fail to attain their daily goals.[8]

Carbohydrates

Carbohydrate intake is slowly increased postoperatively. The specific type of carbohydrate consumed is vital to ensure success as well as avoid undesirable complications. In particular, ingestion of simple carbohydrates, such as sugar, can contribute to rapid gastric emptying, diarrhea, or abdominal discomfort, otherwise known as dumping syndrome. Emphasis should be placed on educating patients to read nutrition labels, in order to limit the total amount of sugar to less than 7 g per 100-g serving and avoid foods with sugar alcohols due to laxative effect.

Fat

In the initial postoperative period, total intake of fat is usually low due to the gradual progression from a liquid to solid diet. Over time, as the variety and tolerability of foods increase, the percentage of kilocalories from fat also increases. Patients who maintain a higher protein, lower fat diet generally achieve better weight loss due to lower total caloric intake. Some experts have suggested no more than 25% of total calories be derived from fat following bariatric surgery, to promote optimal weight loss.[11] Therefore, patient education to avoid calorically dense foods and adhere to an appropriate distribution of calories will likely facilitate improved weight loss success and help avoid weight regain.

Hydration

Decreased fluid intake in the early postoperative period can lead to dehydration. This is especially common after restrictive procedures as patients adapt to the smaller gastric potential volume and have difficulty drinking the necessary fluid. Dehydration in this setting can be challenging to correct with oral fluids as the reduced gastric capacity limits how quickly patients are able to drink. Patient education of the signs of dehydration is imperative, including thirst, fatigue, muscle cramps, dizziness, and decreased urine output. If patients develop severe dehydration and cannot adequately replete themselves, parenteral fluids may be necessary.

Patients should aim to achieve fluid intake of at least 1.5 liters per day. It is important to counsel patients to wait 30 minutes before and/or after meals to consume liquids in order to avoid gastrointestinal discomfort. Caffeinated beverages, such as coffee and tea, should be avoided immediately following surgery as caffeine can potentiate gastric acid secretion resulting in gastroesophageal reflux. Also, caffeine can lead to increased urine output, which may potentiate dehydration. Consumption of carbonated beverages may lead to cramping, bloating, and vomiting, and thus should be avoided, especially during the first 6 months postoperatively.

Following any bariatric surgery, vomiting and/or diarrhea can quickly lead to dehydration. These patients may need hospital admission for aggressive fluid resuscitation. In cases involving LAGB, the band may need to be deflated completely to promote adequate oral rehydration as well as to prevent band slippage during episodes of vomiting.

Nutritional Deficiencies

Micronutrient deficiencies are more common in RYGB and BPD ± DS due to the alteration in intestine anatomy; however, they can occur in all types of bariatric procedures. The most common deficiencies include iron, vitamin B_{12}, thiamine, folate, and the fat-soluble vitamins A, D, E, and K. General recommendations for routine nutritional supplementation in all patients undergoing a malabsorptive procedure include the following[10] (Table 18-1):

- 1 to 2 chewable daily multivitamins, which include iron (40 to 65 mg), folic acid (400 mcg), thiamine (400 mcg), vitamin A (1 mg), vitamin E (100 to 300 mg), and vitamin K (65 to 80 mg)
- 1200 to 1500 mg elemental calcium (as calcium citrate, divided dose)
- Vitamin D at least 3000 IU/day; goal 25-hydroxyvitamin D > 30
- B_{12} > 350 mcg/day

Iron

Iron is important in the oxidative and reductive activities in cellular respiration, involved in erythrocyte function, and heme utilization. Iron deficiency is the most common micronutrient deficiency after bariatric surgery. In order to absorb iron, it needs to be reduced to the ferrous state by gastric acid. It is then primarily absorbed in the duodenum and proximal jejunum. Postoperatively, the mechanism by which iron deficiency occurs is 2-fold. First, after a restrictive procedure, where a portion of the stomach is removed, there is reduced gastric hydrochloric acid production. Second, in procedures with a malabsorptive component, there is less intestinal surface area to absorb iron. Iron deficiency anemia is therefore more common and can be more severe after combination procedures. It is also more common in menstruating women following combination procedures.[9]

Table 18-1

Standard Preventative Nutrition Supplementation[10]

SUPPLEMENT	RECOMMENDED SUPPLEMENTAL DOSE
Chewable multivitamin (one that includes 40 to 65 mg iron, 400 mcg folic acid, 400 mcg thiamine, 1 mg vitamin A, 100 to 300 mg vitamin E, and 65 to 80 mg vitamin K)	2 tablets by mouth daily for sleeve gastrectomy, RYGB, and BPD ± DS 1 tablet by mouth daily for LAGB
Elemental calcium (calcium citrate preferred)	1200 to 1500 mg by mouth daily
Vitamin D_3	3000 IU by mouth daily and titrate as needed to maintain normal range
Vitamin B_{12}	At least 350 mcg/day and titrate as needed to maintain normal range May be administered orally daily, intranasal weekly, intramuscularly monthly or every 6 months

To achieve the recommended daily goal, patients undergoing a procedure with a malabsorptive component may need to take an iron supplement in addition to the iron found in a standard daily multivitamin. Treatment regimens for deficient patients include oral ferrous sulfate, fumarate, or gluconate to provide up to 150 to 200 mg of elemental iron daily. Vitamin C supplementation may be added simultaneously to increase iron absorption. Intravenous iron infusion (preferably with ferric gluconate or sucrose) may be needed for patients with severe intolerance to oral iron or refractory deficiency due to severe iron malabsorption.

Vitamin B_{12}

Vitamin B_{12} or cobalamin, a water-soluble vitamin, serves as a cofactor in many processes required for normal nerve cell activity as well as DNA replication. It is bound to protein from which it is cleaved by pepsin in the stomach and subsequently bound to R factor. In the duodenum, cobalamin is exposed to pancreatic proteases, which separate it from R factor after which it binds to gastric-produced intrinsic factor. This complex is acted upon by a specific receptor in the terminal ileum that facilitates absorption. Symptoms of B_{12} deficiency include macrocytic anemia, peripheral neuropathy, leukopenia, glossitis, thrombocytopenia, paresthesia, and neuropathy.[7] Vitamin B_{12} deficiency is seen in up to one-third of RYGB patients[12] due to the reduced pepsin and inadequate secretion of intrinsic factor.[13] It may also occur due to bacterial overgrowth as a result of reduced motility of the bypassed small intestine. If preoperative cobalamin stores are replete, a deficiency may not present for years following surgery.

Baseline and postoperative evaluation for vitamin B_{12} deficiency is recommended in all bariatric surgeries and annually in those with procedures that exclude parts of the stomach, such as with the RYGB, sleeve gastrectomy, and BPD ± DS.

All bariatric surgery patients should have at least 350 mcg daily of preventive B_{12} supplementation. Oral high-dose supplementation with crystalline vitamin B_{12} at a dosage of 1000 mcg daily or more may be used to maintain normal vitamin B_{12} levels. Intranasal vitamin B_{12}, 500 mcg weekly, may also be considered parenteral (intramuscular or subcutaneous) B_{12} supplementation;

1000 mcg per month to 1000 to 3000 mcg every 6 to 12 months is indicated if B_{12} sufficiency cannot be maintained using oral or intranasal routes. If bacterial overgrowth is suspected, an empiric course of antibiotic therapy can be used.

Folate

Folate is needed to synthesize DNA, repair DNA, and act as a cofactor in many biologic reactions, including cell division and growth. Folate is absorbed both in the proximal small intestine and the jejunum. Folate deficiency can lead to macrocytic anemia, thrombocytopenia, leukopenia, and glossitis. Deficiency is preventable with a standard daily multivitamin, which typically includes at least 400 mcg. Women of childbearing age should have additional supplementation to reduce the risk of fetal neural tube defects. Due to the inability to tolerate high-residue foods, such as green, leafy vegetables, folic acid deficiency may present in patients undergoing restrictive procedures as well as combined and malabsorptive procedures.

Thiamine

Vitamin B_1, or thiamine, is a water-soluble vitamin that plays a role in oxidative metabolism and is a coenzyme in several neurologic and cardiac pathways. Thiamine is primarily absorbed in the proximal small intestine.[14] The body's storage of thiamine is limited, about 18 days[15]; therefore, symptoms of a deficiency can occur as early as a few weeks postoperatively.[16] Particularly vulnerable patients include those who experience persistent vomiting.[17,18] It is important to note that thiamine deficiency may occur in purely restrictive procedures, not only those with a malabsorptive component.[19]

A high degree of suspicion must be maintained when evaluating patients who have undergone bariatric surgery and present with ophthalmoplegias (nystagmus), ataxia, or mental status changes. These symptoms may characterize Wernicke encephalopathy, which must be attended to promptly with thiamine replacement to avoid permanent neurologic damage, such as Korsakoff syndrome.

Other complications of thiamine deficiency include peripheral neuritis and cardiac dysfunction.[14]

Most cases of thiamine deficiency can be prevented with a daily multivitamin that includes 400 mcg of B_1. Screening for thiamine deficiency and/or empiric thiamine supplementation should be considered in post-bariatric surgery patients with rapid weight loss, protracted vomiting, parenteral nutrition, excessive alcohol use, neurologic changes, or heart failure. Mild deficiency can be treated with intravenous thiamine, 100 mg daily, for 7 to 14 days. Patients with severe thiamine deficiency, suspected or established, should be treated with intravenous thiamine 500 mg daily for 3 to 5 days, followed by 250 mg daily for 3 to 5 days or until resolution of symptoms. Treatment with 100 mg daily per oral should then be considered, usually indefinitely or until risk factors have resolved.[10]

Calcium and Vitamin D

Vitamin D is essential for the regulation of serum calcium levels, which is essential for bone health. Dietary vitamin D uptake occurs in the jejunum and ileum. Active transport of calcium occurs in the duodenum and proximal jejunum, but passive absorption may occur along the entire small intestine. Both hypocalcemia and vitamin D deficiency are more common in obese patients than nonobese people, notwithstanding surgery. This may be due to a combination of reduced exposure to sunlight, low physical activity, and increased storage of calcium in adipose tissue with reduced bioavailability.

Postoperatively, reduced absorption of both calcium and vitamin D may occur. Vitamin D deficiency leads to reduced intestinal absorption of calcium and phosphorus, which may lead to secondary hyperparathyroidism. This results in increased resorption of calcium from bone with a resultant risk of metabolic bone pathology. In addition, post-surgical patients may not tolerate dairy, which can lead to reduced intake. Calcium and vitamin D supplementation should be routinely advised for all patients. Calcium carbonate is not bioavailable without gastric acid; therefore, calcium citrate is recommended in patients who have undergone RYGB, BPD ± DS, and sleeve gastrectomy. All patients should be counseled on the importance of life-long supplementation including calcium citrate 1500 mg daily plus cholecalciferol 3000 IU daily. Severe vitamin D deficiency may require high doses of D_2 or D_3 oral supplementation up to 50,000 IU 1 to 3 times a week.[10]

Markers of metabolic bone disease can be observed as early as 3 months postoperatively. Routine monitoring should include serum levels of calcium, vitamin D, phosphorus, parathyroid hormone, and alkaline phosphatase. In addition, dual-energy x-ray absorptiometry for bone density should be performed yearly until stable.

Vitamin C

Vitamin C, ascorbic acid, when deficient, may lead to scurvy. This is uncommon following bariatric procedures in patients who consume fruits and vegetables. Patients with iron deficiency, who fail to respond to oral iron, may benefit from supplementation of vitamin C because this will enhance absorption of iron from both dietary sources and supplements.

Vitamin A

Vitamin A levels tend to be low after procedures with a malabsorptive component as a result of poor intake and fat malabsorption. Vitamin A deficiency may cause night blindness as well as other ocular complications. Although rare, monitoring is necessary following BPD ± DS every 6 to 12 months.

Vitamin K

Vitamin K deficiency may also occur after procedures with a malabsorptive component. Routine screening for vitamin K deficiency is not recommended but should be considered in the setting of other fat-soluble vitamin deficiencies, coagulopathy, and hepatopathy.[10]

Zinc

Zinc is an essential mineral with a role as a cellular antioxidant and is essential in the structure and metabolic activity of proteins. It is absorbed primarily in the jejunum. Signs of zinc deficiency include hair loss, pica, dysgeusia, and erectile dysfunction. All patients should take a daily multivitamin that includes 8 mg of elemental zinc. Serum monitoring of zinc levels is not recommended unless suspicious symptoms are present. Zinc supplementation in high doses of 50 mg daily or more can interfere with intestinal absorption of copper; therefore, patients receiving prolonged zinc supplementation should be monitored for copper deficiency.[20] Patients treated for zinc deficiency or who are using supplemental zinc for hair loss should receive 1 mg of copper for each 8 to 15 mg of zinc.

Copper

Copper is another essential mineral. It is important for the production of erythrocytes and an important cofactor for enzymes involved in erythrocyte and nerve function. Copper deficiency can occur in patients with prolonged emesis leading to anemia and demyelinating neuropathy. Copper supplementation of 2 mg should be included as part of the standard post-surgical multivitamin. Routine copper screening is not indicated following bariatric surgery but should be evaluated in patients with anemia, neutropenia, myeloneuropathy, and impaired wound healing. Mild to moderate deficiency can be treated with oral copper sulfate or gluconate 3 to 8 mg/day until levels normalize and symptoms resolve. In severe deficiency, treatment can be initiated with intravenous copper.[10]

Selenium

Selenium is a trace mineral important in the function of the thyroid gland as well antioxidant defense. It is absorbed in the duodenum and proximal jejunum. Selenium deficiency has been linked to skeletal muscle dysfunction and cardiomyopathy.[21] Routine monitoring is not necessary; however, levels should be checked in patients who have undergone a malabsorptive bariatric surgical procedure with unexplained anemia or fatigue, persistent diarrhea, cardiomyopathy, or metabolic bone disease. Selenium deficiency can be managed with oral supplementation. Care must be taken as the optimal range for dietary intake of selenium is narrow. Selenium toxicity may occur with excess intake. Symptoms of toxicity include nausea, emesis, diarrhea, hair loss, and mental status changes, among others (Table 18-2).

Dietary Advancement and Eating Behaviors After Bariatric Surgery

Patients who undergo bariatric surgery will require a staged progression of nutrition intake specific to the type of surgery performed. Adherence to the gradual dietary progression will minimize dumping syndrome and vomiting, which may lead to anastomotic damage and gastroesophageal reflux.

In general, the immediate postoperative diet focuses on adequate protein intake as well as hydration. Postoperatively, day 1 is typically limited to water and quickly advanced to clear liquids on postoperative day 2 or 3. Full liquids with protein-rich formulations are added at this time as well. If able, patients may be discharged on this diet to further advance as an outpatient guided by a trained registered dietician.

Following LABG, patients are able to tolerate a normal diet relatively soon as the band is initially placed deflated and is not filled until 6 weeks postoperatively. Patients should be able to advance to a restricted, healthy, and regular diet by postoperative week 6 prior to adjustments. After filling, the patient will resume full liquids for 2 to 3 days then advance. As the band is tightened, patients may begin to experience food intolerances and/or vomiting. General principles for patients undergoing LAGB include eat slowly (1 ounce over 10 minutes), eat small meals, wait at least 30 minutes after eating in order to consume liquids, and stop eating when satiated.

Advancing the diet following an RYGB and sleeve gastrectomy is similar. Typically the time to a healthy solid food diet is greater than 5 weeks postoperative. The BPD ± DS procedure may require 12 weeks or more until a long-term diet is achieved. A focus on protein and adequate hydration remains paramount when composing a long-term diet plan for these procedures. Additionally, as the post-surgical pouch is not capable of digestion in the same manner as the original stomach, patients are advised to chew food extensively. This also helps to maximize absorption once food moves from the pouch.

RYGB patients are at risk of dumping syndrome. Dumping syndrome occurs when food passes too rapidly into the small intestine. Early dumping syndrome, occurring 30 minutes following a meal, is characterized by abdominal bloating, discomfort, nausea, cramping, diaphoresis, flushing, lightheadedness, flatulence, and diarrhea. This is a result of fluid shift into the intestine due to hyperosmolar contents as well as enhanced release of gastrointestinal hormones. The later stages of dumping syndrome appear 1 to 3 hours after a meal as a result of reactive hypoglycemia. Prevention involves avoidance of high sugar content foods, consumption of small frequent meals, eating slowly, chewing food thoroughly, and drinking liquids in between meals.

Table 18-2
Screening and Surveillance for Nutritional Deficiencies

DEFICIENCY	SIGNS AND SYMPTOMS	SCREENING AND SURVEILLANCE SCHEDULE				COMMENTS
		LAGB	*LSG*	*RYGB*	*BPD-DS*	
Calcium	Tetany, paresthesias, muscle cramps, Trousseau's sign, Chvostek's sign, seizures, prolonged QT, hypotension, heart failure, arrhythmia	Included in comprehensive metabolic panel obtained with each visit				Preventive supplementation necessary
Vitamin D	May be asymptomatic, bone demineralization, weakness, bone pain	Preop	Preop	Preop, postop every 3 to 6 months for the first year, then annually	Preop, postop every 3 months for the first year, then every 6 to 12 months	Preventive supplementation necessary May lead to hypocalcemia, hypophosphatemia, and secondary hyperparathyroidism
		If repletion is necessary check 2 months following treatment prior to starting maintenance dose				
Vitamin B_{12}	May be asymptomatic, megaloblastic anemia, paresthesias, ataxia, weakness, spasticity, clonus, memory loss, irritability, dementia, increased risk of osteoporosis	Preop and postop	Preop, postop, and annually	Preop, postop every 3 to 6 months for the first year, then annually	Preop, postop every 3 months for the first year, then every 3 to 6 months depending on symptoms	Preventive supplementation necessary Prevalence increases after postoperative year 1 Consider bacterial overgrowth treatment if suspected
		If repletion is necessary check every 3 to 6 months as appropriate				

(continued)

Table 18-2 (continued)

Screening and Surveillance for Nutritional Deficiencies

DEFICIENCY	SIGNS AND SYMPTOMS	SCREENING AND SURVEILLANCE SCHEDULE				COMMENTS
		LAGB	*LSG*	*RYGB*	*BPD-DS*	
Folic acid	Megaloblastic anemia, thrombocytopenia, leukopenia, glossitis, and elevated homocysteine levels	Preop, postop, and with any specific findings especially in patients who have undergone a combination procedure				Preventive supplementation necessary Stores can deplete within months Special consideration to women of childbearing age and need for additional supplementation
Iron	Anemia, fatigue, weakness, pica, restless leg syndrome	Preop, postop, and PRN	Preop, postop, and PRN	Preop, postop every 3 to 6 months for the first year, then annually	Preop, postop every 3 months for the first year, then every 3 to 6 months depending on symptoms	Preventive supplementation necessary Consider vitamin C supplementation for increased iron absorption Consider intravenous iron infusion for oral intolerance or refractory deficiency Usually seen in menstruating women May develop early or several years postoperative
Copper	Anemia, neutropenia, myeloneuropathy, impaired wound healing	Routine screening not recommended Consider screening any with specific findings especially in patients who have undergone a combination procedure				Consider supplementation in patients who are undergoing treatment for zinc deficiency as this may cause copper deficiency

(continued)

Table 18-2 (continued)

Screening and Surveillance for Nutritional Deficiencies

DEFICIENCY	SIGNS AND SYMPTOMS	SCREENING AND SURVEILLANCE SCHEDULE				COMMENTS
		LAGB	*LSG*	*RYGB*	*BPD-DS*	
Zinc	Hair loss, dysgeusia, hypogonadism, or erectile dysfunction in males	Routine screening not recommended	Routine screening not recommended	Annually or PRN	Annually or PRN	
Selenium	Anemia, fatigue, persistent diarrhea, cardiomyopathy, metabolic bone disease	Routine screening not recommended. Consider screening any with specific findings especially in patients who have undergone a combination procedure.				
Thiamine	Confusion, nystagmus, ataxia, ophthalmoplegia, neuropathy, encephalopathy, heart failure	Routine screening not recommended in those taking appropriate preventive supplementation Consider screening or empiric supplementation in patients with rapid weight loss, protracted vomiting, parenteral nutrition, excessive alcohol use or symptoms				Neurologic deficits have been reported as soon as 1 to 3 months after bariatric surgery May consider treatment for small bowel bacterial overgrowth in recurrent cases
Vitamin A	Night blindness, xerophthalmia, keratomalacia, hyperkeratosis, phrynoderma	None	None	Optional	Initial visit and every 6 to 12 months thereafter	
Vitamin K	Easy bruising, mucosal bleeding, melena, hematuria	Routine screening not recommended				

It is imperative all bariatric surgery patients are taught to recognize signs of satiety and encouraged to make long-term lifestyle changes to their eating habits. Patients should receive continued nutrition education and monitoring. Any difficulty adhering to the long-term diet plan must be addressed by the medical team.

Immediate Postoperative Complications Affecting Nutrition

All the bariatric procedures are associated with the possibility of postoperative complications. These may range from esophageal or gastric perforation, band slippage with obstruction, anastomotic leaks, fistula formation, bowel obstruction to prolonged mechanical ventilation, hemorrhage, or wound infection. All of these may prevent initiation of enteral nutrition. Often, this patient population has preexisting malabsorption and malnutrition prior to presentation and hence parenteral nutrition should not be delayed.[22] Special attention should be given to intravenous replacement of potassium and essential vitamins, including thiamine, and minerals.

Nutrition in Pregnancy Following Bariatric Surgery

It is generally recommended to postpone conception at least 1 year after surgery due to the significant decrease in caloric intake and rapid weight loss. Women of childbearing age should be counseled on appropriate contraceptive choices including nonoral contraception for those who have undergone a malabsorptive procedure. Following this period, pregnancy after bariatric surgery appears to be safe. Bariatric surgery is effective in reducing complications such as gestational diabetes mellitus, gestational hypertensive disorders, and fetal macrosomia, but may result in an increase in neonates born small-for-gestational age. Pre-pregnancy assessment of micronutrient status is important to identify and correct any deficiencies, particularly folic acid, as early deficiency is associated with fetal malformations. Additionally, iron requirement increases significantly during pregnancy, and this needs to be addressed appropriately with oral supplementation. Iron supplements should be taken between meals to decrease gastric irritation and to increase absorption. Pregnant patients should have nutritional surveillance with laboratory screening every trimester to include iron, folate, B_{12}, calcium, and fat-soluble vitamins. Patients who have undergone an LABG may need band adjustments to allow for appropriate weight gain.[9]

References

1. Saltzman E, Karl JP. Nutrient deficiencies after gastric bypass surgery. *Annu Rev Nutr.* 2013;33:183-203.
2. Dodsworth A, Warren-Forward H, Baines S. A systematic review of dietary intake after laparoscopic adjustable gastric banding. *J Hum Nutr Diet.* 2011;24(4):327-341.
3. Deitel M, Gagner M, Erickson AL, Crosby RD. Third International Summit: current status of sleeve gastrectomy. *Surg Obes Rel Dis.* 2011;7(6):749-759.
4. Hess DS, Hess DW, Oakley RS. The biliopancreatic diversion with the duodenal switch: results beyond 10 years. *Obes Surg.* 2005;15(3):408-416.
5. Kushner R. Managing the obese patient after bariatric surgery: a case report of severe malnutrition and review of the literature. *JPEN J Parenter Enteral Nutr.* 2000;24(2):126-132.
6. Sarwer DB, Dilks RJ, West-Smith L. Dietary intake and eating behavior after bariatric surgery: threats to weight loss maintenance and strategies for success. *Surg Obes Rel Dis.* 2011;7(5):644-651.
7. Andreu A, Moize V, Rodriguez L, Flores L, Vidal J. Protein intake, body composition, and protein status following bariatric surgery. *Obes Surg.* 2010;20(11):1509-1515.

8. Shikora SA, Kim JJ, Tarnoff ME. Nutrition and gastrointestinal complications of bariatric surgery. *Nutr Clin Pract.* 2007;22(1):29-40.
9. Mechanick JI, Kushner RF, Sugerman HJ, et al. American Association of Clinical Endocrinologists, the Obesity Society, and American Society for Metabolic and Bariatric Surgery medical guidelines for clinical practice for the perioperative nutritional, metabolic, and nonsurgical support of the bariatric surgery patient. *Obesity (Silver Spring, MD).* 2009;17(Suppl 1):S1-S70, v.
10. Mechanick JI, Youdim A, Jones DB, et al. Clinical practice guidelines for the perioperative nutritional, metabolic, and nonsurgical support of the bariatric surgery patient—2013 update: cosponsored by American Association of Clinical Endocrinologists, the Obesity Society, and American Society for Metabolic and Bariatric Surgery. *Surg Obes Rel Dis.* 2013;9(2):159-191.
11. Marinari GM, Murelli F, Camerini G, et al. A 15-year evaluation of biliopancreatic diversion according to the Bariatric Analysis Reporting Outcome System (BAROS). *Obes Surg.* 2004;14(3):325-328.
12. Mallory G. Maximum nutrition, minimum calories. *Obes Surg.* 1992;2(4):375-378.
13. Love AL, Billett HH. Obesity, bariatric surgery, and iron deficiency: true, true, true and related. *Am J Hematol.* 2008;83(5):403-409.
14. Feldman M, Friedman LS, Brandt LJ. *Sleisenger and Fordtran's Gastrointestinal and Liver Disease Pathophysiology/ Diagnosis/Management.* 10th ed. Philadelphia, PA: Saunders/Elsevier; 2015.
15. Sechi G, Serra A. Wernicke's encephalopathy: new clinical settings and recent advances in diagnosis and management. *Lancet Neurol.* 2007;6(5):442-455.
16. Al-Fahad T, Ismael A, Soliman MO, Khoursheed M. Very early onset of Wernicke's encephalopathy after gastric bypass. *Obes Surg.* 2006;16(5):671-672.
17. Aasheim ET. Wernicke encephalopathy after bariatric surgery: a systematic review. *Ann Surg.* 2008;248(5):714-720.
18. Singh S, Kumar A. Wernicke encephalopathy after obesity surgery: a systematic review. *Neurology.* 2007;68(11):807-811.
19. Milone M, Di Minno MN, Lupoli R, et al. Wernicke encephalopathy in subjects undergoing restrictive weight loss surgery: a systematic review of literature data. *Eur Eat Disord Rev.* 2014;22(4):223-229.
20. Shankar P, Boylan M, Sriram K. Micronutrient deficiencies after bariatric surgery. *Nutrition.* 2010;26(11-12):1031-1037.
21. Brolin RE, Leung M. Survey of vitamin and mineral supplementation after gastric bypass and biliopancreatic diversion for morbid obesity. *Obes Surg.* 1999;9(2):150-154.
22. Ecklund MM. Meeting the nutritional needs of the bariatric patient in acute care. *Crit Care Nurs Clin North Am.* 2004;16(4):495-499.

19

Medical Management of the Patient After Bariatric Surgery

Reevaluating Diabetes

Sangeeta Rao Kashyap, MD

Bariatric surgery is rapidly gaining approval as a treatment for severe obesity, especially when complicated by type 2 diabetes. In Centers of Excellence, postoperative care is usually administered by the patient's endocrinologist and multidisciplinary obesity teams and involves long-term evaluation of comorbidity status, weight regain, and multiple nutritional deficiencies. In the private sector particularly, patients who are self-funding for surgery often do not choose to stay in follow-up, and high attrition rates remain a major challenge. Although many observational studies document the effectiveness of bariatric surgery to treat diabetes in the setting of morbid obesity, recent studies document that a growing number of patients (25% to 40%) with type 2 diabetes do not achieve "biochemical remission" of hyperglycemia defined as normal glycemic control (hemoglobin A1c [HbA1c] < 6% or < 42 mmol/mol) without the need for diabetic medications,[1] or are unable to sustain this effect long term despite initial success with weight loss.[2-4]

Although the definition of diabetes remission is highly variable and controversial, Buse et al[1] propose partial remission of hyperglycemia to consist of an HbA1c below 6.5% (48 mmol/mol) without the need for diabetes medications and nonremission status as HbA1c > 7% (53 mmol/mol) with or without the need for medications. Remission of diabetes cannot and should not be defined merely in terms of restoring a "normal" A1c, particularly as this definition overlaps with the American Diabetes Association definition of prediabetes, and in a patient achieving this A1c on say insulin, he or she would be described as having good control, not partial remission. Many would also object to this definition because diabetes is more than just hyperglycemia, and little is known about the natural history of micro- and macrovascular disease after bariatric surgery. However, according to the remission definition criteria proposed by Buse et al, complete remission rates for diabetes at 23 months in a retrospective review of 1006 patients undergoing bariatric surgery was 34.4% overall.[5] In another series of 177 superobese patients with diabetes, 43% of patients who initially underwent diabetes remission after gastric bypass redeveloped diabetes.[4] A larger retrospective series from multiple sites demonstrated that 68% of 4434 patients with diabetes followed experienced initial complete remission within 5 years after gastric bypass surgery.[6] Among these, 35% redeveloped diabetes within 5 years. Thus, the median duration of remission was 8.3 years in this series. Moreover, the reemergence of hyperglycemia following initial weight

Forse RA, Apovian CM, eds.
Bariatric Surgery: What Every Provider Needs to Know (pp 229-237).

loss is more commonly observed following banding, sleeve gastrectomy, and other gastric restrictive procedures than with gastric bypass and biliopancreatic diversion (BPD) procedures, and is typically associated with advanced duration and severity of diabetes preoperatively and inadequate weight loss and/or weight regain related effects.[2,3,7,8] Advanced stage of type 2 diabetes is characterized by severe impairments in insulin secretion due to pancreatic beta-cell failure requiring the use of exogenous insulin. Clinical application of glucagon-like peptide (GLP) agonists to improve hyperglycemia and optimize weight loss in select bariatric patients (ie, post-lap banding) seems logical, but experimental evidence for their use is currently lacking for the bariatric population. Although the relapse rates for diabetes control following various procedures are merely estimates, given the lack of adequate follow-up in observational reports, little information regarding long-term management of diabetes following bariatric surgery is available. Therefore, based on our clinical experience we provide a rationale for long-term clinical management of residual diabetes following various bariatric procedures, and propose a clinical approach for the use of antidiabetic agents based on the known pathophysiologic effects of bariatric procedures on diabetes.

Effects of Bariatric Procedures on Diabetes Control and Diabetes Pathophysiology

Energy restriction and weight loss are key components of diabetes management that may induce biochemical diabetes remission. A very low calorie diet (not surgically induced) for as little as 1 week resulted in biochemical reversal of type 2 diabetes in humans that was associated with normalization of beta-cell function, reduction in hepatic glucose production, and was linked to diminished pancreatic and liver triacylglycerol.[9] Two meta-analyses of bariatric surgery studies demonstrated that surgery results in marked total body weight loss (15% to 25%) with restoration of normal glycemic control in a majority of individuals with type 2 diabetes (78% on average), resulting in discontinuation for the need for diabetic medications (defined as remission of type 2 diabetes).[2] Overall, 87% of participants achieved improved glucose control with fewer antidiabetic medications following bariatric surgery.[2] Sjostrom et al[10] reported an improvement in the rate of recovery from diabetes at 2 and 10 years following bariatric surgery vs conventional medical treatment in the Swedish Obesity Study cohort; however, the rate of recovery from diabetes dropped from 72% at 2 years to 36% at 10 years following surgery, implying a ~50% relapse rate of for diabetes recovery. Aside from biochemical remission of hyperglycemia, a 10-year follow-up study of BPD demonstrated reduction in renal and possible cardiovascular complications in people with diabetes.[11] Diabetes complication rates following other bariatric procedures are not known, but clinical trials are underway at several major medical centers (clinicaltrials.gov). Two recent randomized control trials demonstrated diabetes remission rates of 75% in severely obese (body mass index [BMI] = 42 kg/m^2) and ~40% in moderately obese (BMI = 36) patients after gastric bypass, with greater relapse rates noted after sleeve gastrectomy during the second year of follow-up despite comparable weight loss to gastric bypass.[12,13]

The 2 major types of bariatric surgery that were originally conceived consist of purely gastric restrictive procedures (laparoscopic adjustable gastric banding [LAGB], sleeve gastrectomy, vertical gastroplasty) and intestinal bypass procedures (Roux-en-Y gastric bypass [RYGB], BPD). Classification of these procedures was initially based on the proposed mechanism for weight loss; however, it is now recognized that both types of procedures produce a variety of neurohormonal effects by altering nutrient-intestinal flow that blur the distinction between these proposed categories. Gastric-restrictive operations limit gastric volume and hence restrict the intake of energy/calories by inducing satiety and facilitate total body weight loss in the range of 10% to 20%. Multiple studies, including a randomized controlled trial, have shown remission of type 2 diabetes with LAGB (vs conventional medical therapy) that is primarily mediated by weight loss and improved

Table 19-1

Possible Factors Associated With Diabetes Nonremission or Reemergence

- Older age
- Male gender
- Lower preoperative BMI
- Diabetes duration > 10 years
- Insulin use
- Inadequate weight loss and weight regain
- Surgery type: LAGB vs sleeve gastrectomy vs RYGB vs BPD
- Severity of preoperative beta-cell dysfunction (ie, hyperglycemia)
- Inadequate incretin stimulation following surgery?

Adapted from Schauer PR, Burguera B, Ikramuddin S, et al. Effect of laparoscopic Roux-en Y gastric bypass on type 2 diabetes mellitus. *Ann Surg.* 2003;238:467-484 and Chikunguwo SM, Wolfe LG, Dodson P, et al. Analysis of factors associated with durable remission of diabetes after Roux-en-Y gastric bypass. *Surg Obes Relat Dis.* 2010;6:254-259.

insulin sensitivity, both of which occur several months following surgery in patients with early duration of diabetes. In contrast, intestinal bypass procedures (RYGB, BPD) result in enforced caloric restriction from surgical gastric restriction that is comparable to LAGB/vertical gastroplasty. In addition, they have an added component of malabsorption related to shortening of the small intestine with greater (82% to 99%) remission rates of diabetes as compared to gastric restrictive operations in patients with longer duration of disease, including those treated with insulin. Hence, a dose-dependent effect of weight loss on diabetes remission has been noted across the spectrum of bariatric procedures (Table 19-1).[3] In addition, the rate of remission of type 2 diabetes over time also differs between gastric restrictive and intestinal bypass procedures in that following RYGB and BPD, diabetes remission is observed days following surgery, prior to significant weight loss.[14] This is not typically observed following gastric restrictive procedures.[3,15] The sleeve gastrectomy procedure involves gastric restriction but some studies suggest that it may produce changes in gut hormones and glucose homeostasis similar to that of RYGB in patients with diabetes.[16]

Patients with long duration (> 10 years), poorly controlled diabetes who require insulin therapy have been observed to achieve diabetes remission less frequently. Schauer et al[7] examined the effects of RYGB on type 2 diabetes in morbidly obese patients and reported that patients with the shortest duration (5 years) of diabetes, its mildest form (diet controlled), and the greatest weight loss after surgery were those most likely to achieve complete resolution of their diabetes. Preoperative glycemic control also impacted the rate of diabetes resolution. They pointed out that patients with the more severe forms of type 2 diabetes according to duration and insulin use showed significantly less weight loss than those who had milder forms. The study of 191 patients after 5 years of follow-up indicated that 65% treated by oral agents and 27% treated by insulin achieved an euglycemic status, eliminating the requirement for antidiabetic medications. The team also observed that type 2 diabetes patients had an overall lower excess weight loss (EWL) than nondiabetic patients, as did Dixon et al,[17] who investigated the use of gastric banding. In the Schauer et al study,[7] EWL was significantly lower in patients using oral agents (57%) or insulin (59%) vs those with impaired fasting glucose (73%) and on a diet only (65%). Also postoperative

HbA1c levels in patients using insulin were significantly higher than in patients with impaired fasting glucose: 6.0% (42 mmol/mol) vs 5.0% (30 mmol/mol), respectively ($p < .001$).

Improvement of glycemic control following bariatric surgery must be considered after various time periods. In most cases, a dramatic lowering in glucose levels has been observed days to weeks following surgery, before major weight loss but in the setting of enforced caloric restriction.[14,18] Persistent cases of diabetes after this initial period gradually improve in parallel with weight loss.[17] Patients who undergo RYGB and BPD procedures improve sooner and maintain glucose control for longer periods than do patients treated by banding or sleeve gastrectomy procedures. However, compared with patients following a very low calorie diet who achieved similar weight loss, patients who underwent RYGB have increased secretion of insulin, c-peptide, GLP-1, and gastric inhibitory peptide (GIP) after oral glucose challenge consistent with an incretin effect.[18] Overstimulation of the incretin axis (primarily GLP-1) has been noted to underlie exaggerated prandial insulin responses leading to post-RYGB hypoglycemia[19] that may be reversed by gastrostomy tube feeds,[20] suggesting that altered nutrient-intestinal transit rather than beta-cell hyperplasia[21] may be responsible for this underrecognized condition. Blocking the GLP-1 receptor with exendin (9-39) by Salehi et al[22] was shown to reduce post-prandial insulin secretion by half following RYGB, suggesting that GLP-1 is the major intestinal hormone related to increased prandial insulin secretion. Recently, Van der Schueren et al have noted high intersubject variability in GLP-1 levels 1 and 2 years after RYGB in diabetes, suggesting that other factors maybe at play other than intestinal exclusion that modulate GLP-1 levels involved with long-term glucose control.[23]

Massive weight loss may play an important role in consolidating the long-term antidiabetic impact of bariatric procedures.[24] However, metabolic improvements in cohort with lower BMI are also noted following gastric bypass.[25] Satiety hormones such as ghrelin and peptide YY are favorably altered following gastric bypass but not after gastric restriction and have been proposed to be linked to sustained post-surgical weight loss.[26-28] However, whether these satiety hormones have an impact on glucose regulation (insulin secretion/sensitivity) in type 2 diabetes following bariatric surgery is still unclear. Insulin sensitivity increases markedly after gastric bypass and is accompanied by elevated adiponectin levels, reduced free fatty acid levels, enhanced insulin signaling in key target tissues, and reduced intramuscular and hepatic fat.[29-33] It remains unclear if weight loss alone or incretin-related effects on beta-cell function are the dominant mechanism related to long-term diabetes remission. Other gut hormones, including peptide YY and oxyntomodulin,[34] may also be responsible for increased prandial insulin secretion, and further scale studies are needed. Other contributing mechanisms to improved glucose metabolism following RYGB include increased recirculation of bile salts following gastric bypass that may link to improved glucose and lipid levels.[35] Gut microbiota is altered in obesity and may be involved with altered entero-insular responses after gastric bypass.

Reemergence of Diabetes Following Bariatric Surgery: Clinical Considerations

Factors associated with diabetes nonremission based on observational clinical studies are noted in Table 19-1. Nonremission or reemergence of diabetes following gastric restrictive procedures particularly is increasingly recognized, and although studies examining the mechanistic links are lacking, clinical observations suggest that inadequate weight loss and weight gain to be factors for suboptimal control of diabetes following these procedures.[36,37] Suboptimal weight loss and weight regain have been associated with noncompliance with dietary and lifestyle recommendations, variations in presurgical weight loss, and occasionally surgical failure.[38] Prevention of weight gain requires optimizing patient selection criteria, consideration of benefits of bypass vs LAGB or sleeve gastrectomy procedures, and adherence to scheduled visits. Psychological factors such as uncontrolled depression, eating disorders, and previous history of sexual abuse have also been linked to weight regain and inadequate weight loss and warrant evaluation and continuing treatment.[39] Post-surgical adherence to scheduled visits and compliance is also a major factor related to success of weight loss maintenance.[37] The factors associated with redevelopment of type 2 diabetes mellitus following gastric bypass are related to poor baseline beta-cell function in patients characterized by advanced duration (ie, insulin requiring) and severity of type 2 diabetes (ie, hyperglycemia) in older aged individuals.[4,7] The incidence of residual or worsening type 2 diabetes following RYGB in one small study of 42 participants with type 2 diabetes was noted to be 26% 3 years following surgery and was associated with a lower preoperative BMI.[40] Although much of the literature has focused on biochemical remission following bariatric surgery, little information about the effects of surgery on long-term diabetes complications exist. The importance of ongoing and continuous surveillance for micro- and macrovascular complications in post-surgical patients is warranted.

Diabetes Therapies for Residual Diabetes Following Bariatric Surgery

Although decision points for intervention with pharmacotherapy need to be individualized to the patient, Figure 19-1 provides a proposed clinical algorithm for type 2 diabetes management following various bariatric procedures based on pathophysiological effects of the various types of procedures on type 2 diabetes. Nonremission of hyperglycemia is noted by HbA1c > 7% or 53 mmol/mol that necessitates the use of antidiabetic medications. Initial preoperative assessment of type 2 diabetes should include documentation of type 1, latent onset autoimmune diabetes, or type 2 diabetes given the increasing prevalence of obesity in all classifications of diabetes. The determination of c-peptide and autoimmune status is helpful in particular clinical scenarios where a primary beta-cell defect is suspected. Indicators of diabetes severity and poor residual pancreatic beta-cell function include duration of disease greater than 10 years, use of insulin, poor glycemic control despite oral agents, and presence of microvascular complications. Diabetes nonremission following LAGB and sleeve gastrectomy procedures needs to be considered in the setting of inadequate weight loss or weight regain and progressive beta-cell failure without weight regain as shown in Figure 19-1. The treatment of residual diabetes following LAGB/sleeve gastrectomy procedures should target glycemic control and weight loss with diabetes agents that are weight losing or neutral agents. Metformin remains the first-line agent for type 2 diabetes mellitus in that it improves insulin sensitivity by suppressing hepatic gluconeogenesis and increases muscle/liver glucose uptake by increasing AMP-activated protein kinase activity. Insulin sensitivity is improved to a greater extent following gastric bypass than gastric restrictive procedures, thus the use of metformin for glycemic control seems reasonable following gastric restrictive procedures, especially in the setting of weight gain. In contrast, use of thiazolidinediones may hamper weight loss efforts despite increasing insulin sensitization. A recent report indicated accelerated absorption and bioavailability of metformin following gastric bypass and indicated that a reduced dose of metformin may be required for achieving glycemic control.[41] Sulfonylureas improve insulin secretion and in the early postoperative period following bariatric surgery may precipitate hypoglycemia and precipitate dumping symptoms. Therefore, caution is warranted for the use of these agents early in the postoperative course. However, in patients with relapse of glycemic control years following gastric restrictive procedures, the addition of sulfonylureas to metformin would enhance insulin secretion and restore glycemic control by targeting pancreatic beta-cell failure. For those patients who do not respond to sulfonylurea, insulin therapy is indicated with the introduction of basal insulin followed by the addition of prandial insulin as indicated by the level of glycemic control.

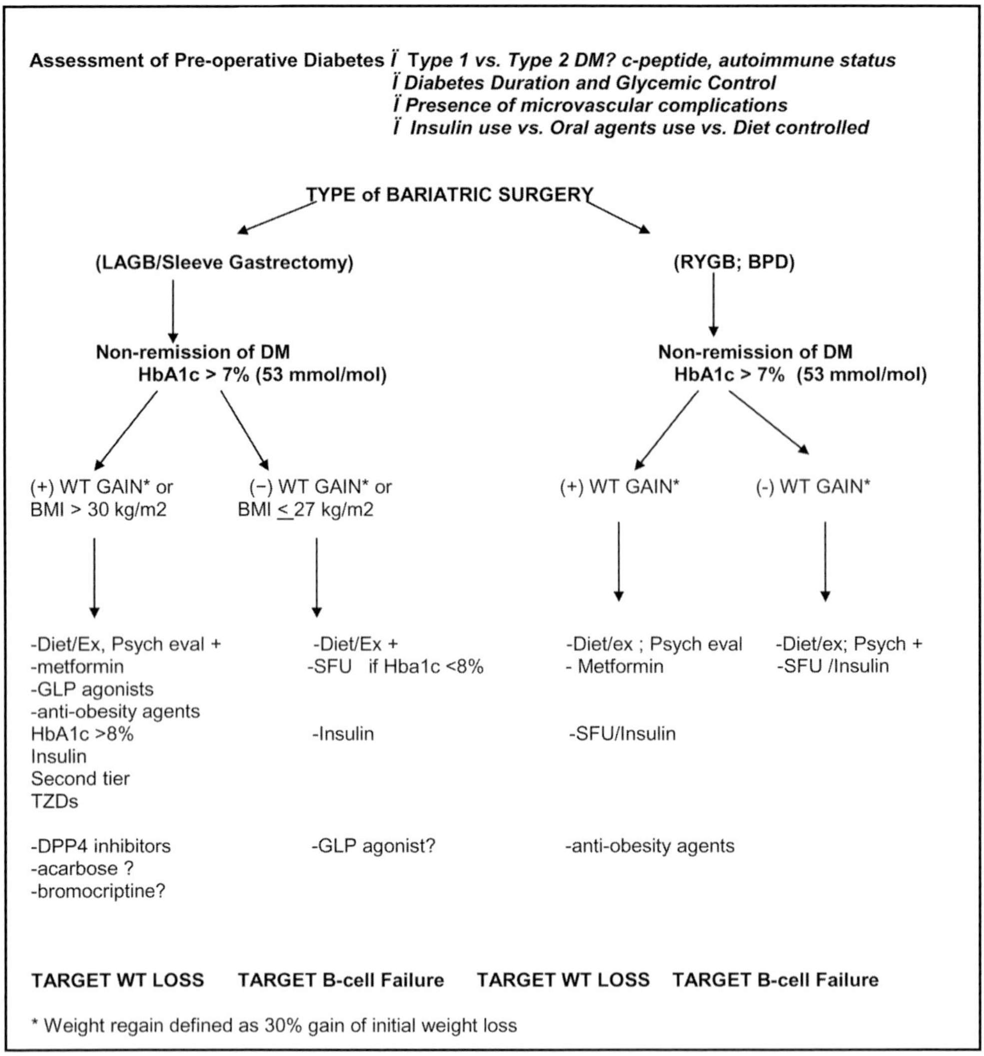

Figure 19-1. Proposed clinical approach to management of residual diabetes following bariatric surgery procedures.

Incretin analogs (ie, dipeptidyl peptidase 4 [DPP-4] inhibitors and GLP-agonists) enhance glucose dependent insulin secretion and offer advantages for weight loss in patients with obesity and type 2 diabetes but evidence for their use in bariatric patients is currently lacking. Although glucose-lowering effects are greater with GLP-1 agonists (-1% HbA1c) than DPP-4 inhibitors (-0.5% to 0.7% HbA1c),[42] weight loss is greater with GLP-agonists, exenatide, and liraglutide.[43] A clinical trial of exenatide 10 mg bid in participants with obesity and type 2 diabetes resulted in a 10-lb reduction in 1 year.[44] In the multicenter randomized trial with liraglutide, liraglutide demonstrated a dose-dependent reduction in weight of up to 3 to 5 kg in participants with type 2 diabetes.[43] Given that incretin stimulation of insulin secretion is partially responsible for the improvement in glucose levels acute following gastric bypass, the long-term adjunctive use of GLP-1 analogs in LAGB/sleeve gastrectomy and bypass patients is clearly enticing and warrants further clinical investigation. Conversely, it could be that diabetes recurrence and weight regain relate not to inadequate GLP-1 stimulation, but to the fact that this axis is less important or overridden by other factors in patients who fail. Hence, greater understanding of the pathophysiology underlying diabetes relapse is needed in addition to clinical trial data to show that hyperaugmentation of GLP-1 levels may be effective in sustaining glycemic control.

Sodium glucose transport 2 inhibitors (ie, canagliflozin) may be useful in post-bariatric patients with residual diabetes because these agents do not rely on pancreatic beta-cell function and result in renal excretion of glucose. The additional benefits of these agents result in modest blood pressure and weight lowering. No clinical trials have examined the use of these agents in post-bariatric patients, but clinical experience at our center suggests utility of these agents.

Use of Anti-Obesity Agents in Post-Bariatric Surgical Patients With Type 2 Diabetes

Special consideration of the use of recently approved anti-obesity agents is clearly indicated for patients with significant weight regain. Extended release phentermine/topiramate and lorcaserin were approved by the Food and Drug Administration in 2012 and result in weight loss of 5% to 10% for patients with moderate obesity with comorbidities including type 2 diabetes. Both drugs inhibit appetite and may benefit patients who experience post-surgical weight regain. It is currently not known if anorectic agents as these would be more effective than lifestyle measures and/or hypoglycemic agents to regulate glucose levels in patients with diabetes post-bariatric surgery. Further studies related to these agents are warranted.

Although diabetes nonremission is a recognized condition post-bariatric surgery, evidence-based data to make clinical recommendations are lacking. Based on our clinical experience, diabetes relapse following gastric bypass in the absence of weight regain is likely related to beta-cell exhaustion. In addition to diet and exercise counseling, targeting beta-cell failure with a trial of sulfonylureas and subsequent addition of insulin is indicated. However, caution is placed with the use of sulfonylureas and short-acting insulin and potential of hypoglycemia, given the insulin-sensitizing and incretin-related effects of gastric bypass in patients with diabetes. Revisional bariatric surgery is associated with additional morbidity, but may be considered for select surgical failure cases. As the number of bariatric surgery procedures performed for obesity and type 2 diabetes grows, additional research into the adjunctive use of medications for long-term diabetes control is clearly warranted. A greater understanding of the pathophysiology underlying diabetes relapse following various procedures is also warranted. Clinical trials examining the efficacy and safety of alternative diabetes agents (ie, GLP agonists, acarbose, bromocriptine) in addition to lifestyle counseling following various surgical procedures should be considered. Most importantly, continued monitoring of long-term diabetes complications is warranted regardless of initial remission status.

References

1. Buse JB, Caprio S, Cefalu WT, et al. How do we define cure of diabetes? *Diabetes Care.* 2009;32:2133-2135.
2. Buchwald H, Avidor Y, Braunwald E, et al. Bariatric surgery: a systematic review and meta-analysis. *JAMA.* 2004;292:1724-1737.
3. Buchwald H, Estok R, Fahrbach K, et al. Weight and type 2 diabetes after bariatric surgery: systematic review and meta-analysis. *Am J Med.* 2009;122:248-256.
4. Chikunguwo SM, Wolfe LG, Dodson P, et al. Analysis of factors associated with durable remission of diabetes after Roux-en-Y gastric bypass. *Surg Obes Relat Dis.* 2010;6:254-259.
5. Pournaras DJ, Aasheim ET, Sovik TT, et al. Effect of the definition of type II diabetes remission in the evaluation of bariatric surgery for metabolic disorders. *Br J Surg.* 2012;99:100-103.
6. Arterburn DE, Bogart A, Sherwood NE, et al. A multisite study of long-term remission and relapse of type 2 diabetes mellitus following gastric bypass. *Obes Surg.* 2013;23(1):93-102.
7. Schauer PR, Burguera B, Ikramuddin S, et al. Effect of laparoscopic Roux-en Y gastric bypass on type 2 diabetes mellitus. *Ann Surg.* 2003;238:467-484.

8. Pournaras DJ, Aasheim ET, Sovik TT, et al. Effect of the definition of type II diabetes remission in the evaluation of bariatric surgery for metabolic disorders. *Br J Surg.* 2012;99:100-103.
9. Lim EL, Hollingsworth KG, Aribisala BS, Chen MJ, Mathers JC, Taylor R. Reversal of type 2 diabetes: normalisation of beta cell function in association with decreased pancreas and liver triacylglycerol. *Diabetologia.* 2011;54:2506-2514.
10. Sjostrom L, Lindroos AK, Peltonen M, et al. Lifestyle, diabetes, and cardiovascular risk factors 10 years after bariatric surgery. *N Engl J Med.* 2004;351:2683-2693.
11. Iaconelli A, Panunzi S, De GA, et al. Effects of bilio-pancreatic diversion on diabetic complications: a 10-year follow-up. *Diabetes Care.* 2011;34:561-567.
12. Schauer PR, Kashyap SR, Wolski K, et al. Bariatric surgery versus intensive medical therapy in obese patients with diabetes. *N Engl J Med.* 2012;366:1567-1576.
13. Kashyap SR, Bhatt DL, Wolski K, et al. Metabolic effects of bariatric surgery in patients with moderate obesity and type 2 diabetes: analysis of a randomized control trial comparing surgery with intensive medical treatment. *Diabetes Care.* 2013;36(8):2175-2182.
14. Pories WJ, Swanson MS, MacDonald KG, et al. Who would have thought it? An operation proves to be the most effective therapy for adult-onset diabetes mellitus. *Ann Surg.* 1995;222:339-350.
15. Kashyap SR, Daud S, Kelly KR, et al. Acute effects of gastric bypass versus gastric restrictive surgery on beta-cell function and insulinotropic hormones in severely obese patients with type 2 diabetes. *Int J Obes (Lond).* 2010;34(3):462-471.
16. Peterli R, Wolnerhanssen B, Peters T, et al. Improvement in glucose metabolism after bariatric surgery: comparison of laparoscopic Roux-en-Y gastric bypass and laparoscopic sleeve gastrectomy: a prospective randomized trial. *Ann Surg.* 2009;250:234-241.
17. Dixon JB, O'Brien PE, Playfair J, et al. Adjustable gastric banding and conventional therapy for type 2 diabetes: a randomized controlled trial. *JAMA.* 2008;299:316-323.
18. Laferrere B, Teixeira J, McGinty J, et al. Effect of weight loss by gastric bypass surgery versus hypocaloric diet on glucose and incretin levels in patients with type 2 diabetes. *J Clin Endocrinol Metab.* 2008;93:2479-2485.
19. Goldfine AB, Mun EC, Devine E, et al. Patients with neuroglycopenia after gastric bypass surgery have exaggerated incretin and insulin secretory responses to a mixed meal. *J Clin Endocrinol Metab.* 2007;92:4678-4685.
20. McLaughlin T, Peck M, Holst J, Deacon C. Reversible hyperinsulinemic hypoglycemia after gastric bypass: a consequence of altered nutrient delivery. *J Clin Endocrinol Metab.* 2010;95:1851-1855.
21. Service GJ, Thompson GB, Service FJ, Andrews JC, Collazo-Clavell ML, Lloyd RV. Hyperinsulinemic hypoglycemia with nesidioblastosis after gastric-bypass surgery. *N Engl J Med.* 2005;353:249-254.
22. Salehi M, Prigeon RL, D'Alessio DA. Gastric bypass surgery enhances glucagon-like peptide 1-stimulated postprandial insulin secretion in humans. *Diabetes.* 2011;60:2308-2314.
23. Van der Schueren BJ, Homel P, Alam M, et al. Magnitude and variability of the glucagon-like peptide-1 response in patients with type 2 diabetes up to 2 years following gastric bypass surgery. *Diabetes Care.* 2012;35:42-46.
24. Weyer C, Hanson K, Bogardus C, Pratley RE. Long-term changes in insulin action and insulin secretion associated with gain, loss, regain and maintenance of body weight. *Diabetologia.* 2000;43:36-46.
25. Lomanto D, Lee WJ, Goel R, et al. Bariatric surgery in Asia in the last 5 years (2005-2009). *Obes Surg.* 2012;22(3):502-506.
26. Cummings DE, Weigle DS, Frayo RS, et al. Plasma ghrelin levels after diet-induced weight loss or gastric bypass surgery. *N Engl J Med.* 2002;346:1623-1630.
27. Korner J, Inabnet W, Conwell IM, et al. Differential effects of gastric bypass and banding on circulating gut hormone and leptin levels. *Obesity (Silver Spring).* 2006;14:1553-1561.
28. le Roux CW, Aylwin SJ, Batterham RL, et al. Gut hormone profiles following bariatric surgery favor an anorectic state, facilitate weight loss, and improve metabolic parameters. *Ann Surg.* 2006;243:108-114.
29. Diab DL, Yerian L, Schauer P, et al. Cytokeratin 18 fragment levels as a noninvasive biomarker for nonalcoholic steatohepatitis in bariatric surgery patients. *Clin Gastroenterol Hepatol.* 2008;6:1249-1254.
30. Alexandrides TK, Skroubis G, Kalfarentzos F. Resolution of diabetes mellitus and metabolic syndrome following Roux-en-Y gastric bypass and a variant of biliopancreatic diversion in patients with morbid obesity. *Obes Surg.* 2007;17:176-184.
31. Bikman BT, Zheng D, Pories WJ, et al. Mechanism for improved insulin sensitivity after gastric bypass surgery. *J Clin Endocrinol Metab.* 2008;93:4656-4663.
32. Polyzogopoulou EV, Kalfarentzos F, Vagenakis AG, Alexandrides TK. Restoration of euglycemia and normal acute insulin response to glucose in obese subjects with type 2 diabetes following bariatric surgery. *Diabetes.* 2003;52:1098-1103.
33. Navaneethan SD, Kelly KR, Sabbagh F, Schauer PR, Kirwan JP, Kashyap SR. Urinary albumin excretion, HMW adiponectin, and insulin sensitivity in type 2 diabetic patients undergoing bariatric surgery. *Obes Surg.* 2010;20:308-315.
34. Laferrere B, Swerdlow N, Bawa B, et al. Rise of oxyntomodulin in response to oral glucose after gastric bypass surgery in patients with type 2 diabetes. *J Clin Endocrinol Metab.* 2010;95:4072-4076.

35. Patti ME, Houten SM, Bianco AC, et al. Serum bile acids are higher in humans with prior gastric bypass: potential contribution to improved glucose and lipid metabolism. *Obesity (Silver Spring).* 2009;17:1671-1677.
36. Lee WJ, Ser KH, Chong K, et al. Laparoscopic sleeve gastrectomy for diabetes treatment in nonmorbidly obese patients: efficacy and change of insulin secretion. *Surgery.* 2010;147:664-669.
37. Heber D, Greenway FL, Kaplan LM, Livingston E, Salvador J, Still C. Endocrine and nutritional management of the post-bariatric surgery patient: an Endocrine Society Clinical Practice Guideline. *J Clin Endocrinol Metab.* 2010;95:4823-4843.
38. Himpens J, Dobbeleir J, Peeters G. Long-term results of laparoscopic sleeve gastrectomy for obesity. *Ann Surg.* 2010;252:319-324.
39. Fujioka K, Yan E, Wang HJ, Li Z. Evaluating preoperative weight loss, binge eating disorder, and sexual abuse history on Roux-en-Y gastric bypass outcome. *Surg Obes Relat Dis.* 2008;4:137-143.
40. DiGiorgi M, Rosen DJ, Choi JJ, et al. Re-emergence of diabetes after gastric bypass in patients with mid- to long-term follow-up. *Surg Obes Relat Dis.* 2010;6:249-253.
41. Padwal RS, Gabr RQ, Sharma AM, et al. Effect of gastric bypass surgery on the absorption and bioavailability of metformin. *Diabetes Care.* 2011;34:1295-1300.
42. Pratley RE, Nauck M, Bailey T, et al. Liraglutide versus sitagliptin for patients with type 2 diabetes who did not have adequate glycaemic control with metformin: a 26-week, randomised, parallel-group, open-label trial. *Lancet.* 2010;375:1447-1456.
43. Buse JB, Rosenstock J, Sesti G, et al. Liraglutide once a day versus exenatide twice a day for type 2 diabetes: a 26-week randomised, parallel-group, multinational, open-label trial (LEAD-6). *Lancet.* 2009;374:39-47.
44. Defronzo RA, Ratner RE, Han J, Kim DD, Fineman MS, Baron AD. Effects of exenatide (exendin-4) on glycemic control and weight over 30 weeks in metformin-treated patients with type 2 diabetes. *Diabetes Care.* 2005;28:1092-1100.

20

Hypertension Following Bariatric Surgery
Pathophysiology, Follow-Up, and Treatment

Venkata M. Alla, MD and Dennis Esterbrooks, MD

The prevalence of hypertension (HTN) in adults with obesity is approximately 50% to 70%. This is almost twice that in normal-weight adults.[1-3] Furthermore, with increasing severity (grades) of obesity, the prevalence of HTN increases and control of blood pressure (BP) worsens. HTN is a key mediator of the adverse health consequences of obesity and directly contributes to the excess cardiovascular morbidity and mortality in this patient population.[1,2] In this chapter, we briefly review the etiopathogenic mechanisms of obesity-related HTN (Obesity-HTN), the impact of bariatric surgery on the course of Obesity-HTN, pre- and post-surgical factors impacting course of HTN, and, finally, some of the management issues pertaining specifically to this selected population.

Obesity-Hypertension: Etiopathogenesis

Obesity-HTN is multifactorial in etiology, resulting from a complex interplay of neurohormonal, metabolic, hemodynamic, and structural perturbations in multiple organ systems. Patients with obesity have increased activity of the renin-angiotensin-aldosterone system (RAAS) and sympathetic nervous system (SNS) compared to the normal-weight population.[4-7] Proposed mechanisms for elevated SNS activity include modulation of baroreceptor sensitivity by insulin, free fatty acids and adipokines, and intermittent hypoxia resulting from obstructive sleep apnea and hypoventilation.[7] Alteration in kidney structure and function is another major contributor to Obesity-HTN. Obesity leads to abnormal renal salt and fluid handling leading to increased circulatory volume and volume-dependent HTN. Long-standing obesity also results in chronic glomerular hyperfiltration, proteinuria, and glomerulopathy, all of which lead to progressive chronic kidney disease and further elevations in systemic BP.[4,7] Abnormal endothelial function, increased secretion of proinflammatory and mineralocorticoid-like factors by adipocytes, and the paracrine effects of

Forse RA, Apovian CM, eds.
Bariatric Surgery: What Every Provider Needs to Know (pp 239-245).

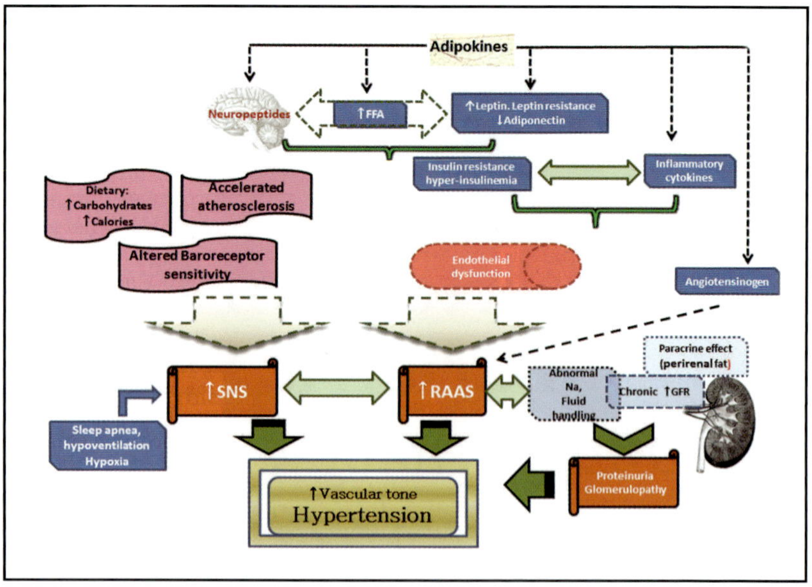

Figure 20-1. Schematic figure showing the potential neurohormonal mediators of Obesity-HTN.

perirenal adipocytes are additional mediators of Obesity-HTN.[4] These multiple interconnected pathways that contribute to the development and progression of Obesity-HTN are depicted schematically in Figure 20-1. In addition, it is now being recognized that HTN itself perpetuates obesity leading to further progression of the aforementioned alterations and further increases in BP.

Impact of Bariatric Surgery on Obesity-Hypertension: Mechanisms and Long-Term Efficacy

Bariatric surgery has been shown to produce significant and sustained weight loss compared to dietary interventions with or without pharmacotherapy.[8] Rapid weight loss occurs in the first 6 months following surgery, with a more gradual loss up to 1 year.[9] Subsequently, there is a gradual weight gain in the majority of patients. Despite this increase, in the Swedish Obese Subjects (SOS) study, patients in the surgery group had 16% lower weight compared to baseline at 10-year follow-up.[9] Similarly, bariatric surgery favorably impacts total mortality, cardiovascular events, and diabetes in the long term.[9,10] In contrast, there have been conflicting reports regarding the efficacy of bariatric surgery on long-term BP reduction and incident HTN, despite definite early improvements.[11]

Unarguably, HTN improves in the immediate and intermediate terms in the majority of patients undergoing bariatric surgery, irrespective of the type of surgery.[11-15] In a large meta-analysis of more than 22,000 patients, Buchwald et al demonstrated that bariatric surgery led to resolution of HTN in approximately 66% and significant improvement (without resolution) in another 16%.[14] While the most direct impact of bariatric surgery on BP is mediated through weight loss, multiple other mechanisms that are wholly or partly independent of weight loss also contribute to improvements in BP. Bariatric surgery reverses a majority of the metabolic and hormonal abnormalities that are thought to mediate Obesity-HTN. Increase in adiponectin, decrease in leptin, improvements in insulin resistance, and downregulation of RAAS and SNS occur within weeks following bariatric surgery even before significant weight loss has occurred.[16] Reduction in the severity of obstructive sleep apnea and consequent decrease in nocturnal hypoxemia reduces SNS activation and BP. In addition, bariatric surgery delays progression of chronic kidney disease by decreasing glomerular hyperfiltration and proteinuria, results in favorable histologic changes in the arterial wall, and improves endothelial function.[17] Finally, it has been shown that bariatric surgery is associated with a significant improvement in physical and social quality of life indices and decrease in pain and disability due to arthritis.[18] Intuitively, these factors could increase the patient's willingness and ability to exercise, thereby leading to improvements in BP. However, there has been no study assessing the direct contribution of these factors to the post-surgical improvements in HTN and cardiovascular risk.

In contrast to the early and intermediate-term results, the beneficial effects of bariatric surgery on BP were not sustained at 10-year follow-up in the SOS study.[9] Furthermore, the 10-year incidence of HTN was not significantly different between the surgery and control groups (49% vs 41%). One potential explanation for this discrepancy is the differential effects of the various types of bariatric surgery on long-term BP. Notably, only 5% of the patients in the surgery arm of the SOS study underwent gastric bypass, with the majority of them undergoing vertical banded gastroplasty or gastric banding (purely restrictive procedures). In a subgroup analysis of only patients who underwent gastric bypass, there was a more favorable long-term impact on BP. Other studies in patients who underwent exclusively gastric bypass procedures have corroborated this finding.[15] This suggests that that long-term resolution, incidence, and course of HTN are more favorable with gastric bypass compared to purely restrictive surgeries. This is further supported by the demonstration of larger improvements in the neurohormonal, metabolic, and inflammatory mediators of Obesity-HTN in patients undergoing mixed (diversionary + restrictive) procedures compared to purely restrictive procedures.[19] Finally, one important issue warrants caution in the interpretation of the results of all the aforementioned studies. A majority of the studies have used office BP recordings to estimate the impact of bariatric surgery on HTN rather than ambulatory BP recordings, which are more accurate and have a higher correlation with clinical outcomes.

Predictors of Resolution and Recurrence of Hypertension Following Bariatric Surgery

A complex analysis of patients in the SOS study revealed that the strongest predictors of elevated BP in the long term were duration of follow-up and ongoing weight gain during follow-up.[11] The other predictors were amount of early weight loss and inclusion weight (presurgery). A weight increase of 1 kg/year during late follow-up had a 2-fold greater impact on final systolic or diastolic BP compared to 1 kg of weight loss during the first year following surgery or 1 kg difference in body weight at inclusion. Compared with 1 kg/year weight change during late follow-up, additional follow-up of 1 year had a 4-fold greater impact on the final systolic BP and a 2- to 3-fold greater impact on the final diastolic BP. Though other studies have suggested that age at the time of surgery was an important predictor of BP on follow-up, this was not the case in the SOS study. Another major determinant of late recurrence is the type of bariatric surgery performed, with sustained and significantly greater reductions noted in patients undergoing diversion or mixed (diversion + restriction) procedure compared to those undergoing purely restrictive surgery.

While the precise reasons for recurrent HTN during late follow-up remain unclear, there are a few potential explanations. Patients undergoing bariatric surgery are relatively young, with the median age in most studies being 40 to 55 years. Therefore, late recurrence of HTN could be a result of progressive arteriosclerosis and increased arterial stiffness known to occur with advancing age. It is known that patients with obesity have premature arteriosclerosis and atherosclerosis predisposing them to early-onset systolic HTN.[20] Alternatively, recurrence of HTN could be due to gradual weight gain following surgery. Notably, in the SOS study, even small increments in weight predicted HTN recurrence despite the overall weight being below the presurgical weight.[9,11] Finally, a high prevalence of occult micronutrient deficiencies (calcium, magnesium, potassium, zinc, and vitamin D) has been demonstrated in patients following bariatric surgery.[21] These micronutrients are known modulators of vascular homeostasis and BP, and their deficiency could predispose patients to recurrent HTN, though this has not been addressed in any prior study.[22]

Perioperative and Long-Term Management of Hypertension in the Bariatric Surgery Population

Preoperative assessment and control of comorbid disorders, such as diabetes, HTN, and obstructive airway disease, and comprehensive cardiovascular risk stratification are essential for minimizing perioperative mortality and morbidity in patients undergoing bariatric surgery. While there are no data specific to bariatric surgery, it is well known that preoperative BP control is a predictor of perioperative outcomes in patients undergoing noncardiac surgeries in general. Patients with suboptimal control of BP in the preoperative period are at higher risk of exaggerated intraoperative BP fluctuation and perioperative ischemia. This risk can be minimized by adequate treatment of HTN in the preoperative period. Initiation or uptitration of beta-blockers may be the more preferred option given their established benefits in preventing perioperative myocardial infarction, atrial fibrillation, and availability of intravenous formulations allowing easy transition between enteral and parenteral administration. While clonidine and calcium channel blockers are not known to prevent perioperative myocardial infarction or atrial fibrillation, they do have readily available transdermal and intravenous formulations allowing easy transition and titration intra- and postoperatively. Diuretics and angiotensin-converting enzyme (ACE) inhibitors are less preferred in the pre- and perioperative period as they increase the risk of perioperative hypotension and kidney injury. It is important to remember that inappropriate cuff size and inaccurate cuff placement can be a common problem in severely obese patients, resulting in inaccuracies in the noninvasive measurement of BP. It is therefore preferable to use an arterial line for close monitoring of BP in the intraoperative and immediate postoperative period in patients undergoing bariatric surgery.

Three important issues need elaboration with respect to the long-term management of BP in post-bariatric surgery patients. First, despite significant improvements in BP during the first year following surgery, complete resolution of HTN is uncommon and a majority of patients would need antihypertensive medications in the long term, underscoring the need for close clinical follow-up. The next important issue is the impact of altered gastrointestinal anatomy, physiology, and function on the pharmacokinetics and efficacy of common antihypertensive medications. Depending on the type of bariatric surgery performed, absorption and kinetics of medications become unpredictable based on changes in gastric/intestinal pH, gastric and intestinal dwell times, and site and length of bowel segment resected or bypassed. In general, the aforementioned factors are more likely to impact the sustained release or long-acting formulations and hence these should be avoided where possible. Even among the regular-release formulations, the site of absorption, optimal pH required, percent absorption, and time to peak absorption vary widely across classes of drugs and across individual drugs and formulations within the same class. Unfortunately, these issues have not been adequately explored, and therefore, definite recommendations cannot be made. The clinician should be mindful of these variables when evaluating a post-bariatric surgery patient with difficult to control BP and carefully review the pharmacology of the antihypertensive regimen.

Lastly, while the basic strategies for treating HTN in the post-bariatric surgery patient do not differ from other patients with HTN, physicians need to bear in mind issues like pathophysiology of Obesity-HTN, adverse effects of individual classes of drugs, and the differential efficacy of antihypertensives in obese vs lean hypertensives. Though limited data suggest that ACE inhibitors and angiotensin receptor blockers (ARB) may be more effective than diuretics or calcium channel blockers in reducing ambulatory BP and that combined alpha- and beta-blockers might be superior to pure beta-blockers for reducing BP in patients with obesity, all traditional classes of drugs largely appear to have comparable efficacy.[23,24] Therefore, therapeutic choices should be made on the presence of specific comorbidities (beta-blockers for patients with myocardial infarction; ACE inhibitors/ARBs for patients with left ventricular dysfunction), tolerability, and anticipated adverse effects in any individual patient. Table 20-1 summarizes trials assessing the comparative efficacy of different drugs in obese populations. Impaired insulin sensitivity, dyslipidemia, and electrolyte disturbances associated with beta-blockers and thiazide diuretics can be deleterious in patients with obesity in whom these conditions are highly prevalent.[25] Therefore, it would be prudent not to use these 2 classes of drugs as the initial choice. In contrast, ACE inhibitors/ARBs do not have the aforementioned adverse metabolic effects, have reno-protective effects, and favorably impact cardiac remodeling. Hence, based on available evidence and our personal experience, this class of drugs is the preferred initial choice. Calcium channel blockers are generally devoid of major metabolic effects and are generally well tolerated, and aldosterone blockers have been shown to be particularly effective in patients with obesity with difficult to control HTN. Hence, these could be used as second- and third-line agents, respectively.

Summary

HTN is very prevalent in patients with obesity undergoing bariatric surgery and is a mediator of obesity-related morbidity and mortality. Bariatric surgery, irrespective of the type of procedure, is effective in reducing BP in the short and intermediate term. However, diversionary and mixed procedures are superior to purely restrictive surgeries in the magnitude of initial reduction and in their ability to result in sustained improvements in BP, and this needs to be factored into the decision-making process while selecting the type of surgery. The strongest predictors of recurrent HTN are the duration of follow-up and ongoing weight increase during follow-up. Hence, the importance of a healthy lifestyle and the critical need to avoid weight gain cannot be overemphasized. Irrespective of the type of surgery and the early BP response, continued surveillance of all patients is necessary to assess for reemergence of HTN and other adverse cardiovascular risk markers. However, more diligent follow-up is required in those at higher risk, such as patients who undergo purely restrictive surgery; have smaller magnitude of initial weight loss, android obesity, or metabolic syndrome; and ongoing weight gain. Finally, despite the absence of convincing data supporting the superiority of any particular drug class, ACE inhibitors/ARBs may be preferable in these patients in view of their favorable metabolic effects.

References

1. Flegal KM, Carroll MD, Ogden CL, Curtin LR. Prevalence and trends in obesity among US adults, 1999-2008. *JAMA*. 2010;303(3):235-241.
2. Thomas F, Bean K, Pannier B, Oppert JM, Guize L, Benetos A. Cardiovascular mortality in overweight subjects: the key role of associated risk factors. *Hypertension*. 2005;46(4):654-659.
3. Bramlage P, Pittrow D, Wittchen HU, et al. Hypertension in overweight and obese primary care patients is highly prevalent and poorly controlled. *Am J Hypertens*. 2004;17(10):904-910.
4. Kotsis V, Stabouli S, Papakatsika S, Rizos Z, Parati G. Mechanisms of obesity-induced hypertension. *Hypertens Res*. 2010;33(5):386-393.
5. Esler MD, Eikelis N, Lambert E, Straznicky N. Neural mechanisms and management of obesity-related hypertension. *Curr Cardiol Rep*. 2008;10(6):456-463.
6. Straznicky NE, Eikelis N, Lambert EA, Esler MD. Mediators of sympathetic activation in metabolic syndrome obesity. *Curr Hypertens Rep*. 2008;10(6):440-447.
7. Hall JE. The kidney, hypertension, and obesity. *Hypertension*. 2003;41(3 Pt 2):625-633.

Table 20-1

Randomized Trials Comparing the Efficacy of Various Antihypertensive Drugs in Obese Patients

STUDY	SAMPLE SIZE (N)	MEAN BMI KG/M2	FOLLOW-UP (WEEKS)	STUDY DRUGS	MAIN RESULTS	COMMENTS
Reisin et al[26]	232	32	12	Lisinopril vs HCTZ	BP lowering similar (office and ambulatory)	Blood sugars higher and potassium lower with HCTZ; Blacks responded better to HCTZ and Whites to lisinopril
Grassi et al[27]	127	33	12	Candesartan vs HCTZ	BP lowering similar	↑ Insulin sensitivity and ↓ muscle sympathetic nerve activity in candesartan arm
Jordan et al[28]	132	33	12	Valsartan vs atenolol (add on HCTZ 12.5 to 25 after 4 weeks)	Systolic BP reduction similar; diastolic BP reduction was better and need for add on HCTZ was lower with atenolol	↑ Insulin sensitivity with valsartan
Jordan et al[29]	489	34	8	Aliskiren vs Irbesartan vs Amlodipine (all were on HCTZ)	BP control was similar in all combination arms	Adverse events were highest with amlodipine (peripheral edema)
Raij et al[24]	412 Ambulatory BP sub-study: 111	NA	16	Valsartan/HCTZ vs amlodipine/HCTZ	Similar reduction in office BP	Ambulatory BP was better in valsartan arm

BP = blood pressure, HCTZ = hydrochlorthiazide.

8. Padwal R, Klarenbach S, Wiebe N, et al. Bariatric surgery: a systematic review and network meta-analysis of randomized trials. *Obes Rev.* 2011;12(8):602-621.
9. Sjostrom L, Lindroos AK, Peltonen M, et al. Lifestyle, diabetes, and cardiovascular risk factors 10 years after bariatric surgery. *N Engl J Med.* 2004;351(26):2683-2693.
10. Sjostrom L, Peltonen M, Jacobson P, et al. Bariatric surgery and long-term cardiovascular events. *JAMA.* 2012;307(1):56-65.
11. Sjostrom CD, Peltonen M, Sjostrom L. Blood pressure and pulse pressure during long-term weight loss in the obese: the Swedish Obese Subjects (SOS) intervention study. *Obes Res.* 2001;9(3):188-195.
12. Carson JL, Ruddy ME, Duff AE, Holmes NJ, Cody RP, Brolin RE. The effect of gastric bypass surgery on hypertension in morbidly obese patients. *Arch Intern Med.* 1994;154(2):193-200.
13. Foley EF, Benotti PN, Borlase BC, Hollingshead J, Blackburn GL. Impact of gastric restrictive surgery on hypertension in the morbidly obese. *Am J Surg.* 1992;163(3):294-297.
14. Buchwald H, Avidor Y, Braunwald E, et al. Bariatric surgery: a systematic review and meta-analysis. *JAMA.* 2004;292(14):1724-1737.
15. Adami G, Murelli F, Carlini F, Papadia F, Scopinaro N. Long-term effect of biliopancreatic diversion on blood pressure in hypertensive obese patients. *Am J Hypertens.* 2005;18:780-784.
16. Ashrafian H, le Roux CW, Darzi A, Athanasiou T. Effects of bariatric surgery on cardiovascular function. *Circulation.* 2008;118(20):2091-2102.
17. De Ciuceis C, Porteri E, Rizzoni D, et al. Effects of weight loss on structural and functional alterations of subcutaneous small arteries in obese patients. *Hypertension.* 2011;58(1):29-36.
18. Kolotkin RL, Crosby RD, Gress RE, Hunt SC, Adams TD. Two-year changes in health-related quality of life in gastric bypass patients compared with severely obese controls. *Surg Obes Relat Dis.* 2009;5(2):250-256.
19. Appachi S, Kelly KR, Schauer PR, et al. Reduced cardiovascular risk following bariatric surgeries is related to a partial recovery from "adiposopathy." *Obes Surg.* 2011;21(12):1928-1936.
20. Wildman RP, Mackey RH, Bostom A, Thompson T, Sutton-Tyrrell K. Measures of obesity are associated with vascular stiffness in young and older adults. *Hypertension.* 2003;42(4):468-473.
21. Shankar P, Boylan M, Sriram K. Micronutrient deficiencies after bariatric surgery. *Nutrition.* 2010;26(11-12):1031-1037.
22. Houston MC, Harper KJ. Potassium, magnesium, and calcium: their role in both the cause and treatment of hypertension. *J Clin Hypertens (Greenwich).* 2008;10(7 Suppl 2):3-11.
23. Wofford MR, Anderson DC Jr, Brown CA, Jones DW, Miller ME, Hall JE. Antihypertensive effect of alpha- and beta-adrenergic blockade in obese and lean hypertensive subjects. *Am J Hypertens.* 2001;14(7 Pt 1):694-698.
24. Raij L, Egan BM, Zappe DH, Purkayastha D, Samuel R, Sowers JR. Office and ambulatory blood pressure-lowering effects of combination valsartan/hydrochlorothiazide vs. hydrochlorothiazide-based therapy in obese, hypertensive patients. *J Clin Hypertens (Greenwich).* 2011;13(10):731-738.
25. Cooper-DeHoff RM, Wen S, Beitelshees AL, et al. Impact of abdominal obesity on incidence of adverse metabolic effects associated with antihypertensive medications. *Hypertension.* 2010;55(1):61-68.
26. Reisin E, Weir MR, Falkner B, Hutchinson HG, Anzalone DA, Tuck ML for the Treatment in Obese Patients With Hypertension (TROPHY) Study Group. Lisinopril versus hydrochlorothiazide in obese hypertensive patients: a multicenter placebo-controlled trial. *Hypertension.* 1997;30(1 Pt 1):140-145.
27. Grassi G, Seravalle G, Dell' Oro R, et al. Comparative effects of candesartan and hydrochlorothiazide on blood pressure, insulin sensitivity, and sympathetic drive in obese hypertensive individuals: results of the CROSS study. *J Hypertens.* 2003;21:1761-1769.
28. Jordan J, Engeli S, Boschmann M. Hemodynamic and metabolic responses to valsartan and atenolol in obese hypertensive patients. *J Hypertens.* 2005;23:2313-2318.
29. Jordan J, Engeli S, Boye SW, Le Breton S, Keefe DL. Direct renin inhibition with aliskiren in obese patients with arterial hypertension. *Hypertension.* 2007;49(5):1047-1055.

21

Medical Management of the Patient After Bariatric Surgery

Reevaluating Nonalcoholic Fatty Liver Disease and Dyslipidemia

Lalita Khaodhiar, MD and Karen C. McCowen, MB, MRCPI

Important complications of obesity include nonalcoholic fatty liver disease (NAFLD) and dyslipidemia. While the former is more clearly directly related to obesity and in particular central distribution of obesity, in both conditions insulin resistance is an important contributor to the pathogenesis. Medical therapy of NAFLD is poor, other than weight loss. Dyslipidemia does improve with weight loss, although there are many other contributing influences upon dyslipidemia, such that it is not uncommon in lean individuals. One might anticipate a better effect of bariatric surgery upon NAFLD compared to dyslipidemia, but in both cases these conditions need reevaluation at regular intervals after surgery.

Nonalcoholic Fatty Liver Disease

In parallel with the worldwide obesity epidemic is an explosion of cases of NAFLD. NAFLD is a catch-all designation for a set of hepatic disorders of fat infiltration in microvesicles, common in obesity and insulin resistance. NAFLD is also particularly linked to type 2 diabetes, and each predicts the development of the other.[1] A requirement for the diagnosis is lack of significant alcohol intake in the preceding years, although this remains poorly defined. The spectrum of fat infiltration ranges from simple steatosis all the way to cirrhosis. Fat accumulation is the initial lesion; subsequently, an inflammatory infiltrate in a subset—steatohepatitis (NASH)—might eventually lead to fibrosis, considered an irreversible stage. Certainly early on, this disorder is reversible with lifestyle modification and weight loss. Since nonsurgical weight loss is so poorly sustained over the long term, an important question is the effectiveness of bariatric surgery as a treatment for NAFLD.

Forse RA, Apovian CM, eds.
Bariatric Surgery: What Every Provider Needs to Know (pp 247-256).

Prevalence

Currently, NAFLD is the third most common chronic liver disease requiring transplantation in the United States and predicted to be the leading cause of cirrhosis in the near future. As much as 30% of the US population is estimated to have liver steatosis on ultrasound[2]; what proportion of these have NASH is unknown. One disturbing study of US servicemen and their families (mean age 55 years) reported a 50% prevalence of steatosis on ultrasound. In those with steatosis who underwent liver biopsy, about 30% had NASH (approximately 12% of the total group).[3] Physicians generally only seek to diagnose NAFLD when unexplained transaminitis is present. Neither liver enzyme concentrations nor ultrasound imaging are sensitive measures of NAFLD. The gold standard for accurate diagnosis is a liver biopsy; notably, patients with completely normal liver enzymes may demonstrate steatohepatitis on biopsy. Thus, the development of cirrhosis might be silent.

Diagnosis

Much of the published literature on NAFLD progression or reversal with therapy is flawed by lack of liver biopsy data, although bariatric surgery generally allows the opportunity to perform liver biopsies. Ultrasound, computed tomography, and magnetic resonance imaging (MRI) scanning are all sensitive techniques that can easily diagnose fat accumulation in the liver. However, they distinguish simple steatosis from NASH rather poorly. Newer imaging modalities such as MR elastography, MR spectroscopy, and ultrasound elastography are promising in this regard and should allow more widespread detection in larger populations. Biomarkers of inflammation (such as TNF-α, interleukin-6 [IL-6], and C-reactive protein), of apoptosis, and of hepatic fibrosis are all being studied as surrogate markers of NASH.[4] Guidelines from the American College of Gastroenterology recommend use of the NAFLD Fibrosis Score.[5] This is based on 6 readily available variables (age, body mass index [BMI], hyperglycemia, platelet count, albumin, AST/ALT ratio), and it is calculated using the published formula (http://nafldscore.com). In a meta-analysis of 13 studies consisting of more than 3000 patients, a score of ≤ 1.455 had 90% sensitivity and 60% specificity to exclude advanced fibrosis whereas a score of >0.676 had 67% sensitivity and 97% specificity to identify the presence of advanced fibrosis.[6]

Pathophysiology

The pathophysiology of NAFLD appears linked to the presence and severity of insulin resistance. In general, fat accumulation in the liver depends on a delicate balance between 2 opposing forces. On one side, insulin resistance in adipose tissue results in enhanced release of free fatty acids leading to increased liver uptake. The prevailing hyperinsulinemia leads to upregulation of genes that regulate de novo lipogenesis. This is a paradox, since these latter pathways do not exhibit insulin resistance. Therefore, excessive liver triglyceride synthesis occurs. However, the increased fat accumulation is not balanced by increased beta-oxidation or export of lipids, both of which are relatively impaired in conditions of insulin resistance. Progression to inflammatory infiltrate might also be linked to peripheral fat stores, which are a source of proinflammatory cytokines. Oxidative stress may contribute by allowing production of excessive reactive oxidative species and free radicals via mitochondrial and peroxisomal pathways in the liver, thereby causing hepatocyte injury, inflammation, and fibrosis.

Obstructive sleep apnea (OSA) is a syndrome of repetitive nocturnal desaturations caused by some form of upper airway collapse and cessation of breathing that results in repeated hypoxemia. OSA has recently been investigated as either an underlying cause of or permissive for NAFLD. Morbid obesity is a strong risk factor for OSA, and both conditions are associated with increases in markers of inflammation. The links between OSA and NAFLD are not fully recognized but emerging evidence suggests that OSA may contribute to the underlying pathophysiology. In a recent paper, 101 morbidly obese French participants underwent standard sleep studies, followed by a liver biopsy at the time of bariatric surgery. Classical NAFLD histology was noted on the biopsy, and the severity of the fibrotic lesions (but not simple steatosis) was significantly greater in those in the highest tertile of intermittent hypoxia score, independent of age, obesity, and insulin sensitivity.[7] Weaker evidence of a potential etiologic link between OSA and NAFLD has been seen in studies examining only transaminases (a poor substitute for the diagnosis of NAFLD). In 40 obese men with OSA, morning transaminases were significantly higher than evening values. This difference disappeared after institution of continuous positive airway pressure (CPAP) therapy to treat the OSA and was maintained out to at least 6 months.[8] The biological basis for suspecting a link between intermittent hypoxemia and NAFLD is fairly solid, even though not all studies found that CPAP improved liver function. Hypoxemia has been shown to upregulate certain transcription factors that are involved in lipogenesis, and NF-kappaB, also induced by hypoxemia, promotes liver inflammation.

Classification

There are various different classification systems for NAFLD based on liver biopsy findings. The pathology resembles alcoholic liver disease. The most commonly used is a semiquantitative assessment of 4 features: fat accumulation in the form of triacylglycerol, hepatocyte ballooning, lobular inflammatory infiltrate with necrosis, and fibrosis. Fibrosis is staged histologically from 0 to 4, with a score of at least 2 implying advanced fibrosis and a score of 4 consistent with cirrhosis.[9] Hepatocellular carcinoma can develop in noncirrhosis NASH, as well as in end-stage liver disease. In contrast, in alcoholic liver disease, generally only patients with cirrhosis are at risk of liver cancer.

Weight Loss

Theoretically, lifestyle modification can reverse NAFLD, but is poorly sustained even in research trials. A threshold weight loss of 5% appears necessary to effect pathological change. Greater weight loss has been shown to reverse features of NASH, such as lobular inflammation, as well as NAFLD activity score. Exercise alone without energy restriction also reduces liver fat, but the data are more sparse. Aside from weight loss, medical therapy for NAFLD is poorly established. Even prospective trials of the insulin sensitizers metformin and thiazolidinedione drugs have been disappointing; metformin has been suggested in observational studies to reduce the risk of hepatocellular carcinoma in patients with NAFLD but otherwise does not effect marked improvements in liver function. In the Diabetes Prevention Project trial, more than 2100 patients were randomized to either placebo or metformin for a mean of 3.2 years. In the placebo group, the ALT rose throughout the study, but rose less in the metformin group. Statistical adjustment for weight loss obliterated the difference between the groups, although the clinical relevance is unclear since ALT in both groups remained in the normal range.[10] Given how poor a substitute serum markers are for diagnosis of NAFLD, the scientific relevance is also questionable.

Pioglitazone can improve liver histology but is ineffective in the treatment of liver fibrosis; glucagon-like peptide-1 (GLP-1) inhibitors in various classes appear to reduce hepatic lipogenesis and enhance lipid oxidation, but there have been no published reports on these drugs specifically targeting NAFLD. This class of incretin drugs is attractive for NAFLD therapy, since GLP-1 receptors have been demonstrated on hepatocytes. Vitamin E, currently the only approved treatment for pediatric populations, has been shown to improve histology (and was better than pioglitazone) but again does not reverse fibrosis.[11,12] Placement of an intragastric balloon for 6 months is a technique that has been associated with decreased food intake and results in weight loss. In a recent Italian study of 130 obese patients in whom a balloon was placed for 6 months, 75% were deemed "responders" (BMI decrease of >3.5 kg/m^2) and were studied further. At 6 months, ultrasound detection of severe steatosis was reduced from 52% of participants to 4% only.[13]

Hence, the natural question is the effect of decent and sustained weight reduction via bariatric surgery on the pathology of NAFLD. The Cochrane Database report on this topic was stymied by an utter lack of randomized clinical trials or quasirandomized clinical studies that fulfilled the inclusion criteria.[14] They noted 21 prospective or retrospective cohort studies prior to 2010, in which improvement on steatosis or inflammation scores was reported. However, 4 studies also described some deterioration in the degree of fibrosis. Indeed, there are many prospective studies in which participants underwent liver biopsy at the time of the initial surgery and a follow-up biopsy after weight loss. The results are remarkably consistent in showing a dramatic reduction in steatosis and steatohepatitis. The degree of resolution can be as high as 90%, and the type of bariatric surgery (pure restriction vs mixed restriction/malabsorption) is not clearly the determining factor of success. A review in 2012 discussed all of the literature published in this regard and is notable for the similarity between the studies.[15] The different types of surgery are also discussed. Since that time, 2 studies of Roux-en-Y gastric bypass (RYGB) have been published. Tai et al reported on 21 patients, in whom the mean BMI dropped from 44 to 28. Again, a marked improvement in histology including fibrosis was noted.[16] Moretto et al described 78 patients, with a mean excess weight loss of 82%. At baseline, 44% had evidence of fibrosis, and many reversed. Some developed de novo fibrosis, such that at the endpoint of the study, the prevalence of fibrosis was 31%.[17]

In some but not all studies, the degree of resolution of NAFLD is proportional to the amount of weight that is lost. Thus, RYGB might appear to be more effective at improving liver histology, but often this difference disappears after accounting for its better weight loss. However, the proportion of patients with progression of fibrosis after RYGB seems very small. In contrast, for vertical banded gastroplasty, Stratopoulos et al reported on 216 patients. In 40% with fibrosis, there was no change despite weight loss. In 12% fibrosis progressed, although there were no participants who developed cirrhosis.[18] Kral et al reported on their experience with 104 patients who underwent biliopancreatic diversion (BPD). In this group, 33% had no change in fibrosis and 40% even had progression.[19] In patients in whom fibrosis continues to progress, substantial and sustained weight loss are usually noted, which is not distinguishable from patients who reverse or stabilize. Occasional and rare cases of fulminant steatohepatitis are reported after bariatric surgery, possibly contributed to by rapid and massive weight loss. One hypothesis to explain this is the massive release of fatty acids from peripheral depots with an influx into the liver. None of these patients can be clearly identified prior to surgery. There are no trials reporting differences in NAFLD between a group undergoing bariatric surgery and those whose treatment was limited to medical weight loss. The Swedish obesity cohort has published comparisons between medical and surgical weight loss in their parallel groups, but no data on liver biopsy or noninvasive evaluation of NAFLD have been reported.

Contributors to Nonalcoholic Fatty Liver Disease Improvement After Bariatric Surgery

What is the trigger for the improvements in NAFLD? After surgery, insulin sensitivity improves, and plasma insulin concentrations are reduced. This reverses the processes of lipogenesis and improves fatty acid disposal. An overall lower fat mass should result in a decline in inflammatory cytokine concentrations. Sleep apnea and hence intermittent hypoxemia both improve after bariatric surgery, with complete resolution in some patients.

The concentrations of gastrointestinal hormones are very different before and after surgery, and whether this impacts resolution of steatosis has not been investigated. For example, ghrelin, a stomach-derived peptide that rises with fasting and promotes food intake, rises after energy restriction related to a diet, thus promoting maintenance of the BMI. After gastric bypass, in contrast, ghrelin levels can be inappropriately lower, which might permit the better weight loss after surgery vs simple caloric deficient diets. Whether ghrelin has any impact on fat metabolism in the liver is unknown. Adiponectin and peptide YY rise after bariatric surgery.

Klein et al have performed one of the only studies of metabolism in patients with NAFLD before and after RYGB.[20] Seven participants participated in paired liver biopsies (before and average 1 year post surgery). At the 1-year mark, 29% of the body weight had been lost, and glucose and insulin concentrations were reduced; homeostasis model showed large improvement in insulin sensitivity. In stable isotope studies, hepatic glucose production and adipose tissue lipolysis were reduced by 50% despite a 70% reduction in circulating insulin concentrations. Liver chemistries were unchanged; however, hepatic steatosis was substantially reduced on biopsy. The mild inflammation and fibrosis that had been present were unaltered. There was a remarkable reduction in expression of genes that regulate fibrosis, such as TGF-β 1 (a major fibrogenic factor) and of chemokines that are proinflammatory such as IL-8 and monocyte chemoattractant protein-1.

Cytochrome P450 (enzyme CYP2E1) may play a role in the pathogenesis of NAFLD and in particular NASH through induction of oxidative stress and lipid peroxidation. NAFLD and NASH are associated with increased systemic lipid peroxidation levels and elevated hepatic CYP2E1 activity. Hepatic malondialdehyde concentrations are a marker of lipid peroxidation. Malondialdehyde and CYP2E1 were both strikingly reduced in livers of patients who underwent bariatric surgery after mean of 15 months, in parallel with BMI reductions, and improved hepatic histology.[21]

Summary

There are no prospective trials comparing the effects of bariatric surgery with medical weight loss on outcome of NAFLD, nor are there likely to be, given the requirement for paired liver biopsies to assess progression vs regression. Noninvasive surrogate markers of different stages of NAFLD will help in this regard. Whether the beneficial effects of bariatric surgery on NAFLD are independent of the degree of weight loss is currently unknown. Given that insulin sensitivity can improve so much shortly after gastric bypass and well before weight loss, there is reason to suppose that manipulation of incretins such as occurs after surgery might have relevant effects on NAFLD independent of weight loss.

Dyslipidemia

Dyslipidemia is a known risk factor for the development of atherosclerosis and coronary artery disease. In the worldwide INTERHEART study of patients from 52 countries, 9 potentially modifiable factors accounted for over 90% of the population-attributable risk of a first myocardial infarction including smoking, dyslipidemia, hypertension, diabetes, abdominal obesity, psychosocial factors, daily consumption of fruits and vegetables, regular alcohol consumption, and regular physical activity.[22] Dyslipidemia is usually defined as total cholesterol, low-density lipoprotein cholesterol (LDL-C), triglyceride or Lp(a) levels above the 90th percentile, or high-density lipoprotein cholesterol (HDL-C) or apo A-1 levels below the 10th percentile for the general population. The dyslipidemia of obesity commonly consists of fasting hypertriglyceridemia with increased plasma, very low-density lipoprotein (VLDL), reduced HDL-C, and the presence of small, dense LDL particles. Prevalence of dyslipidemia varies among the population studied and up to 50% of morbidly obese patients who undergo bariatric surgery have been reported to have dyslipidemia.[23] Generally, abnormal lipoprotein metabolism is often familial. However, in the majority of patients, inheritance is polygenic and the expression of dyslipidemia is strongly influenced by other factors, such as the saturated fat and cholesterol content of the diet and obesity. This polygenic type of dyslipidemia is the major source for atherosclerotic cardiovascular disease and plays a significant role in the excess morbidity and mortality among patients with obesity.

Randomized controlled studies consistently show that lipid-lowering treatment with statins reduces cardiovascular disease morbidity and mortality.[24] In a prospective controlled study of obese subjects, bariatric surgery has been shown to reduce overall mortality, when compared with conventional treatment of matched controls.[25] The most common causes of death in these obese subjects were myocardial infarction and cancer. Bariatric surgery is associated with beneficial effects on diabetes and cardiovascular risk factors including the improvement in lipid profiles. Nonetheless, the extent of lipid improvement varies with different bariatric procedures. The meta-analysis by Buchwald et al showed the biggest improvements in dyslipidemia with BPD or BPD with duodenal switch (BPD-DS) procedures (99.1% of patients evaluated) and with RYGB (96.9% of patients).[26] Reduction of triglyceride levels are consistently seen both immediately and after long-term follow-up with all surgical procedures.

Roux-en-Y Gastric Bypass

Jamal at el reported an improvement of serum total cholesterol (TC), triglycerides, and LDL-C profiles within 6 months after RYGB in 94 patients with a diagnosis of dyslipidemia. The HDL-C levels improved more slowly, reaching desirable levels within 12 months after surgery. All patients were able to discontinue lipid-lowering medications by the end of the study (6 years).[27] Similarly, Nguyen et al found that within 1 year, 82% patients who required lipid-lowering medications pre-operatively were able to discontinue their medications.[23] The 66% excess weight loss with RYGB shown in that study was associated with a 16% decrease in total cholesterol levels, a 63% decrease in triglyceride levels, a 31% decrease in LDL-C levels, and a 39% increase in HDL-C levels.[23] A sustained improvement in cardiovascular risk factors has been shown as long as 6 to 10 years after RYGB despite some weight regain. A recent study showed that at 6 years after RYGB, patients who underwent RYGB surgery lost 27.7% of their initial body weight, LDL-C decreased by 9 mg/dL, TC decreased by 13.7 mg/dL, and HDL-C increased by 11 mg/dL.[28] Remission of low HDL-C, high LDL-C, and high triglyceride levels were observed in 67%, 53%, and 71% of the patients, respectively. In the Swedish Obese Subjects (SOS) study, there was a 28% reduction in triglyceride levels and a 12% reduction in TC levels in patients who underwent RYGB at 10 years postoperatively.[29]

Gastric Banding

In general, gastric banding is associated with lesser weight loss and less improvement of some comorbidities as compared to RYGB.[30] The meta-analysis by Buchwald et al showed a 71% improvement in hyperlipidemia in patients who underwent gastric banding compared to 97% in patients who had RYGB.[26] Triglyceride levels are reduced by only 16% to 25% after gastric banding compared to 50% to 60% after RYGB.[26,30] At 10 years postoperatively, HDL-C increased by 20% vs 47% and TC decreased by 5% vs 13% when compared to RYGB.[26]

Laparoscopic Sleeve Gastrectomy

Laparoscopic sleeve gastrectomy (LSG) is a newer procedure being done with increasing frequency. Limited data show that in patients undergoing LSG, BMI reduction and the improvement in most of the weight-related comorbidities lies between the results of gastric banding and RYGB. The first report from the American College of Surgeons, which included 109 hospitals, showed that the average reduction in BMI in patients who underwent LSG was 8.75 at 6 months and 11.87 at 1 year compared to 5.02 and 7.05 at 6 months and 1 year after gastric banding, and 10.82 and 15.34 at 6 months and 1 year after RYGB. For patients who had hyperlipidemia at baseline, 35% had their hyperlipidemia resolve 1 year after LSG, compared to 33% for gastric banding and 66% for RYGB.[31] In contrast, one center study found similar remission rates between LSG and RYGB for hyperlipidemia (63% and 56%) at 1 year postoperatively.[32]

Table 21-1

Adult Treatment Panel III Classification of LDL, Total, and HDL Cholesterol

LDL CHOLESTEROL, MG/DL (MMOL/L)	
< 100 (2.58)	Optimal
100 to 129 (2.58 to 3.33)	Near or above optimal
130 to 159 (3.36 to 4.11)	Borderline high
160 to 189 (4.13 to 4.88)	High
≥ 190 (4.91)	Very high
TOTAL CHOLESTEROL, MG/DL (MMOL/L)	
< 200 (5.17)	Desirable
200 to 239 (5.17 to 6.18)	Borderline high
≥ 240 (6.20)	High
HDL CHOLESTEROL, MG/DL (MMOL/L)	
< 40 (1.03)	Low
≥ 60 (1.55)	High

Adapted from the Adult Treatment Panel III, http://www.nhlbi.nih.gov/

Mechanism of Lipid Improvements After Weight Loss Surgery

The exact mechanisms for the improvements in lipid profiles seen after weight loss surgery are not clear. An increase in hepatic insulin sensitivity partly induced by energy restriction is likely responsible for some of the changes. A weight loss induced improvement in peripheral insulin sensitivity follows later on.[33] Insulin resistance leads to abnormal metabolism of triglyceride-rich lipoproteins, which includes both increased hepatic secretion and impaired clearance of VLDL and intestinally derived chylomicrons. Interestingly, Brolin et al reported no differences in lipid profiles between patients who maintained their weight loss for 5 years postoperatively compared to those who regained the weight back.[34] This suggests that weight loss may not be the primary mechanism for lipid improvement. GLP-1, a hormone secreted during meal absorption that plays a key role in the control of plasma glucose, has been implicated as a candidate hormone for regulating intestinal lipid metabolism. Increases in GLP-1 have been shown after malabsorptive procedures (RYGB and BPD) and may play a role in the improvements in lipid metabolism.[35]

In the SOS cohort, HDL-C response to surgery-induced weight loss over time also showed large inter-individual variation. It has been postulated that the heterogeneity in HDL-C response to bariatric surgery-induced weight loss may be caused in part by a genetic predisposition. Certain candidate genes, such as cholesteryl ester transfer protein, hepatic lipase, and lipoprotein lipase, have been found to influence plasma HDL-C levels in individuals with obesity, and the associations persist even after considerable weight loss due to bariatric surgery. However, none of the genes studied to date have demonstrated an association with surgery-induced changes in HDL-C levels.[36]

Treatment of Dyslipidemia After Weight Loss Surgery

Lipid profiles should be followed after surgery and lipid abnormalities should be treated according to the National Cholesterol Education Program (NCEP) guidelines[37] (Tables 21-1 and 21-2).

Table 21-2

ATP III LDL-Cholesterol Goals and Cutpoints for Therapeutic Lifestyle Changes and Drug Therapy in Different Risk Categories

RISK CATEGORY	LDL-C GOAL	LDL-C LEVEL AT WHICH TO INITIATE THERAPEUTIC LIFE-STYLE CHANGES	LDL-C LEVEL AT WHICH TO CONSIDER DRUG THERAPY
CHD or CHD risk equivalent (10-year risk > 20%)*	< 100 mg/dL (2.58 mmol/L)	≥ 100 mg/dL (2.58 mmol/L)	≥ 130 mg/dL (3.36 mmol/L); drug optional at 100 to 129 mg/dL (2.58 to 3.33 mmol/L)•
2 or more risk factors (10-year risk ≤ 20%)△	≤ 130 mg/dL (3.36 mmol/L)	≥ 130 mg/dL (3.36 mmol/L)	10-year risk 10% to 20%: > 130 mg/dL (3.36 mmol/L) 10-year risk < 10%: ≥ 160 mg/dL (4.13 mmol/L)
0 to 1 risk factor◊	≤ 160 mg/dL (4.13 mmol/L)	≥ 160 mg/dL (4.13 mmol/L)	≥ 190 mg/dL (4.91 mmol/L); LDL-cholesterol lowering drug optional at 160 to 189 mg/dL (4.13 to 4.88 mmol/L)

* CHD risk equivalents defined in text. Ten-year risk defined by Framingham risk score (see text).

• Some authorities recommend use of LDL-C lowering drugs in this category if LDL-C < 100 mg/dL (2.58 mmol/L) cannot be achieved by therapeutic lifestyle changes. Others prefer use of drugs that primarily modify triglycerides and HDL-C (eg, nicotinic acid or fibrate). Clinical judgment may also call for deferring drug therapy in this subcategory.
△ Risk factors that modify LDL-C goals include cigarette smoking; hypertension (blood pressure 140/90 mm Hg or on antihypertensive medication); low HDL-C (<40 mg/dL [1.03 mmol/L]); family history of premature CHD (CHD in male first-degree relative <55 years or CHD in female first-degree relative <65 years); age (men 45 years; women 55 years). HDL-C 60 mg/dL (1.55 mmol/L) counts as a negative risk factor; its presence removes one risk factor from the total count.

◊ Almost all people with 0 to 1 risk factor have a 10-year risk < 10%; thus, 10-year risk assessment in people with 0 to 1 risk factor is not necessary.

CHD = coronary heart disease.

Adapted from the Adult Treatment Panel III, http://www.nhlbi.nih.gov/

Lipid-lowering therapy should be continued for LDL-C, non-HDL-C, and triglyceride levels that remain above the desired goal after surgery. Since drastic improvements in lipid profiles are usually seen after surgery, particularly after malabsorptive procedures, the need and the doses of lipid-lowering medications should be periodically reevaluated.

Summary

Triglycerides decrease, LDL-C decreases, and HDL-C increases after RYGB, gastric banding, LGS, BPD, and BPD-DS procedures. The biggest improvements in dyslipidemia were seen with BPD, BPD-DS, and RYGB. Many patients were able to discontinue lipid-lowering medications within 1 year after surgery. Weight loss and improvement of hepatic insulin sensitivity most likely play some role in the improvement of lipid profiles after weight loss surgery.

References

1. Williams KH, Shackel NA, Gorrell MD, McLennan SV, Twigg SM. Diabetes and nonalcoholic fatty liver disease: a pathogenic duo. *Endocr Rev.* 2013;34(1):84-129.
2. Browning JD, Szczepaniak LS, Dobbins R, et al. Prevalence of hepatic steatosis in an urban population in the United States: impact of ethnicity. *Hepatology.* 2004;40(6):1387-1395.
3. Williams CD, Stengel J, Asike MI, et al. Prevalence of nonalcoholic fatty liver disease and nonalcoholic steatohepatitis among a largely middle-aged population utilizing ultrasound and liver biopsy: a prospective study. *Gastroenterology.* 2011;140(1):124-131.
4. Yang HR. Noninvasive diagnosis of pediatric nonalcoholic fatty liver disease. *Korean J Pediatr.* 2013;56(2):45-51.
5. Chalasani N, Younossi Z, Lavine JE, et al. The diagnosis and management of non-alcoholic fatty liver disease: practice guideline by the American Gastroenterological Association, American Association for the Study of Liver Diseases, and American College of Gastroenterology. *Gastroenterology.* 2012;142(7):1592-1609.
6. Musso G, Gambino R, Cassader M, Pagano G. Meta-analysis: natural history of non-alcoholic fatty liver disease (NAFLD) and diagnostic accuracy of non-invasive tests for liver disease severity. *Ann Med.* 2011;43(8):617-649.
7. Aron-Wisnewsky J, Minville C, Tordjman J, et al. Chronic intermittent hypoxia is a major trigger for non-alcoholic fatty liver disease in morbid obese. *J Hepatol.* 2012;56(1):225-233.
8. Chin K, Nakamura T, Takahashi K, et al. Effects of obstructive sleep apnea syndrome on serum aminotransferase levels in obese patients. *Am J Med.* 2003;114(5):370-376.
9. Kleiner DE, Brunt EM, Van Natta M, et al. Design and validation of a histological scoring system for nonalcoholic fatty liver disease. *Hepatology.* 2005;41(6):1313-1321.
10. Krakoff J, Clark JM, Crandall JP, et al. Effects of metformin and weight loss on serum alanine aminotransferase activity in the diabetes prevention program. *Obesity (Silver Spring).* 2010;18(9):1762-1767.
11. Sanyal AJ, Chalasani N, Kowdley KV, et al. Pioglitazone, vitamin E, or placebo for nonalcoholic steatohepatitis. *N Engl J Med.* 2010;362(18):1675-1685.
12. Lavine JE, Schwimmer JB, Van Natta ML, et al. Effect of vitamin E or metformin for treatment of non-alcoholic fatty liver disease in children and adolescents: the TONIC randomized controlled trial. *JAMA.* 2011;305(16):1659-1668.
13. Forlano R, Ippolito AM, Iacobellis A, et al. Effect of the BioEnterics intragastric balloon on weight, insulin resistance, and liver steatosis in obese patients. *Gastrointest Endosc.* 2010;71(6):927-933.
14. Chavez-Tapia NC, Tellez-Avila FI, Barrientos-Gutierrez T, et al. Bariatric surgery for non-alcoholic steatohepatitis in obese patients. *Cochrane Database Syst Rev.* 2010;Jan 20:CD007340.
15. Rabl C, Campos GM. The impact of bariatric surgery on nonalcoholic steatohepatitis. *Semin Liver Dis.* 2012;32(1):80-91.
16. Tai CM, Huang CK, Hwang JC, et al. Improvement of nonalcoholic fatty liver disease after bariatric surgery in morbidly obese Chinese patients. *Obes Surg.* 2012;22(7):1016-1021.
17. Moretto M, Kupski C, da Silva VD, Padoin AV, Mottin CC. Effect of bariatric surgery on liver fibrosis. *Obes Surg.* 2012;22(7):1044-1049.
18. Stratopoulos C, Papakonstantinou A, Terzis I, et al. Changes in liver histology accompanying massive weight loss after gastroplasty for morbid obesity. *Obes Surg.* 2005;15(8):1154-1160.
19. Kral JG, Thung SN, Biron S, et al. Effects of surgical treatment of the metabolic syndrome on liver fibrosis and cirrhosis. *Surgery.* 2004;135(1):48-58.
20. Klein S, Mittendorfer B, Eagon JC, et al. Gastric bypass surgery improves metabolic and hepatic abnormalities associated with nonalcoholic fatty liver disease. *Gastroenterology.* 2006;130(6):1564-1572.
21. Bell LN, Temm CJ, Saxena R, et al. Bariatric surgery-induced weight loss reduces hepatic lipid peroxidation levels and affects hepatic cytochrome P-450 protein content. *Ann Surg.* 2010;251(6):1041-1048.
22. Yusuf S, Hawken S, Ounpuu S, et al. Effect of potentially modifiable risk factors associated with myocardial infarction in 52 countries (the INTERHEART study): case-control study. *Lancet.* 2004;364(9438):937.
23. Nguyen NT, Varela E, Sabio A, Tran CL, Stamos M, Wilson SE. Resolution of hyperlipidemia after laparoscopic Roux-en-Y gastric bypass. *J Am Coll Surg.* 2006;203(1):24-29.
24. Gutierrez J, Ramirez G, Rundek T, Sacco RL. Statin therapy in the prevention of recurrent cardiovascular events: a sex-based meta-analysis. *Arch Intern Med.* 2012;172(12):909-919
25. Sjöström L, Narbro K, Sjöström CD, et al. Effects of bariatric surgery on mortality in Swedish obese subjects. *N Engl J Med.* 2007;357(8):741-752.
26. Buchwald H, Avidor Y, Braunwald E, et al. Bariatric surgery: a systematic review and meta-analysis. *JAMA.* 2004;292(14):1724-1737.
27. Jamal M, Wegner R, Heitshusen D, Liao J, Samuel I. Resolution of hyperlipidemia follows surgical weight loss in patients undergoing Roux-en-Y gastric bypass surgery: a 6-year analysis of data. *Surg Obes Relat Dis.* 2011;7(4):473-479.
28. Adams TD, Davidson LE, Litwin SE, et al. Health benefits of gastric bypass surgery after 6 years. *JAMA.* 2012;308(11):1122-1131.

29. Sjöström L, Lindroos AK, Peltonen M, et al. Lifestyle, diabetes, and cardiovascular risk factors 10 years after bariatric surgery. *N Engl J Med.* 2004;351:2683-2693.
30. Romy S, Donadini A, Giusti V, Suter M. Roux-en-Y gastric bypass vs gastric banding for morbid obesity: a case-matched study of 442 patients. *Arch Surg.* 2012;147(5):460-466.
31. Hutter MM, Schirmer BD, Jones DB, et al. First report from the American College of Surgeons—Bariatric Surgery Center Network: laparoscopic sleeve gastrectomy has morbidity and effectiveness positioned between the band and the bypass. *Ann Surg.* 2011;254(3):410-422.
32. Zhang N, Maffei A, Cerabona T, Pahuja A, Omana J, Kaul A. Reduction in obesity-related comorbidities: is gastric bypass better than sleeve gastrectomy? *Surg Endosc.* 2013;27(4):1273-1280.
33. Poirier P, Cornier MA, Mazzone T, et al. Bariatric surgery and cardiovascular risk factors: a scientific statement from the American Heart Association. *Circulation.* 2011;123(15):1683-1701.
34. Brolin RE, Bradley LJ, Wilson AC, Cody RP. Lipid risk profile and weight stability after gastric restrictive operations for morbid obesity. *J Gastrointest Surg.* 2000;4(5):464-469.
35. Burcelin R, Thorens B; The European Club for the study of GLP-1 (EuCSGLP-1). Incretins: what is known, new and controversial in 2013? *Diabetes Metab.* 2013;39(2):89-93.
36. Sarzynski MA, Jacobson P, Rankinen T, et al. Association of GWAS-based candidate genes with HDL-cholesterol levels before and after bariatric surgery in the Swedish Obese Subjects study. *J Clin Endocrinol Metab.* 2011;96(6):E953-E957.
37. National Cholesterol Education Program (NCEP) Expert Panel on Detection, Evaluation, and Treatment of High Blood Cholesterol in Adults (Adult Treatment Panel III). Third Report of the National Cholesterol Education Program (NCEP) Expert Panel on Detection, Evaluation, and Treatment of High Blood Cholesterol in Adults (Adult Treatment Panel III) final report. *Circulation.* 2002;106:3043-3421.

22

Medical Management of the Patient After Bariatric Surgery

Reevaluating Sleep Apnea

Lee E. Morrow, MD, MSc

Obesity, defined as a body mass index (BMI) > 30 kg/m^2, has increased so rapidly in the past several decades that many consider it to be a global epidemic. Obesity affects men, women, and children of all races and is an important risk factor for the development of multiple comorbidities. One such comorbidity strongly related to obesity is obstructive sleep apnea (OSA). Briefly, OSA is characterized by recurrent episodes of partial or complete airway collapse that lead to ineffective respiratory efforts known as apneas and/or hypopneas. An apneic event requires complete cessation of airflow, while a hypopnea is defined as a 50% reduction in airflow associated with a 3% or greater fall in the oxygen saturation. These events result in recurrent, cyclical arousals, which ultimately fragment normal sleep architecture. The diagnosis and grading of OSA severity uses the apnea-hypopnea index (AHI): patients with AHI values of 5 to 14, 15 to 29, and ≥ 30 events per hour have mild, moderate, and severe disease, respectively.[1] Although historic data report the prevalence of OSA in obese adults between 42% to 48% for men and 8% to 38% in women, several recent studies suggest that these estimates may be significantly underestimated.[2]

Medical sequelae of OSA include systemic hypertension, coronary artery disease, congestive heart failure, arrhythmias, and stroke. Afflicted individuals also routinely report psychosocial dysfunction, cognitive deficits, and impaired quality of life. Not surprisingly, several cohort studies have demonstrated that untreated OSA is an independent risk factor for death.[3] These adverse consequences of disease can be mitigated utilizing strategies to reduce upper airway resistance and prevent airway obstruction. Standard interventions for OSA include continuous positive airway pressure (CPAP), oral appliances, and upper airway surgery. Because noncompliance with these measures is common—and none of these strategies treats comorbid obesity—such prescriptions are essentially temporizing measures.

Because it has been shown that the odds of developing OSA increase by 14% for each kg/m^2 increase in the BMI, weight loss is a central recommendation for the definitive management of OSA.[4] Dietary interventions are generally ineffective for significant, long-term weight reduction. Accordingly, bariatric surgery is viewed by many as the only available option for sustained weight loss for individuals with morbid obesity (BMI ≥ 40 or BMI ≥ 35 with substantial obesity-related comorbidity).[5]

Forse RA, Apovian CM, eds.
Bariatric Surgery: What Every Provider Needs to Know (pp 257-261).

Although there is ample evidence regarding the improvement or resolution of comorbidities such as diabetes and hypertension following bariatric surgery, the literature is somewhat less robust in documenting the effects of operative interventions on OSA. The purpose of this chapter is to summarize our current understanding of the impact of bariatric surgery on OSA and to provide clinicians with guidance regarding repeat sleep symptom evaluation and/or polysomnography (PSG) during postoperative monitoring.

Effects of Bariatric Surgery on Obstructive Sleep Apnea

Early reports regarding the effects of bariatric surgery on OSA symptoms were generally favorable. However, most studies did not routinely repeat PSG, thereby precluding our ability to correlate changes in symptoms and BMI with objective sleep lab measures. While multiple investigators demonstrated that sustained weight loss led to measurable improvement in daytime symptoms, there were minimal data linking these subjective improvements and reductions in BMI to increases in desirable rapid eye movement sleep. These initial studies were further limited by inconsistencies in patient selection, surgical techniques used, lack of randomization, and heterogeneity in the definition and measures of the subjective outcomes studied.

A widely cited meta-analysis by Buchwald and colleagues reported the health outcomes for 22,094 obese individuals who had an average reduction in BMI of 14.2 following bariatric surgery.[5] These investigators determined that 83.6% of patients undergoing various bariatric surgical procedures experienced improvement or resolution of OSA symptoms. Efficacy in improving OSA varied by the specific type of intervention: 94.8% with gastric bypass, 90.7% with gastroplasty, and 68.0% with gastric banding. A limitation to the accuracy of these estimates is the investigators' decision to combine patients with PSG-confirmed OSA, sleep-disordered breathing, and the so-called Pickwickian syndrome into a single group they deemed "representative of OSA." That criticism aside, in the patients with sleep lab-confirmed OSA who had repeat PSG after bariatric surgery, the AHI was reduced from 50.23 to 17.47 events per hour.

Using systematic review and meta-analysis techniques, Greenburg et al demonstrated similarly significant reductions in measures of obesity and severity of OSA following bariatric surgery. These investigators estimated the average reduction of the BMI was equal to 17.5 and the average decrease in AHI was 38.2 events per hour.[6] Although these estimates are both statistically significant and clinically meaningful, the residual AHI after bariatric surgery was 15.8 events per hour. While surgical intervention led to meaningful weight loss and an impressive reduction in the AHI, most patients (77%) continued to suffer from OSA. Such residual disease was more prevalent in patients who were older or whose follow-up weight was more than 100 kg.

A more recent systematic literature review by Sarkhosh et al also demonstrated improvements in OSA post-bariatric surgery.[7] In their analysis of 13,900 patients among 69 published studies (3 randomized controlled trials, 11 nonrandomized controlled trials, and 55 case series), efficacy in treating OSA varied remarkably depending on the surgical intervention. These authors reported improvement/resolution of OSA symptoms in 99.0% of patients undergoing vertical banded gastroplasty, 85.7% with laparoscopic sleeve gastrectomy, 79.2% with Roux-en-Y gastric bypass, 79% with biliopancreatic diversion, and 77.5% with laparoscopic adjustable gastric banding. Only 9 of the included studies included both pre- and postoperative PSG; the remaining studies used subjective measures—including sleep scoring systems—to assess efficacy. The PSG lab-confirmed reductions in AHI averaged 41.6 events per hour with a residual AHI of 15.4 postoperatively.

Several well-designed and rigorously executed longitudinal studies have demonstrated that operative interventions lead to sustained reductions in weight and that such weigh loss is also associated with improvements in OSA symptoms over time.[8,9] One such study followed patients for an average of 90 months and demonstrated an average reduction of the BMI by 19.[10] In this cohort, the prevalence of sleep apnea symptoms was reduced by nearly 50% overall. However, weight regain was substantial in some patients, and this was associated with return and/or eventual worsening of symptoms.

A recent clinical trial randomly assigned 60 OSA patients with a BMI between 35 and 55 to either intensive medical weight loss therapy or bariatric surgery.[11] As with prior studies, surgery resulted in markedly greater reductions in weight loss (27.8 vs 5.1 kg, $p < .001$) and significantly improved physical function scores on the Short Form 36 ($p = .04$). However, the observed post-intervention decreases in AHI were not statistically significantly different between groups (25.5 for surgery vs 14.0 for medical therapy, $p = .18$). Regardless of group assignment, comorbid OSA was prevalent in both groups at the end of study with an average AHI of 39.5 events per hour in surgically managed patients and 43.2 events per hour in medically managed patients. While the sample size in this study may be perceived as potentially inadequate, it was calculated using sound methodologies to provide power of at least 80% to detect a between-group difference of 50% in the AHI.

Reevaluating Obstructive Sleep Apnea After Bariatric Surgery

Collectively, the data reviewed this far support bariatric surgery as a strategy for significant, sustained weight loss with concurrent reductions in OSA symptoms and AHI. However, these data are also uniform in establishing that the majority of patients continue to experience residual OSA despite marked weight loss and irrespective of the surgical intervention provided. This is particularly bothersome as the symptoms of OSA are not directly correlated with the presence or the severity of disease as measured by PSG. Specifically, the lack of daytime somnolence does not definitively indicate resolution/absence of OSA.[12] Many patients with marked weight loss experience benefits that include increased mobility and activity tolerance, and they often erroneously equate such improvements in general well-being to "cure" of their comorbid OSA. This misperception may subsequently lead to noncompliance with CPAP therapy and an increased risk of cardiovascular and metabolic complications.

As such, our present understanding of the effects of bariatric surgery on OSA do not support routine cessation of CPAP or other therapies for OSA regardless of the magnitude of weight loss or perceived change in symptoms.[6,11] Rather, objective measurements of OSA must be incorporated into the routine follow-up care of bariatric surgery patients with comorbid OSA. Neither standardized OSA screening tools (Epworth Sleepiness Scale, STOP BANG Score, etc) nor self-reported symptoms have sufficient sensitivity and specificity to be used as stand-alone OSA assessments.[13] Accordingly, formal PSG testing should be the mainstay of disease monitoring with meaningful weight loss.

Definitive recommendations regarding the timing of repeat sleep testing are lacking. The most recent statement from the Clinical Issues Committee of the American Society for Metabolic and Bariatric Surgery (ASMBS) specifically acknowledge that there is currently no consensus regarding the indications or timing of repeat PSG testing or CPAP titration for individuals who have undergone bariatric surgery.[14] Most clinicians with clinical expertise in this realm generally repeat formal sleep evaluations when goal weight is achieved or once a stable weight is attained. In most patients this will allow for optimization of therapy and increased compliance; for a select few individuals repeat testing may lead to discontinuation of obsolete therapies.

It is also prudent to consider repeat sleep testing in patients with ongoing weight loss who express specific complaints related to their therapy. With partial weight loss CPAP therapy may become excessive and/or uncomfortable—despite its ongoing necessity. In this instance, repeat titration studies increase the likelihood of establishing a therapeutic plan that is simultaneously effective and tolerable. Clinicians must also be attentive to the possibility for worsening or relapse of OSA if a patient who initially improves later experiences significant weight regain. Patients with a history of OSA who experience a 10% increase in weight after achieving their post-procedure nadir merit repeat sleep testing to assess the need for resumption or titration of CPAP.

Given the accumulation of data showing increases in perioperative morbidity and mortality in morbidly obese patients with undiagnosed or inadequately treated OSA who undergo major surgery, PSG is now part of the routine preoperative assessment for bariatric surgery in many centers.[15] The need for PSG is particularly encouraged in patients who are anticipating repeat operations after weight regain. Much of the data supporting these recommendations are extrapolated from studies on morbidly obese patients undergoing a variety of nonbariatric operations. As such, the actual utility of PSG in the setting of initial or repeat bariatric surgery is essentially unknown. Regardless, both of these recommendations are endorsed by the ASMBS.[14]

Reimbursement for PSG in this population is typically not a significant obstacle if indications are documented and 3 or less studies are ordered within a 12-month period. More frequent repeat studies may be indicated in subsets of patients after bariatric surgery, and insurers are typically willing to approve these additional studies if the medical necessity is clearly delineated. The relative ease of getting frequent PSG studies reimbursed likely stems from the observation that bariatric surgery-related weight loss reduces obesity-related claims to insurance companies by 71.6% as early as 4 months following surgery.[16]

Summary

Through the collective experience utilizing bariatric surgery in patients who suffer from comorbid OSA we have established several key observations. Sleep apnea is remarkably common in patients referred for evaluation for bariatric surgery evaluation and successful weight loss results in significant improvements in subjective and objective measures of OSA postoperatively. Accordingly, bariatric surgery should be given strong consideration in the management of OSA among morbidly obese individuals. Because a significant number of patients will have residual disease that merits ongoing therapy—despite marked weight loss and improvement or resolution of symptoms—repeat sleep testing has a role in the longitudinal management of the postoperative patient. The optimal frequency and timing of such studies are not rigorously established. Clinical experience suggests that clinicians should consider repeat PSG when goal weight or stable weight is achieved, if sleep-related symptoms change markedly, when there is a 10% increase in weight, or prior to repeat bariatric surgery.

References

1. Kushida CA, Littner MR, Morgenthaler T, et al. Practice parameters for the indications for polysomnography and related procedures: an update for 2005. *Sleep*. 2005;28:499-521.
2. Young T, Palta M, Dempsey J, et al. The occurrence of sleep-disordered breathing among middle-aged adults. *N Engl J Med*. 1993;328:1230-1235.
3. Marshall NS, Wong KK, Liu PY, et al. Sleep apnea as an independent risk factor for all-cause mortality: the Busselton Health Study. *Sleep*. 2008;31:1079-1085.
4. Pannain S, Mokhlesi B. Bariatric surgery and its impact on sleep architecture, sleep-disordered breathing, and metabolism. *Best Pract Res Clin Endocrinol Metab*. 2010;24:745-761.
5. Buchwald H, Avidor Y, Braunwal E, et al. Bariatric surgery: a systematic review and meta-analysis. *JAMA*. 2004;292:1724-1737.
6. Greenburg DL, Lettieri CJ, Eliasson AH. Effects of surgical weight loss on measures of obstructive sleep apnea: a meta-analysis. *Am J Med*. 2009;122:535-542.
7. Sarkhosh K, Switzer NJ, El-Hadi M, et al. The impact of bariatric surgery on obstructive sleep apnea: a systematic review. *Obes Surg*. 2013;23:414-423.

8. Higa K, Ho T, Tercero F, et al. Laparoscopic Roux-en-Y gastric bypass: 10-year follow-up. *Surg Obes Relat Dis.* 2011;7:516-525.
9. Obeid A, Long J, Kakade M, et al. Laparoscopic Roux-en-Y gastric bypass: long term clinical outcomes. *Surg Endosc.* 2012;26:3515-3520.
10. Laurino Neto RM, Herbella FAM, Tauil RM, et al. Comorbidities remission after Roux-en-Y gastric bypass for morbid obesity is sustained in a long-term follow-up and correlates with weight regain. *Obes Surg.* 2012;22:1580-1585.
11. Chang CL, Marshall NS, Yee BJ, Grunstein RR. Weight loss treatment for obstructive sleep apnea: medical and surgical options. *Eur Respir Monograph.* 2010;5:302-320.
12. Dixon JB, Dixon ME, Anderson ML, et al. Daytime sleepiness in the obese: not as simple as obstructive sleep apnea. *Obesity.* 2007;15:2504-2511.
13. Holty JEC, Parimi N, Ballesteros M, et al. Does surgically induced weight loss improve daytime sleepiness? *Obes Surg.* 2011;21:1535-1545.
14. Clinical Issues Committee, American Society for Metabolic and Bariatric Surgery. *Peri-operative management of obstructive sleep apnea.* March 2012. Available at: http://asmbs.org/wp/uploads/2012/03/PeriopMgmtOSA-May2012.pdf. Accessed May 26, 2015.
15. O'Keefe T, Patterson EJ. Evidence supporting routine polysomnography before bariatric surgery. *Obes Surg.* 2004;14:23-26.
16. Cremieux PY, Ledoux S, Clerici C, et al. The impact of bariatric surgery on comorbidities and medication use among obese patients. *Obes Surg.* 2010;20:861-870.

23

Endoscopy in the Bariatric Patient

Nitin Kumar, MD and
Christopher C. Thompson, MD, MSc, FACG, FASGE

Obesity and its comorbidities are a significant epidemic in the United States and around the world. Lifestyle modification and pharmacologic therapy have been ineffective in controlling this epidemic. Bariatric surgery, while highly effective, can be applied to only a fraction of eligible patients with the current number of bariatric surgeons.[1] Endoscopy can play a role in assessment of symptoms, diagnosis and therapy of disease, revision of bariatric surgery, and primary therapy of obesity. We will describe normal endoscopic findings in patients with bariatric surgery; the incidence, diagnosis, and management of complications after bariatric surgery; endoscopic therapy for weight regain; and endoscopic primary therapies for obesity.

Symptomatic Assessment

Acute or chronic presentation of abdominal pain, nausea, vomiting, fever, and weight regain warrants evaluation in patients who have had bariatric surgery. These symptoms should be evaluated in the context of which type of surgery the patient had and when, history of revision, and presence of risk factors for post-surgical complications. Complete evaluation in symptomatic patients usually warrants endoscopy or cross-sectional imaging.

Endoscopic Evaluation

Each type of bariatric surgery is associated with unique alterations in gastrointestinal tract anatomy and attendant complications and endoscopic findings. In general, endoscopy should be avoided in patients with perforated viscus and when fresh staple lines may be disrupted.

Forse RA, Apovian CM, eds.
Bariatric Surgery: What Every Provider Needs to Know (pp 263-278).

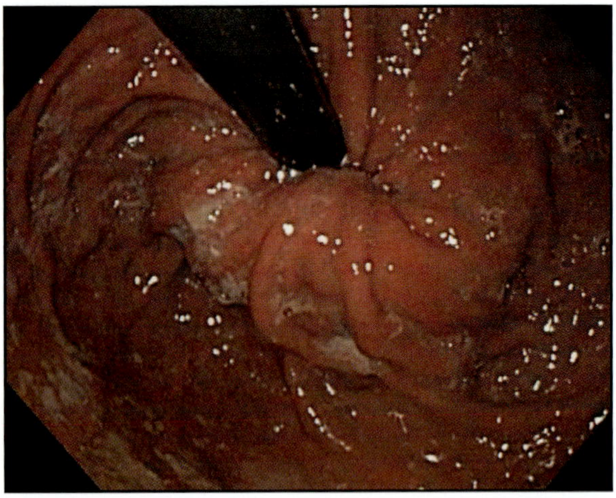

Figure 23-1. View of LAGB on retroflexion and eroded LAGB.

Roux-en-Y Gastric Bypass

Endoscopic examination of the gastrointestinal tract after Roux-en-Y gastric bypass (RYGB) reveals a small gastric pouch, in continuity with the esophagus, with volume of 15 to 30 mL. Staple lines may be visible, and retroflexion may be required to visualize them in entirety. The pouch length can be measured accurately if air insufflation is minimized. The distal pouch contains the end-to-side gastrojejunal anastomosis, which should be approximately 10 to 12 mm in diameter. A double-barrel view should be seen through the anastomosis. The blind limb of jejunum should be approximately 2 cm in length. The Roux limb is typically 60 to 75 cm in length, although it can be as long as 150 cm in long-limb RYGB. The limb should not contain excess retained food or fluid or tight angulation or obstruction characteristic of adhesions or internal hernia. The jejunojejunal anastomosis can eventually be reached, leading to a pancreaticobiliary limb and an alimentary limb. Examination of the pancreaticobiliary limb up to the gastric remnant can be performed using device-assisted enteroscopes.

Laparoscopic Adjustable Gastric Band

The adjustable band is used to create a virtual pouch by constricting the gastric fundus approximately 2 cm distal from the gastroesophageal junction. Endoscopically, the appearance can be consistent with an elongated cardia. In the forward view, a constriction can be seen at the site of the band; on retroflexion, the band appears as a bulging ring around the endoscope below the gastroesophageal junction (Figure 23-1). The site should be carefully assessed for band erosion.

Vertical Banded Gastroplasty

Vertical banded gastroplasty (VBG) entails creation of a vertical gastric channel, approximately 15 mL in volume and 7 cm in length, just distal to the gastroesophageal junction along the lesser curvature. The outlet of the channel, or stoma, is approximately 10 mm in aperture reinforced by a silastic or polypropylene mesh ring. It may be difficult to advance the endoscope through the channel due to its small diameter. However, if the endoscope cannot be advanced straight into the channel at from the gastroesophageal junction, the channel is angulated.[2] Once the endoscope has been advanced through the channel, retroflexion allows visualization of the staple line partition and gastric fundus. The remainder of the gastric and duodenal examination is normal.

Sleeve Gastrectomy

Sleeve gastrectomy (SG) entails creation of a channel along the lesser curvature, with resection of the fundus and gastric body. The endoscopic appearance is long and tubular, often precluding full retroflexion until the antrum is reached. The staple line is visible on the lesser curvature.

Biliopancreatic Diversion With Duodenal Switch

Biliopancreatic diversion (BPD) creates a tubular gastric remnant with volume of approximately 200 mL with end to side anastomosis to the ileum, creating a short common channel.[3] Endoscopically, there is a double-barrel view through the anastomosis. BPD with duodenal switch (BPD-DS) creates a tubular gastric anatomy along the lesser curvature, removing the fundus and greater curvature but leaving the pylorus intact. The duodenum forms an end-to-end anastomosis with the ileum, seen several centimeters distal to the pylorus. The biliopancreatic limb cannot be reached with a standard endoscope after either surgery.

Upper Gastrointestinal Bleeding

Bleeding is more common after RYGB than laparoscopic adjustable gastric band (LAGB), SG, and VBG.[4-7] In patients with RYGB, early bleeding most commonly occurs at the gastrojejunal anastomosis, jejunojejunal anastomosis, or gastric remnant.[8] Bleeding may be extraluminal, resulting in abdominal distention or hypovolemia. Later bleeding after RYGB often occurs in the setting of anastomotic, intestinal, or gastric remnant ulcer. The pouch and gastrojejunal anastomosis can be easily accessed, but the jejunojejunal anastomosis and gastric remnant may be difficult to access. In the immediate postoperative period, endoscopy carries a higher risk of perforation. If endoscopy is performed, insufflation should be minimized and carbon dioxide should be used.[9] If intraluminal bleeding is discovered, epinephrine and endoclips can be used in combination therapy. Electrocautery is not recommended at fresh staple lines. Angiographic intervention may result in bowel ischemia. Surgery may be necessary in refractory cases or to treat extraluminal bleeding.

Ulcer

Patients presenting with epigastric pain, nausea, vomiting, bleeding, or food intolerance should be evaluated for ulcer. Incidence of ulcer after RYGB is up to 20%.[10] Ulcer at the gastrojejunal anastomosis can be associated with *Helicobacter pylori* infection, nonsteroidal anti-inflammatory drug (NSAID) use, tobacco use, alcohol use, diabetes mellitus, bile acid reflux, large pouch, tension on the Roux limb, and foreign body such as suture.[10,11] As the jejunum is particularly susceptible to acid exposure, ulcers on the jejunal side of the anastomosis may be associated with gastrogastric fistula (GGF) or staple line disruption; ischemia may be another factor. In the first 2 weeks after surgery, imaging with gastrografin is recommended for diagnosis; endoscopy must be performed with care. Beyond this period, endoscopy is the preferred diagnostic method. Breath testing for *H pylori* and biopsies of the gastric pouch are not reliable; fecal antigen is recommended for diagnosis and confirmation of eradication.[12] Fluid can be aspirated from the gastric pouch for pH testing, and bile reflux may be visualized. Therapy of anastomotic ulcer should include proton pump inhibitor capsules broken open twice daily and sucralfate solution 1 g 4 times daily. Bile acid binders, such as ursodiol, can be prescribed at 10 g/kg daily, in divided doses. Additionally, other risk factors should be optimized. Tobacco and NSAID use should be discontinued if possible, and glycemic control should be optimized in people with diabetes. GGF should be repaired, and visible nonabsorbable sutures should be removed. Endoscopy should be repeated to assess healing; persistent or deep ulcer may warrant surgical repair. Chronic ulceration can result in stricture formation.

Foreign Body

Chronic pain after bariatric surgery may be due to foreign body, which has been associated with pain even when no inflammation is apparent. Material, including sutures, staples, and bands, inserted during bariatric surgery can result in complications. Embedded suture may result in pain, ulceration, and bezoar formation; in symptomatic patients, excision has proven beneficial in a majority of patients.[13] Large amounts of free suture should be removed even in asymptomatic patients.

Band-Related Complications

Patients with LAGB and VBG may present with band-related complications. In patients with LAGB, gastric prolapse through the band can present with epigastric pain, nausea, vomiting, or reflux. There can be underlying pouch dilation, obstruction, and necrosis. Technique changes have resulted in a decrease in these complications over time.[14] Endoscopically, the pouch may appear enlarged or elongated. The band should be deflated or removed. Erosion of adjustable gastric band through the gastric wall and into the lumen can present with abdominal pain, vomiting, bleeding, and abscess. Infection may present as cellulitis at the access port.[15] Band erosion can also occur after VBG, presenting as abdominal pain and loss of satiety with weight regain. In some cases, eroded bands in patients with LAGB or VGB can be removed endoscopically after transaction. Prior to removal of LAGB, it is important to confirm that the band buckle is endoscopically visible. Cross-sectional imaging should be performed prior to removal to confirm that the band is encapsulated.[16] Band cutting devices and lithotripters have been used to transect bands intraluminally to allow transoral removal.[17] The port must then be removed surgically. Partially eroded bands and mesh have been transected with endoscopic scissors or argon plasma coagulation and removed endoscopically in patients with VBG.[18] To facilitate extraction of partially eroded bands in LAGB and VBG, self-expanding stents have been placed to provoke complete erosion.[19]

Stenosis

Bariatric surgery patients presenting with dysphagia, nausea, vomiting, early satiety, or postprandial abdominal pain should be evaluated endoscopically or radiologically for the presence of stenosis.[20] Endoscopy can be used as a diagnostic tool, identifying etiologic factors such as ulcer. Additionally, therapy can be applied concurrently.

After RYGB, stenosis at the gastrojejunal anastomosis typically occurs 4 to 10 months postoperatively, although delayed presentation may occur in the setting of ulcer or foreign body.[21] NSAID use, smoking, and alcohol use are risk factors for stenosis.[22] Gastrojejunal stenosis has been reported in 3% to 5% of patients after open RYGB and 5% to 12% of patients after laparoscopic RYGB.[23] Stenoses may also develop at the jejunojejunal anastomosis, sites of bowel traversion through the mesocolon, or due to intestinal adhesions. Standard therapy is balloon dilation, which can be used 4 weeks after surgery and may need to be repeated every 2 to 3 weeks until a standard 9.5-mm endoscope can traverse the stenosis.[24] Excessive dilation can result in perforation, which has been reported at 3% to 5%, or weight regain.[25] In the case of dilation of gastrojejunal stenosis, care should be taken to avoid placing the balloon into the blind limb. Foreign body, such as visible suture or staples, should be removed prior to dilation.

Obstruction or stenosis after LAGB may develop due to edema or fibrous reaction to the band; endoscopic dilation may be effective in these cases. Band slippage or rotation, or external adhesions resulting in pouch angulation, warrants band removal or conversion to another type of bariatric surgery.[26] Stenosis after SG usually occurs at the incisura angularis or less commonly at the gastroesophageal junction.[27] Endoscopic balloon dilation or temporary covered metal stent placement may be effective in these cases.[28] VBG is associated with a high stenosis rate, although endoscopic dilation is often successful.

Leak and Fistula

Leak is a serious complication, occurring due to discontinuity of tissue apposition in the postoperative period. Potential etiologies include distal obstruction, excessive anastomotic tension, and tissue ischemia.[29] Diagnosis can be difficult, because fever, leukocytosis, and pain may be absent. Tachycardia, C-reactive protein >22.9, and increased drain output may be present.[30,31] Leaks presenting within 2 days are often mechanical, and leaks presenting later in the first postoperative week may be due to ischemia.[32] Leak occurs in up to 2.6% of patients after open RYGB and up to 5.2% after laparoscopic RYGB, primarily at the gastrojejunal anastomosis, in the gastric pouch, or at the jejunojejunal anastomosis.[33] Mortality rates range from 9% for gastrojejunal leak to 40% for jejunojejunal leak.[34] Less commonly, leaks occur at the jejunal stump or gastric remnant, which may not be apparent on endoscopy or upper gastrointestinal series.[34] Leak occurs in up to 5.1% of patients after SG, primarily just distal to the gastroesophageal junction. Distal stenosis, commonly at the incisura, and delayed gastric emptying are often associated. Endoscopic diagnosis of leak may require use of fluoroscopic contrast, methylene blue, or a bubble test, performed by submerging a surgical drain and insufflating air endoscopically.[35]

Fistula is an abnormal communication between visceral structures. A variety of fistulas present after bariatric surgery, although GGF in the setting of RYGB is most common. GGF allow reflux of acid from the gastric remnant into the pouch, and may present as heartburn, reflux, or ulcer. Additionally, GGF restores continuity of the excluded gastrointestinal tract, negating the bypass and resulting in weight regain.

Management of leak should begin with control of sepsis, organ failure, and abscess or fluid collection if present. Oral intake should be replaced with distal enteral or parenteral nutrition, and broad-spectrum antibiotics should be instituted. Nonoperative management in contained collections results in a high rate of leak resolution.[36] Endoscopic management of both leak and fistula should include dilation of distal stenosis, and endoscopic closure can be attempted. Endoscopic stents, clips, sealants, suturing, and vacuum-assisted drainage have all demonstrated success. These techniques may be more effective when used in conjunction.

Stent placement excludes the leak from the gastrointestinal tract, allowing resumption of enteral nutrition. After a guidewire is advanced (into the Roux limb in RYGB patients or third portion of the duodenum in SG patients), the leak site and gastroesophageal junction should be marked with submucosal contrast injection or external markers. The self-expanding stent should be placed so that its proximal end does not cause globus sensation and its distal end does not impact the enteral wall. Overlapping stents can be placed if needed. The stent should be removed after 2 to 8 weeks. Stent placement can be complicated by pain, nausea, and migration. A meta-analysis of stent placement for therapy of acute bariatric surgery leak found a leak closure rate of 87.8% (95% confidence interval 79.4% to 94.2%).[37] Stent migration was reported in 16.9% of patients and surgical revision was required in 9%.

Endoscopic clips can be used to approximate the edges of the defect in the gastrointestinal tract. One or more clips can be placed after ablation of the defect margin to expose the submucosa, which may assist healing. The Over the Scope Clip ([OTSC] Ovesco) is a nitinol clip placed on a cap at the endoscope tip; it can be used with a grasper accessory to pull the defect edges into the cap. OTSC has demonstrated success rates of 72% to 91% for fistula closure.[38]

Sealants can be placed at the defect site. After ablating the defect margin and removing foreign bodies at the site, fibrin can be injected through a double-lumen catheter to form a plug. Multiple treatments may be necessary, and success rates may be higher with combination endoscopic therapy. Lippert et al reported fistula closure in 36.5% of patients with fibrin alone and 55.7% with combination therapy.[39] Infection and high output can decrease likelihood of success.

Endoscopic suturing has been studied for fistula closure. Suturing devices have been improving, although procedural complexity has limited adoption. StomaphyX (EndoGastric Solutions) has been to close gastric leaks, and the Bard EndoCinch (CR Bard) has been used to repair GGFs with success in fistulas < 10 mm.[40] A newer device, the Apollo OverStitch (Apollo Endosurgery), performs full-thickness suturing. In preliminary study, it has shown early success for GGF.[41]

Vacuum-assisted sponge placement has been used to treat leak and fistula.[42] A feeding tube is inserted intranasally and orally exteriorized. An open-cell sponge, cut to fit within the wound cavity, is attached to the tip of a feeding tube with suture. The sponge is grasped with endoscopic forceps and advanced into the gastrointestinal tract, where it is inserted into the defect. The feeding tube is attached to continuous suction. This method has been used successfully for intrathoracic anastomotic leaks, gastroesophageal anastomotic leaks, and rectal anastomotic fistulas.[43,44] Some patients did develop stenosis requiring dilation.

Pancreaticobiliary Disease

Weight loss after bariatric surgery can predispose patients to gallstone formation.[45] Surgical reconfiguration of gastrointestinal anatomy after certain types of bariatric surgery renders endoscopic procedures for management of biliary and pancreatic disease challenging. Cross-sectional imaging is often useful, given that endoscopic ultrasound is compromised in patients with altered anatomy.

After RYGB and BPD-DS, endoscopic pancreatic or biliary intervention via endoscopic retrograde cholangiopancreatography (ERCP) often requires specialized tools. In RYGB, the papilla can be reached with single- or double-balloon enteroscopy or spiral enteroscopy. The disadvantages of these procedures include long duration, the need to use a forward-viewing endoscope, and inability to use usual accessories. These factors contribute to a lower success rate than in patients with normal anatomy. Alternatively, a percutaneous approach can be used to access the gastric remnant, allowing use of a standard duodenoscope and attendant accessories, potentially allowing shorter procedure duration and higher success rates.[46] This can be performed in the endoscopy suite via pexy of the gastric remnant to the abdominal wall and creation of a gastrostomy tract to allow insertion of the duodenoscope. A fully covered esophageal stent is placed in the gastrostomy tract during the procedure to allow endoscope insertion (Figure 23-2). After completion of ERCP, a percutaneous endoscopic gastrostomy tube can be left in place for 4 to 6 weeks to allow healing of the tract. If surgery is already planned, ERCP can be performed concurrently with laparoscopic access to the gastric remnant via trocar. ERCP after BPD-DS can be performed endoscopically with a transanal approach or through gastrostomy with laparoscopic assistance. In patients with SG, VBG, and LAGB, ERCP can be performed in the routine fashion using standard tools.

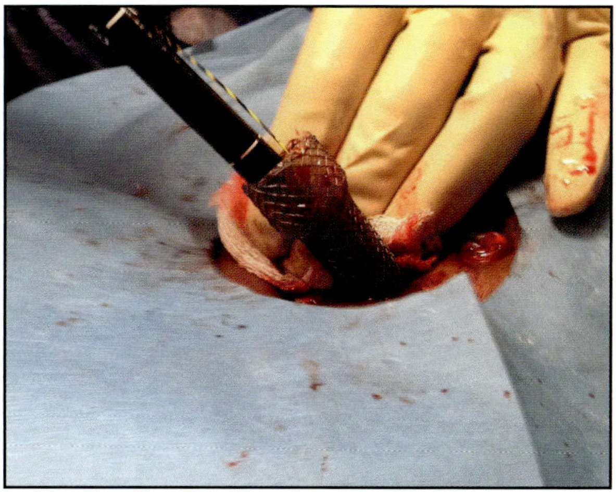

Figure 23-2. Insertion of endoscope during trans-gastric ERCP.

Weight Regain

RYGB has been the most prevalent bariatric surgery in the United States in recent years.[47] RYGB induces excess weight loss (EWL) of 56.7% to 66.5% over 24 months, along with significant improvement in or resolution of diabetes, obstructive sleep apnea, hypertension, and hyperlipidemia. After weight loss for 12 to 18 months, energy equilibrium is reached.[48] However, weight regain occurs in 30% of patients by 24 months, and weight regain of a mean 18 kg has been reported at 2 years.[49] This may result in decreased quality of life, recurrence of comorbidities, and loss of some long-term benefits of bariatric surgery. The mechanism of weight regain is multifactorial, including neurohormonal, physiologic, and anatomic factors. Anatomic factors, including GGF, larger pouch size, and larger gastrojejunal anastomosis aperture, correlate with increased weight regain after RYGB.[50,51] Surgical revision of RYGB is technically challenging and associated with high complication rates surpassing that of primary RYGB.[52] Endoscopic revision of RYGB potentially offers lower risk and cost. Sclerotherapy, tissue plication, and endoscopic suturing have been studied.

Endoscopic sclerotherapy entails injection of sclerosant, such as sodium morrhuate, around the gastrojejunal anastomosis to reduce its aperture and compliance. After injection of a 2-mL test dose at the anastomotic margin and monitoring for a reaction, sclerosant is injected into the submucosa until a bleb is formed. Two-mL aliquots can be injected until 10 to 25 mL has been injected around the anastomosis.[53] Ciprofloxacin should be administered intravenously prior to the procedure and orally in liquid form for 5 days after the procedure. A liquid diet can be started 1 day after the procedure and advanced to a regular diet over 4 weeks. Sclerotherapy should be repeated every 3 months for a total of 2 to 3 sessions. Measurement of anastomotic aperture immediately after the procedure is unreliable due to tissue edema. Sclerotherapy has been shown to arrest or reverse weight regain in 72% to 92% of patients at 12 months. It is likely most effective for gastrojejunal anastomosis aperture < 15 mm. Sodium morrhuate is no longer available, and alternative sclerosants are being investigated.

Tissue plication platforms have demonstrated effectiveness for therapy of dilated gastrojejunal anastomosis and gastric pouch. StomaphyX forms full-thickness tissue plications with polypropylene fasteners. Approximately 20 fasteners can be placed around the anastomotic margin in a circumferential fashion. Studies of patients with body mass index (BMI) of approximately 40 kg/m^2 have demonstrated weight loss of 7.6 kg at 6 months and 19.5% EWL at 1 year.[54,55] The Incisionless Operating Platform ([IOP] USGI Medical) is a multichannel tissue plication platform.[56] One channel is used for a tissue grasper and another for a tissue approximator used to pass a needle

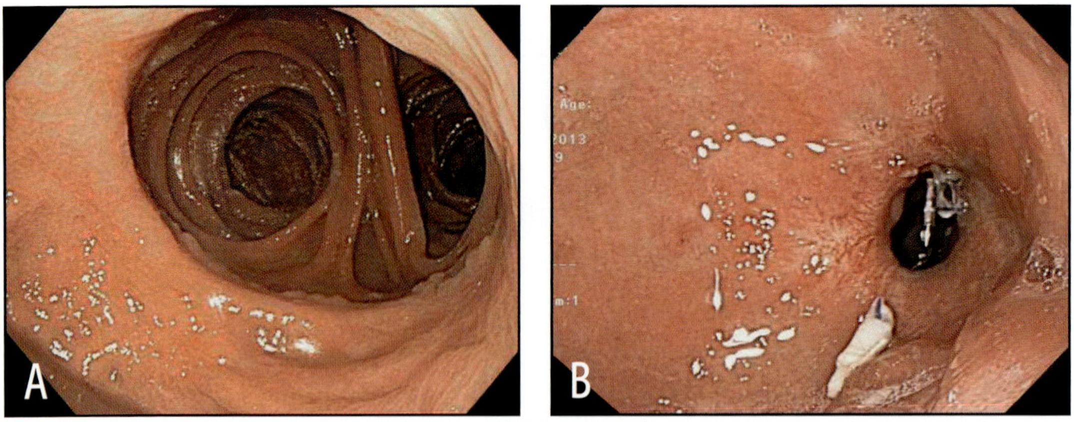

Figure 23-3. Gastrojejunal anastomosis (A) before and (B) 6 months after transoral outlet reduction using the purse-string technique.

through tissue and plicate it with tissue anchors. Another channel contains an ultraslim endoscope for visualization. One prospective study of the Revision Obesity Surgery Endoscopic procedure performed using the IOP demonstrated reduction of gastrojejunal anastomosis aperture by 65% to an average of 16 mm and reduction of gastric pouch length by 36%. At 3 months, average weight loss was 8.8 kg.[57] Another prospective study including 116 patients demonstrated loss of 32% of regained weight after 6 months.[58]

Endoscopic sutured revision of gastrojejunal anastomosis, or transoral outlet reduction (TORe), has evolved since it was first described in 2004.[59] The Bard EndoCinch is a superficial-thickness suturing device. Suction is used to capture mucosa in a hollow capsule at the endoscope tip. A needle is driven through the tissue. TORe begins with ablation of the gastrojejunal anastomosis margin with argon plasma coagulation. Interrupted stitches are placed across the anastomosis to reduce its aperture. RESTORe, a randomized sham-controlled double-blind multicenter trial of superficial-thickness TORe for outlet reduction, resulted in level 1b evidence for effectiveness of TORe.[60] In this study, 77 patients with gastrojejunal anastomosis aperture > 20 mm and BMI of 47.6 underwent TORe using interrupted stitches. Reduction of anastomotic aperture to < 10 mm was achieved in 89% of patients. Complication rate of TORe was similar to the sham group, and no perforations occurred. The TORe group lost significantly more weight than the sham group at 6 months, 3.8% of body weight vs 0.3% in the sham group ($p = .02$). The TORe group demonstrated weight loss or stabilization in 96% of patients during 6-month follow-up. A newer suturing device, the OverStitch (Apollo Endosurgery), is capable of applying full-thickness stitches in interrupted or running fashion under direct visualization. Sutures can be reloaded without removing the device. A tissue retractor can be used via the second channel of the double-channel endoscope. OverStitch has been studied for TORe.[61] Mean gastrojejunal anastomosis aperture was reduced from 26.4 mm to 6 mm, and no adverse events were reported. Patients lost 69.5% of regained weight, or 11.7 kg over 6 months. One-year weight loss was 10.8 kg. Superficial-thickness TORe performed using the EndoCinch and full-thickness TORe using the OverStitch were directly compared in a matched cohort study with 59 patients in each group.[62] Patients were matched by pre-TORe gastrojejunal anastomosis aperture, then BMI, and then age. Weight loss at 6 months was 4.4 ± 0.8 kg in the EndoCinch group vs 10.6 ± 1.8 kg in the OverStitch group ($p < .01$). Weight loss at 1 year was 2.9 ± 1.0 kg in the EndoCinch group vs 8.6 ± 2.5 kg in the OverStitch group ($p < .01$). The interrupted stitch technique used for anastomosis reduction in these studies has since been modified to a full-thickness purse-string technique; studies are ongoing (Figure 23-3).

PRIMARY THERAPY FOR OBESITY

Endoscopic procedures offer the potential to treat obesity in patients with BMI below the threshold for bariatric surgery, to optimize patients for bariatric surgery, and to address metabolic disease. Endoscopic procedures may offer lower invasiveness, reversibility, and lower cost; these characteristics may allow them to be repeated at regular intervals if needed. Current primary endoscopic therapies are restrictive, space-occupying, or malabsorptive. Restrictive procedures include endoscopic gastroplasty and restrictive implants. Space-occupying devices include the intragastric balloon. Malabsorptive devices prevent contact of food with segments of the small intestine.

Restrictive Procedures

Endoscopic restrictive procedures reduce gastric volume by placement of sutures or tissue anchors. The EndoCinch has been studied for transoral gastroplasty in adults and adolescents. A study of 64 adults with average BMI of 39.9 (divided into Group 1 with BMI $\geq$ 40, 33 patients; Group 2 with BMI 35 to 40, 19 patients; and Group 3 with BMI $<$ 35, 12 patients) reported no serious adverse events, although the study was not approved by an institutional review board.[63] One-year follow-up included 94% of patients. The study reported 39.6 ± 11.3% EWL at 3 months and 58.1 ± 19.9% EWL at 1 year. A subsequent study in 21 adolescents aged 13 to 17 with mean BMI of 36.2 reported 63.8% EWL at 6 months, 67.3% EWL at 12 months, and 61.5% EWL at 18 months.[64]

The EndoCinch was subsequently improved and renamed the RESTORe system. This device has the capability to reload suture without endoscope removal, as well as the capability to perform full-thickness suturing. A 2-center study using the device for transoral gastroplasty in 18 patients reported no significant complications.[65] An average 6 plications were used to reduce gastric volume. Mean procedure time was 125 ± 23 minutes. At 1-year follow-up, mean weight loss was 11.0 ± 10 kg, or 27.7 ± 21.9% EWL. Half of patients experienced over 30% EWL. Average waist circumference decreased by 12.6 ± 9.5 cm. Significant decreases in systolic blood pressure (15.2 mm Hg) and diastolic blood pressure (9.7 mm Hg) were reported. Partial or complete release of plications was reported in 13/18 patients on follow-up endoscopy.

The TransOral GAstroplasty ([TOGA] Satiety Inc) device is a flexible endoscopic stapler that uses vacuum to appose the gastric walls and then performs full-thickness stapled tissue apposition. The device requires removal for reloading. The device is used to create a partition parallel to the lesser curvature, forming a sleeve. One study of TOGA in 21 patients with mean BMI of 43.3 reported no serious adverse events.[66] Pain, nausea, vomiting, and transient dysphagia were reported. Partially or fully intact sleeves were noted at 6 months, with gaps present in 13 of 21 patients. At 6-month follow-up, average weight loss was 12 kg, with 24.4% EWL. A subsequent study using a second-generation device, and with retreatment to create additional distal restrictions as needed, included 11 patients.[67] No serious adverse events were noted. Average weight loss was 17.5 kg at 3 months. At 6 months, average weight loss was 24.0 kg with decrease in mean BMI from 41.6 to 33.1. A subsequent multicenter study including 67 patients (of which 53 completed follow-up) reported 41.3% EWL in patients with BMI $<$ 40 and 52.2 % EWL in patients with BMI $\geq$ 40.[68] Additionally, there was a significant decrease in hemoglobin A1c ([HbA1c] from 7.0% to 5.7%), and significant improvements in high-density lipoprotein and triglyceride levels. One case of respiratory insufficiency and one case of asymptomatic pneumoperitoneum were reported.

The Trans-oral Endoscopic Restrictive Implant System ([TERIS] Barosense) is a diaphragm with a 10-mm orifice. This implantable device is stapled into the gastric cardia. One study of 13 patients reported 12 successful placements and 1 failure due to gastric perforation.[69] Additionally, 2 cases of pneumoperitoneum were reported. The procedure was modified after these adverse events, and no further complications were seen. Procedure time was 142 minutes on average. Three-month follow-up revealed weight loss of 16.9 kg or 22.2% EWL. During this period, median BMI decreased from 42.1 to 37.9.

Space-Occupying Devices

Space-occupying devices include balloons and polymers placed into the stomach. These devices result in volume displacement and gastric distention, and may also induce changes in gastric motility.[70] Additionally, there may be hormone effects (eg, cholecystokinin may be released due to gastric distention, resulting in pyloric constriction and delay in gastric emptying). Although the intragastric balloon was first approved for use in the United States in 1985, this technology has not been widely adopted in the United States. Although more commonly used in Europe, balloons have found a role as a bridge to definitive therapy.

The BioEnterics Intragastric Balloon ([BIB] Allergan) is an endoscopically implanted silicone elastomer balloon.[70] The device is resistant to gastric acid for 6 months. It is filled with saline and methylene blue dye, which results in a urine color change in the event of balloon perforation. The BIB has been studied more extensively than other endoscopic bariatric therapies. A meta-analysis including 3698 patients found weight loss of 14.7 kg, or 32.1% EWL, resulting in BMI decrease of 5.7 during 6-month placement.[71] Severe complications included bowel obstruction in 0.8% of patients and gastric perforation in 0.1% of patients. Overall, 4.2% of patients had removal of the balloon before 6-month therapy was complete. A retrospective study of 2515 patients with mean BMI of 44.4 undergoing BIB placement reported BMI decrease of 9.0 during 6-month therapy.[72] In addition to weight loss, there was significant improvement or normalization of HbA1c in 87.2% of diabetic patients.

A study of long-term weight trend after BIB removal included 500 patients with initial mean BMI of 43.7.[73] Success was defined as EWL of at least 20% at the time of removal. Eighty-three percent of patients met this criteria, with average weight loss of 23.9 ± 9.1 kg and BMI decrease of 8.3. At 5 years, 41% of the cohort was available. Average weight loss was 7.3 ± 5.4 kg and BMI decrease was 2.5. Twenty-three percent of patients met criteria for success, with weight loss of at least 20% EWL.

The BIB has demonstrated success as a bridge to RYGB.[74] Of 60 super-superobese patients with average BMI of 66.5 ± 3.4, 23 underwent BIB placement for 155 ± 62 days. During this period, the BIB group experienced BMI decrease of 5.5 ± 1.3. The BIB group also demonstrated significant improvement in systolic blood pressure and gamma-glutamyl transpeptidase. At the time of RYGB, the BIB group had significantly shorter operative time for RYGB (146 ± 47 vs 201 ± 81 minutes). There were significantly fewer major adverse events, including conversion to laparotomy, intensive care unit stay longer than 2 days, and hospital stay longer than 2 weeks, in the BIB group (2 vs 13). Weight loss 1 year after RYGB was similar between groups.

The effectiveness of repeat BIB placement was studied in a prospective trial.[75] Of 118 patients, 8 had BIB reinsertion immediately after completion of therapy, 11 had BIB replacement after a balloon-free interval, and 99 did not have BIB replacement. The second balloon placement resulted in less weight loss than the first placement (9.0 kg vs 14.6 kg) and less EWL (18.2% vs 49.3%). By the third year of follow-up, there was no additional weight loss in patients who had second balloon placement. A study of second balloon placement within 1 month of balloon removal in 112 patients reported BMI loss of 2.5 with second balloon vs 6.5 with the first balloon.

The metabolic improvements occurring after BIB placement were studied prospectively in 130 patients.[76] Of these, 10 patients required balloon removal prior to completing therapy. A 1000 to 1200 kcal/day diet was maintained during the 6-month follow-up period. Metabolic comorbidities improved significantly, with decrease in prevalence of hyperglycemia from 50% to 12% and decrease in hypertriglyceridemia from 58% to 19%. In patients with fall in BMI of more than 3.5, prevalence of severe hepatic steatosis decreased from 52% to 4%. However,

50% of patients regained weight during the follow-up period of an average 22 months. Another randomized prospective trial including 21 patients studied histologic improvement in nonalcoholic steatohepatitis.[77] Patients were randomized to BIB or sham endoscopy, and all patients were placed on the American Heart Association diet. Three out of 11 patients in the BIB group required early removal due to vomiting and discomfort. The control group experienced BMI decrease of 0.8 vs decrease of 1.6 in the BIB group. After 6-month treatment, the BIB group demonstrated significantly lower nonalcoholic fatty liver disease activity score (2 vs 4), as well as a trend toward improvement in median steatosis score. However, there was no improvement in hepatocellular ballooning, lobular inflammation, or fibrosis. There was no significant change in ALT or AST in either group.

The effect of intragastric balloon therapy on depression has been studied in 100 consecutive females classified as depressed (65 patients) or nondepressed (35 patients) as classified using the Beck Depression Inventory.[78] Baseline characteristics were similar between groups. The depressed and nondepressed groups experienced similar weight loss (39.3% EWL and 36.1% EWL, respectively). Depression score decreased from 20.3 ± 8.5 to 7.9 ± 5.6 in the depressed group during intragastric balloon therapy, with resolution of depression in 70.8%. The rate of severe depression declined from 27.7% to 1.5%.

Other intragastric balloons have been studied. The Heliosphere BAG, which is filled with 950 mL of air, has been compared with the saline-filled BIB.[79] The randomized trial of 60 patients with mean BMI of 46.3 reported BMI decrease of 5.7 in the BIB group vs 4.2 in the Heliosphere BAG group. Balloon extraction at the end of therapy was characterized by significantly longer extraction time and significantly more extraction discomfort in the Heliosphere BAG group. A nonrandomized study compared 6-month therapy with BIB (19 patients, mean BMI 45.6 ± 9) with Heliosphere BAG (13 patients, mean BMI 45.0 ± 8).[80] BIB therapy resulted in higher weight loss (19.0 kg vs 13.0 kg) and EWL (38.3% vs 21.9%). One patient in the BIB group required early removal at 1 month for persistent nausea and vomiting, and another patient died 13 days after BIB placement due to cardiac arrest after aspiration of gastric contents.

The Duo intragastric balloon (Reshape) includes 2 spheres filled with 900 mL of saline. This design prevents migration if one balloon deflates. A prospective trial including 3 centers allocated 21 patients to the balloon group and 9 patients to the control group; both groups also received diet and exercise counseling.[81] Four of 21 patients in the balloon group required readmission for nausea, and 2 patients had gastritis at balloon removal. After 48 weeks, 25% of the control group reached the 25% EWL goal vs 30% of the balloon group.

The Transpyloric Shuttle (BAROnova) is made of a sphere attached to a smaller cylinder by a flexible tether. The cylinder is small enough to enter the duodenal bulb with peristalsis, while the sphere intermittently occludes the pylorus to reduce gastric emptying rate. Although removal requires endoscopy, placement can be performed with transoral catheter. A nonblinded single-center prospective trial including 20 patients with mean BMI of 36.0 reported 3-month weight loss of 8.9 ± 5.2 kg and $31.3 \pm 15.7\%$ EWL.[82] At 6 months, weight loss was 14.6 ± 5.7 kg and $50.0 \pm 26.4\%$ EWL. Two of 20 patients required early removal due to persistent gastric ulcer.

The SatiSphere (Endosphere) is an implant rather than a balloon. It is a preformed memory wire that conforms to the shape of the duodenum, anchoring itself in the distal stomach and in the duodenum. With the device in place, food travels through the duodenum more slowly, resulting in altered satiety hormone levels and glucose metabolism. A trial of 31 patients with mean BMI of 41.3 compared 21 implanted patients with 10 control patients.[83] Device migration was reported in 10 of 21 implanted patients, requiring emergency surgery in 2 patients. Of patients completing the trial, weight loss was 6.7 kg vs 2.2 kg in controls after 3 months. Glucose absorption was delayed, and insulin and glucagon-like peptide-1 kinetics were altered.

Malabsorptive Devices

Bypass of the small intestine is hypothesized to contribute to improvement in metabolic parameters after bariatric surgical procedures such as RYGB and BPD-DS. Placement of endoluminal malabsorptive devices allow bypass of absorption in the small intestine.

The EndoBarrier duodenal-jejunal bypass liner (GI Dynamics) is a nickel-titanium implant and 60-cm polymer sleeve. It extends from the duodenal bulb into the jejunum, preventing food from contacting those portions of the small intestinal mucosa. Pancreatic and biliary secretions travel along the outside of the sleeve, first making contact with food in the jejunum. A multicenter randomized trial of EndoBarrier allocated 30 patients with mean BMI 48.9 to EndoBarrier and 11 patients with mean BMI 47.4 to diet control only.[84] Four of 30 EndoBarrier patients required removal due to migration, obstruction, pain, or anchor dislocation, although no serious adverse events were reported. BMI decreased significantly more in the EndoBarrier group, 5.5 vs 1.9 in the control group. Seven of 8 diabetic patients in the EndoBarrier group had improvement in diabetes. An open-label randomized multicenter trial enrolled 25 patients for EndoBarrier therapy, with successful implantation in 21 patients; implantation was unsuccessful in patients with small duodenal bulb.[85] A sham arm including 26 patients underwent sham endoscopy and implantation. Seven of 21 EndoBarrier patients experienced adverse events requiring explantation, including 3 patients with hematemesis. Weight loss after 3 months was significantly higher in the EndoBarrier group: 8.2 ± 1.3 kg vs 2.0 ± 1.1 kg in the sham group. Another randomized trial included 25 EndoBarrier patients and 14 control patients, with all patients undergoing baseline diet and lifestyle counseling.[86] Adverse events, including bleeding, migration, and obstruction, were reported in 20% of the EndoBarrier group. At 3 months, the EndoBarrier group experienced 22% EWL vs 5% in the control group.

An open-label prospective trial of 1-year outcomes after EndoBarrier implantation enrolled 42 patients.[87] Of these, 39 patients with mean BMI 43.7 ± 5.9 had successful implantation, and 3 patients could not be implanted due to short duodenal bulb. Fifteen of 39 patients required explantation due to anchor movement in 8 patients, device obstruction in 3 patients, abdominal pain in 2 patients, acute cholecystitis in 1 patient, and 1 patient request. The 24 patients who had EndoBarrier for 1 year experienced average weight loss of 22.1 ± 2.1 kg, BMI loss of 9.1 ± 0.9, and 47.0 ± 4.4% EWL. Significant decrease in waist circumference from 120.5 ± 6.8 cm to 96.0 ± 2.6 cm was reported. Statistically significant improvement was reported in the prevalence of metabolic syndrome (from 83.3% to 41.6%), as well as in blood pressure, HbA1c, total cholesterol, low-density lipoproteins, and triglycerides.

The metabolic effects of EndoBarrier in type 2 diabetes were studied in a randomized sham-controlled trial.[88] Twelve patients with mean BMI of 38.9 and HbA1c of 9.2% underwent EndoBarrier implantation, and 6 patients with mean BMI of 39.0 and HbA1c of 9.0% had sham endoscopy. All patients had diet and lifestyle counseling, with a controlled low-calorie diet during follow-up. Additionally, glucose self-monitoring was required, and sulfonylurea dose was cut in half at the time of device implantation. HbA1c fell by 2.4 ± 0.7% in the EndoBarrier patients vs a fall of 0.8 ± 0.4% in the sham patients; the result did not achieve statistical significance. However, postprandial plasma glucose was reduced significantly more in the EndoBarrier group after 1 week of implantation (19% vs 11%).

A modified version of the EndoBarrier with a flow-restricting 4-mm proximal opening, intended to slow gastric emptying, was studied in 10 patients with average BMI of 40.8.[89] Endoscopic balloon dilation of the restrictive orifice was required in 8 patients who developed abdominal pain, nausea, and vomiting. After 3 months, average weight loss was 16.7 ± 1.4 kg. Eighty-four percent of patients had delayed gastric emptying at 3 months, but this generally improved after explantation.

Summary

With the growing cohort of patients with bariatric surgery, endoscopic diagnosis and treatment of gastrointestinal disease and post-surgical complications in these patients has become commonplace. Endoscopic revision of RYGB has acquired level 1 evidence for effectiveness. Endoscopic primary bariatric therapies continue to build evidence for safety and long-term efficacy in the treatment of obesity and metabolic disease.

References

1. Buchwald H, Oien DM. Metabolic/bariatric surgery worldwide. *Obes Surg.* 2009;19:1605-1611.
2. Sataloff DM, Lieber CP, Seinige UL. Strictures following gastric stapling for morbid obesity. Results of endoscopic dilatation. *Am Surg.* 1990;56(3):167-174.
3. Mathus-Vliegen EM. The role of endoscopy in bariatric surgery. *Best Pract Res Clin Gastroenterol.* 2008;22(5):839-864.
4. Podnos YD, Jimenez JC, Wilson SF, et al. Complications after laparoscopic gastric bypass: a review of 3464 cases. *Arch Surg.* 2003;138:957-961.
5. Iannelli A, Dainese R, Piche T, et al. Laparoscopic sleeve gastrectomy for morbid obesity. *World J Gastroenterol.* 2008;14:821-827.
6. Papakonstantinou A, Terzis L, Stratopoulos C, et al. Bleeding from the upper gastrointestinal tract after Mason's vertical banded gastroplasty. *Obes Surg.* 2000;10:582-584.
7. Belachew M, Belva PH, Desaive C. Long-term results of laparoscopic adjustable gastric banding for the treatment of morbid obesity. *Obes Surg.* 2002;12(4):564-568.
8. Rabl C, Peeva S, Prado K, et al. Early and late abdominal bleeding after Roux-en-Y gastric bypass: sources and tailored therapeutic strategies. *Obes Surg.* 2011;21(4):413-420.
9. Kumar N, Thompson CC. Endoscopic management of complications after gastrointestinal weight loss surgery. *Clin Gastroenterol Hepatol.* 2013;11(4):343-353.
10. Keith JN. Endoscopic management of common bariatric surgical complications. *Gastrointest Endosc Clin N Am.* 2011;21(2):275-285.
11. Azagury DE, Abu Dayyeh BK, Greenwalt IT, Thompson CC. Marginal ulceration after Roux-en-Y gastric bypass surgery: characteristics, risk factors, treatment, and outcomes. *Endoscopy.* 2011;43(11):950-954.
12. Gisbert JP, de la Morena F Abraira V. Accuracy of monoclonal stool antigen test for the diagnosis of H. pylori infection: a systematic review and meta-analysis. *Am J Gastroenterol.* 2006;101:1921-1930.
13. Ryou M, Mogobgab O, Lautz DB, et al. Endoscopic foreign body removal for treatment of chronic abdominal pain in patients after Roux-en-Y gastric bypass. *Surg Obes Relat Dis.* 2010;6:526-531.
14. Singhal R, Bryant C, Kitchen M, et al. Band slippage and erosion after laparoscopic gastric banding: a meta-analysis. *Surg Endosc.* 2010;24(12):2980-2986.
15. Abu-Abeid S, Keidar A, Gavert N, et al. The clinical spectrum of band erosion following laparoscopic adjustable silicone gastric banding for morbid obesity. *Surg Endosc.* 2003;17:861-863.
16. Regusci L, Groebli Y, Meyer JL, et al. Gastroscopic removal of an adjustable gastric band after partial intragastric migration. *Obes Surg.* 2003;13(2):281-284.
17. Offodile AC, Okafor P, Shaikh SN, et al. Duodenal obstruction due to erosion and migration of an adjustable gastric band: a novel endoscopic approach to management. *Surg Obes Relat Dis.* 2010;6(2):206-208.
18. Blero D, Deviere J. Removing foreign bodies in bariatric patient. *Techniques in Gastrointestinal Endoscopy.* 2010;12(3):146-152.
19. Blero D, Eisendrath P, Vandermeeren A, et al. Endoscopic removal of dysfunctioning bands or rings after restrictive bariatric procedures. *Gastrointest Endosc.* 2010;71(3):468-474.
20. Keith JN. Endoscopic management of common bariatric surgical complications. *Gastrointest Endosc Clin N Am.* 2011;21(2):275-285.
21. Nguyen NT, Stevens CM, Wolfe BM. Incidence and outcome of anastomotic stricture after laparoscopic gastric bypass. *J Gastrointest Surg.* 2003;7(8):997-1003.
22. Wetter A. Role of endoscopy after Roux-en-Y gastric bypass surgery. *Gastrointest Endosc.* 2007;66(2):253-255.
23. Espinel J, De-la-Cruz JL, Pinedo E, et al. Stenosis in laparoscopic gastric bypass: management by endoscopic dilation without fluoroscopic guidance. *Rev Esp Enferm Dig.* 2011;103(10):508-510.
24. Peifer KJ, Shiels AJ, Azar R, et al. Successful endoscopic management of gastrojejunal anastomotic strictures after Roux-en-Y gastric bypass. *Gastrointest Endosc.* 2007;66:248-252.

25. Go MR, Muscarella P, Needleman BJ, et al. Endoscopic management of stomal stenosis after Roux-en-Y gastric bypass. *Surg Endosc.* 2004;18(1):56-59.
26. Obstein KL, Thompson CC. Endoscopy after bariatric surgery (with videos). *Gastrointest Endosc.* 2009;70(6):1161-1166.
27. Sataloff DM, Lieber CP, Seinige UL. Strictures following gastric stapling for morbid obesity. Results of endoscopic dilatation. *Am Surg.* 1990;56:167-174.
28. Schneider BE, Villegas L, Blackburn GL, et al. Laparoscopic gastric bypass surgery: outcomes. *J Laparoendosc Adv Surg Tech A.* 2003;13(4):247-255.
29. Fernandez AZ. Experience with over 3000 open and laparoscopic bariatric procedures: multivariate analysis of factors related to leak and resultant mortality. *Surg Endosc.* 2004;18:193-197.
30. Gonzalez R, Sarr MG, Smith CD, et al. Diagnosis and contemporary management of anastomotic leaks after gastric bypass for obesity. *J Am Coll Surg.* 2007;204(1):47-55.
31. Warschkow R, Tarantino I, Folie P, et al. C-reactive protein 2 days after laparoscopic gastric bypass surgery reliably indicates leaks and moderately predicts morbidity. *J Gastrointest Surg.* 2012;16(6):1128-1135.
32. Márquez MF, Ayza MF, Lozano RB, et al. Gastric leak after laparoscopic sleeve gastrectomy. *Obes Surg.* 2010;20(9):1306-1311.
33. Morales MP, Miedema BW, Scott JS, de la Torre RA. Management of postsurgical leaks in the bariatric patient. *Gastrointest Endosc Clin N Am.* 2011;21(2):295-304.
34. Lee S, Carmody B, Wolfe L, et al. Effect of location and speed of diagnosis on anastomotic leak outcomes in 3828 gastric bypass cases. *J Gastrointest Surg.* 2007;11(6):708-713.
35. Kumar N, Thompson CC. Endoscopic therapy for postoperative leaks and fistulae. *Gastrointest Endosc Clin N Am.* 2013;23(1):123-136.
36. Thodiyil PA, Yenumula P, Rogula T, et al. Selective nonoperative management of leaks after gastric bypass: lessons learned from 2675 consecutive patients. *Ann Surg.* 2008;248:782-792.
37. Puli SR, Spofford IS, Thompson CC. Use of self-expandable stents in the treatment of bariatric surgery leaks: a systematic review and meta-analysis. *Gastrointest Endosc.* 2012;75(2):287-293.
38. Manta R, Manno M, Bertani H, et al. Endoscopic treatment of gastrointestinal fistulas using an over-the-scope clip (OTSC) device: case series from a tertiary referral center. *Endoscopy.* 2011;43(6):545-548.
39. Lippert E, Klebl FH, Schweller F, et al. Fibrin glue in the endoscopic treatment of fistulae and anastomotic leakages of the gastrointestinal tract. *Int J Colorectal Dis.* 2011;26(3):303-311.
40. Fernandez-Esparrach G, Lautz DB, Thompson CC. Endoscopic repair of gastrogastric fistula after Roux-en-Y gastric bypass: a less-invasive approach. *Surg Obes Relat Dis.* 2010;6(3):282-288.
41. Watson RR, Thompson CC. Applications of a novel endoscopic suturing device in the GI tract [abstract]. *Gastrointest Endosc.* 2011;73(4):AB105.
42. Holle G, Riedel K, von Gregory H, et al. Vacuum-assisted closure therapy: current status and basic research. *Unfallchirurg.* 2007;110:490-504.
43. Weidenhagen R, Gruetzner KU, Wiecken T, et al. Endoscopic vacuum-assisted closure of anastomotic leakage following anterior resection of the rectum: a new method. *Surg Endosc.* 2008;22:1818-1825.
44. Wedemeyer J, Brangewitz M, Kubicka S, et al. Management of major postsurgical gastroesophageal intrathoracic leaks with an endoscopic vacuum-assisted closure system. *Gastrointest Endosc.* 2010;71(2):382-386.
45. Shiffman ML, Sugerman HJ, Kellum JM, et al. Gallstone formation after rapid weight loss: a prospective study in patients undergoing gastric bypass surgery for treatment of morbid obesity. *Am J Gastroenterol.* 1991;86:1000-1005.
46. Baron TH, Song LM, Ferreira LE, et al. Novel approach to therapeutic ERCP after long-limb Roux-en-Y gastric bypass surgery using transgastric self-expandable metal stents: experimental outcomes and first human case study (with videos). *Gastrointest Endosc.* 2012;75(6):1258-1263.
47. Buchwald H, Avidor Y, Braunwald E et al. Bariatric surgery. A systematic review and meta-analysis. *JAMA.* 2004;13:1724-1737.
48. Mitchell JE, Lancaster KL, Burgard MA, et al. Long-term follow-up of patients' status after gastric bypass. *Obes Surg.* 2001;11:464-468.
49. Magro DO, Gelonese B, Delfini R, et al. Long-term weight regain after gastric bypass: a 5-year prospective study. *Obes Surg.* 2008;18(6):648-651.
50. Dayyeh BK, Lautz DB, Thompson CC. Gastrojejunal stoma diameter predicts weight regain after Roux-en-Y gastric bypass. *Clin Gastroenterol Hepatol.* 2011;9(3):228-233.
51. Gumbs AA, Pomp A, Gagner M. Revisional bariatric surgery for inadequate weight loss. *Obes Surg.* 2007;17:1137-1145.
52. Mor A, Keenan E, Portenier D, et al. Case-matched analysis comparing outcomes of revisional versus primary laparoscopic Roux-en-Y gastric bypass. *Surg Endosc.* 2013;27(2):548-552.
53. Spaulding L, Osler T, Patlak J. Long-term results of sclerotherapy for dilated gastrojejunostomy after gastric bypass. *Surg Obes Relat Dis.* 2007;3:623-626.
54. Mikami D, Needleman B, Narula V, et al. Natural orifice surgery: initial US experience utilizing the StomaphyX device to reduce gastric pouches after Roux-en-Y gastric bypass. *Surg Endosc.* 2010;24:223-228.

55. Letiman IM, Virk CS, Avgerinos DV, et al. Early results of trans-oral endoscopic placation and revision of the gastric pouch and stoma following Roux-en-Y gastric bypass surgery. *JSLS 2010*;14:217-220.
56. Seaman DL, Gostout CJ, de la Mora Levy JG, Knipschield MA. Tissue anchors for transmural gut-wall apposition. *Gastrointest Endosc.* 2006;64:577-581.
57. Mullady DK, Lautz DB, Thompson CC. Treatment of weight regain after gastric bypass surgery when using a new endoscopic platform: initial experience and early outcomes (with video). *Gastrointest Endosc.* 2009;70:440-444.
58. Horgan S, Jacobsen G, Weiss GD, et al. Incisionless revision of post-Roux-en-Y bypass stomal and pouch dilation: multicenter registry results. *Surg Obes Relat Dis.* 2010;6:290-295.
59. Thompson CC, Carr-Locke DL, Saltzman J, et al. Peroral endoscopic repair of staple-line dehiscence in Roux-en-Y gastric bypass: a less invasive approach [abstract]. *Gastroenterology.* 2004;126(Suppl 2):A.
60. Thompson CC, Chand B, Chen YK, et al. Endoscopic suturing for transoral outlet reduction increases weight loss after Roux-en-Y gastric bypass surgery. *Gastroenterology.* 2013;145(1):129-137.
61. Jirapinyo P, Slattery J, Ryan MB, et al. Evaluation of an endoscopic suturing device for transoral outlet reduction in patients with weight regain following Roux-en-Y gastric bypass. *Endoscopy.* 2013;45(7):532-536.
62. Kumar N, Lautz DB, Thompson CC. Comparison of a suction-based superficial suturing device with a full-thickness suturing device for transoral outlet reduction: a matched cohort study [abstract]. *Gastrointest Endosc.* 2013;77(5):AB203-AB204.
63. Fogel R, De Fogel J, Bonilla Y, et al. Clinical experience of transoral suturing for an endoluminal vertical gastroplasty: 1-year follow-up in 64 patients. *Gastrointest Endosc.* 2008;68:51-58.
64. Fogel R, De Fogel J. Trans-oral vertical gastroplasty as a viable treatment for childhood obesity: a study of 21 adolescents with up to 18 months of follow-up [abstract]. *Gastrointest Endosc.* 2009;69(5):AB169-AB170.
65. Brethauer SA, Chand B, Schauer PR, Thompson CC. Transoral gastric volume reduction as intervention for weight management: 12-month follow-up of TRIM trial. *Surg Obes Relat Dis.* 2012;8(3):296-303.
66. Deviere J, Ojeda Valdes G, Cuevas Herrera L, et al. Safety, feasibility and weight loss after transoral gastroplasty: first human multicenter study. *Surg Endosc.* 2008;22:589-598.
67. Moreno C, Closset J, Dugardeyn S, et al. Transoral gastroplasty is safe, feasible, and induces significant weight loss in morbidly obese patients: results of the second human pilot study. *Endoscopy.* 2008;40:406-413.
68. Familiari P, Costamagna G, Blero D, et al. Transoral gastroplasty for morbid obesity: a multicenter trial with a 1-year outcome. *Gastrointest Endosc.* 2011;74(6):1248-1258.
69. de Jong K, Mathus-Vliegen EM, Veldhuyzen EA, et al. Short-term safety and efficacy of the Trans-oral Endoscopic Restrictive Implant System for the treatment of obesity. *Gastrointest Endosc.* 2010;72(3):497-504.
70. Evans JT, DeLegge MH. Intragastric balloon therapy in the management of obesity: why the bad wrap? *JPEN J Parenter Enteral Nutr.* 2011;35:25-31.
71. Cervell C, García-Alvarez EE, Sendra-Gutiérrez JM, et al. Safety and effectiveness of the intragastric balloon for obesity. A meta-analysis. *Obes Surg.* 2008;18(7):841-846.
72. Genco T, Bruni B, Doldi SB, et al. BioEnterics Intragastric Balloon: the Italian experience with 2515 patients. *Obes Surg.* 2005;15:1161-1164.
73. Kotzampassi K, Grosomanidis V, Papakostas P, et al. 500 intragastric balloons: what happens 5 years thereafter? *Obes Surg.* 2012;22(6):896-903.
74. Zerrweck C, Maunoury V, Caiazzo R, et al. Preoperative weight loss with intragastric balloon decreases the risk of significant adverse outcomes of laparoscopic gastric bypass in super-super obese patients. *Obes Surg.* 2012;22(5):777-782.
75. Dumonceau JM, François E, Hittelet A, et al. Single vs repeated treatment with the intragastric balloon: a 5-year weight loss study. *Obes Surg.* 2010;20(6):692-697.
76. Forlano R, Ippolito AM, Iacobellis A, et al. Effect of the BioEnterics Intragastric Balloon on weight, insulin resistance, and liver steatosis in obese patients. *Gastrointest Endosc.* 2010;71(6):927-933.
77. Lee YM, Low HC, Lim LG, et al. Intragastric balloon significantly improves nonalcoholic fatty liver disease activity score in obese patients with nonalcoholic steatohepatitis: a pilot study. *Gastrointest Endosc.* 2012;76(4):756-760.
78. Deliopoulou K, Konsta A, Penna S, et al. The impact of weight loss on depression status in obese individuals subjected to intragastric balloon treatment. *Obes Surg.* 2013;23(5):669-675.
79. Giardiello C, Borrelli A, Silvestri E, et al. Air-filled vs water-filled intragastric balloon: a prospective randomized study. *Obes Surg.* 2012;22(12):1916-1919.
80. Caglar E, Dobrucali A, Bal K. Gastric balloon to treat obesity: filled with air or fluid? *Dig Endosc.* 2013;25(5):502-507.
81. Ponce J, Quebbemann BB, Patterson EJ. Prospective, randomized, multicenter study evaluating safety and efficacy of intragastric dual-balloon in obesity. *Surg Obes Relat Dis.* 2013;9(2):290-295.
82. Marinos G, Eliades C, Muthusamy V, et al. First clinical experience with the TransPyloric Shuttle (TPS) device, a non-surgical endoscopic treatment for obesity: results from a 3-month and 6-month study [abstract]. *SAGES.* 2013.

83. Sauer N, Rösch T, Pezold J, et al. A new endoscopically implantable device (SatiSphere) for treatment of obesity: efficacy, safety, and metabolic effects on glucose, insulin, and GLP-1 levels. *Obes Surg.* 2013;23(11):1727-1733.
84. Schouten R, Rijs CS, Bouvy ND, et al. A multicenter, randomized efficacy study of the EndoBarrier Gastrointestinal Liner for presurgical weight loss prior to bariatric surgery. *Ann Surg.* 2010;251(2):236-243.
85. Gersin KS, Rothstein RI, Rosenthal RJ, et al. Open-label, sham-controlled trial of an endoscopic duodenojejunal bypass liner for preoperative weight loss in bariatric surgery candidates. *Gastrointest Endosc.* 2010;71(6):976-982.
86. Tarnoff M, Rodriguez L, Escalona A, et al. Open label, prospective, randomized controlled trial of an endoscopic duodenal-jejunal bypass sleeve versus low calorie diet for pre-operative weight loss in bariatric surgery. *Surg Endosc.* 2009;23(3):650-656.
87. Escalona A, Pimentel F, Sharp A, et al. Weight loss and metabolic improvement in morbidly obese subjects implanted for 1 year with an endoscopic duodenal-jejunal bypass liner. *Ann Surg.* 2012;255(6):1080-1085.
88. Rodriguez L, Reyes E, Fagalde P, et al. Pilot clinical study of an endoscopic, removable duodenal-jejunal bypass liner for the treatment of type 2 diabetes. *Diabetes Technol Ther.* 2009;11(11):725-732.
89. Escalona A, Yáñez R, Pimentel F, et al. Initial human experience with restrictive duodenal-jejunal bypass liner for treatment of morbid obesity. *Surg Obes Relat Dis.* 2010;6(2):126-131.

24

Imaging of the Gastrointestinal Tract and Bariatric Surgery

Johanna Schubert, MD and Attila Csordas, MD

Morbid obesity is a national health problem in the United States and in many Western industrialized countries with social, economic, and serious medical consequences, such as diabetes, dyslipidemia, hypertension, cardiovascular disease, sleep apnea, and osteoarthritis.[1] Various surgical procedures have been devised that allow considerable weight reduction, extended weight maintenance, and control and reversal of some of the obesity-related health problems. As these procedures become more frequent, it is important for clinicians and radiologists to understand the clinical presentation and radiographic manifestations of potential complications of these interventions.

Bariatric procedures are classified into restrictive and restrictive-malabsorptive procedures. In restrictive procedures, the gastric capacity is reduced, causing early satiety after ingestion of small quantities of food. In restrictive-malabsorptive procedures, the stomach volume is decreased and part of the digestive tract is bypassed, thus causing decreased absorption of calories.[1,2] In this chapter, we discuss the imaging findings relating to the 2 most commonly performed bariatric procedures: laparoscopic Roux-en-Y gastric bypass (RYGB) and laparoscopic adjustable gastric banding, focusing on the role of upper gastrointestinal (UGI) fluoroscopy and computed tomography (CT) in the evaluation of normal postoperative anatomy and gastrointestinal complications.

Roux-en-Y Gastric Bypass

The gold standard of weight loss surgeries is the restrictive-malabsorptive RYGB. Imaging plays a significant role in the (1) preoperative evaluation of bariatric surgery candidates, (2) in the immediate postoperative period to detect surgical technique-related or hospitalization-related complications, and (3) also in the years following the procedure to detect delayed complications and guide treatment (Table 24-1 and Figure 24-1).

Forse RA, Apovian CM, eds.
Bariatric Surgery: What Every Provider Needs to Know (pp 279-299).

TABLE 24-1

IMAGING EVALUATION OF THE ROUX-EN-Y GASTRIC BYPASS

Preoperative imaging	Ultrasound: Rule out gallbladder pathology Myocardial perfusion
Immediate postoperative imaging	Fluoroscopy: Rule out anastomotic leak CT: Rule out abscess, rule out pulmonary embolism, rule out anastomosis breakdown
Delayed imaging	Fluoroscopy: Dehiscence, obstruction, ulcer CT: Fistula, abscess, obstruction Ultrasound: Gallstones Nuclear scintigraphy: Gastric motility

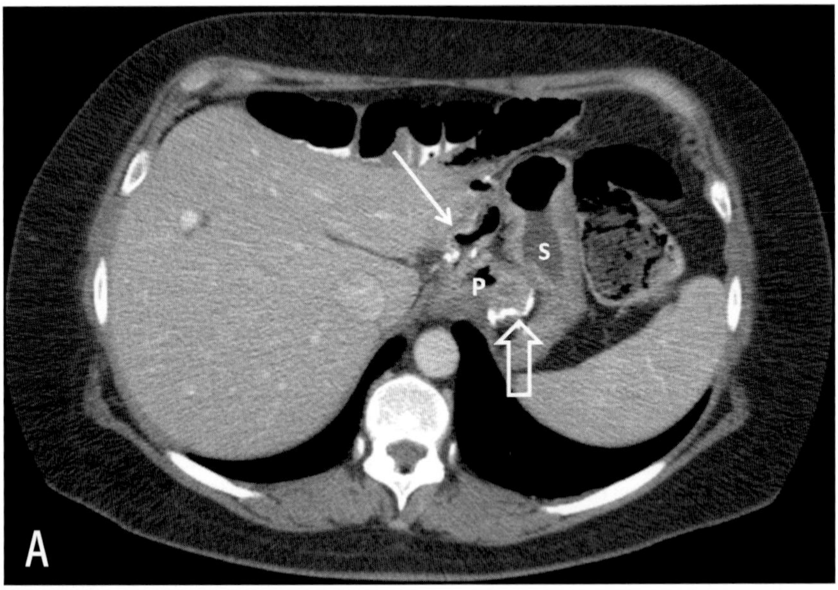

Figure 24-1A. (A-B) Axial and coronal CT of the abdomen showing normal postsurgical changes after Roux-en-Y bypass with staple line (hollow arrow) separating the stomach pouch (P) from the gastric remnant (S) and staples marking the gastrojejunostomy site (arrow). *(continued)*

Preoperative Imaging

Preoperative imaging includes myocardial perfusion study to obtain clearance for surgery and sonographic evaluation of the right upper quadrant to evaluate for gallbladder pathology. If gallstones are identified preoperatively, elective cholecystectomy is performed at the time of the RYGB procedure.

Immediate Postoperative Imaging

The immediate post-surgical evaluation performed on postoperative day 1 consists of a UGI fluoroscopic exam with oral administration of water-soluble contrast material (50 to 100 cc) to evaluate for anastomotic leak, gastric pouch size, stoma size, emptying of the gastric pouch, gastrogastric communication, and patency of the jejunojejunal anastomosis. These patients are at risk for aspiration due to the common postoperative ileus and initial edema at the anastomosis site; therefore, we prefer the use of iohexol as a contrast agent to avoid the complications of a possible

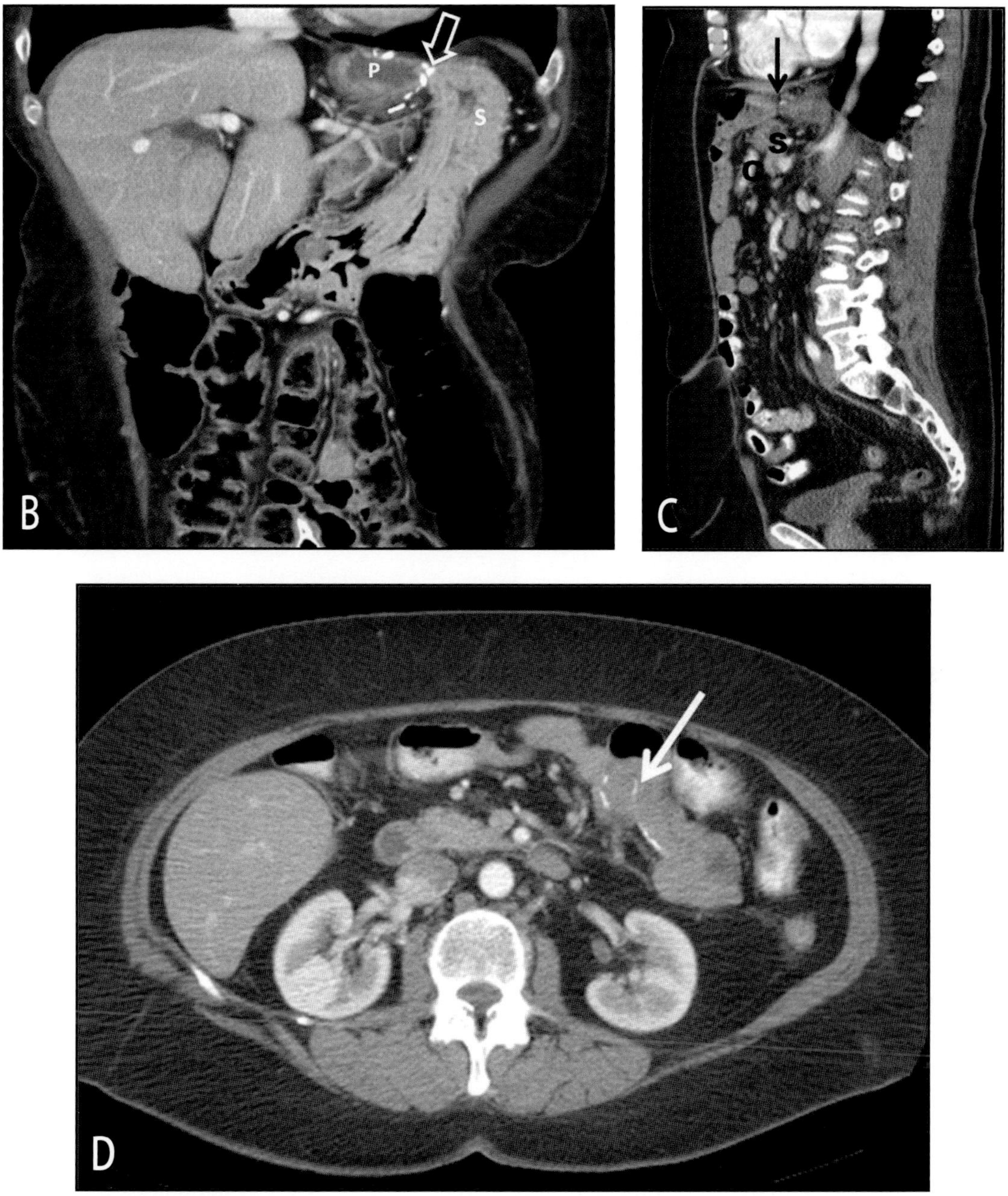

Figure 24-1B-D (continued). (A-B) Axial and coronal CT of the abdomen showing normal postsurgical changes after Roux-en-Y bypass with staple line (hollow arrow) separating the stomach pouch (P) from the gastric remnant (S) and staples marking the gastrojejunostomy site (arrow). (C) Sagittal view of the abdomen and pelvis demonstrating the antecolic approach: jejunum pulled up to the stomach pouch (arrow) anterior to the colon (c) and stomach remnant (s). (D) Axial CT of the abdomen showing the normal enteroenteric anastomosis (arrow).

aspiration. Patient positioning and adequate tissue penetration with fluoroscopy can be often challenging due to the patient body habitus, with patients sometimes reaching the weight limitations of the fluoroscopy table. Ideally images should be obtained in anteroposterior (AP), lateral, and oblique projections in the upright and supine positions; however, typically only an AP standing projection is feasible. If patients reach the weight limitations of the fluoroscopy table, overhead

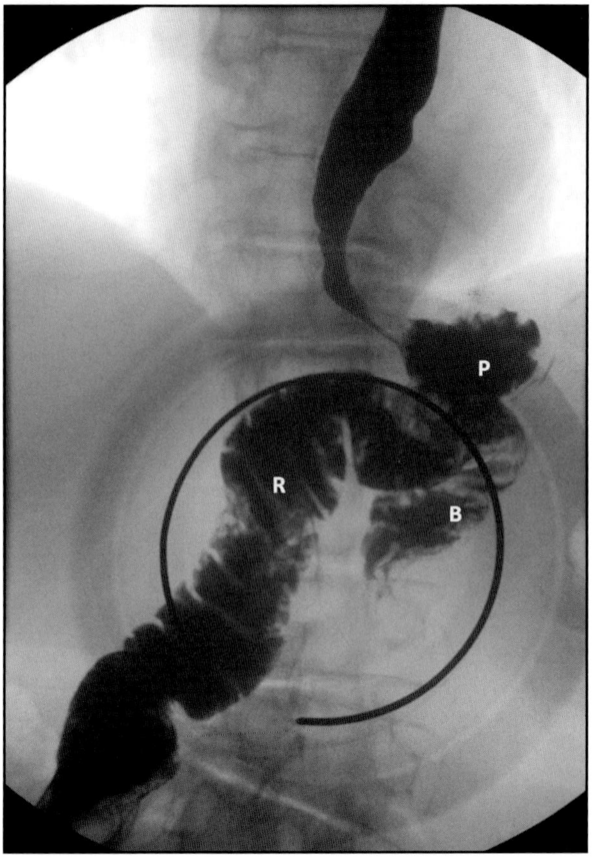

Figure 24-2. Normal UGI status post Roux-en-Y showing the small gastric pouch (P), the Roux limb (R), and the blind jejunal Baker's pouch (B).

images of the upper abdomen can be obtained in the standing position while oral contrast is administered.

Imaging begins with a preliminary abdominal radiograph to identify surgically placed drains, clips, and sutures not to be mistaken for minor leaks on the following contrasted images. This radiograph might also show dilated gas-filled bowel loops suggesting postoperative ileus. Patients typically have the nasogastric tube removed by the time of imaging.

In the upright position the patient is instructed to take 2 to 3 swallows of water-soluble contrast (iohexol) while undergoing fluoroscopy. Frontal and if possible oblique images are performed to evaluate the anastomotic sites and to establish adequacy of the surgical result. In a completely normal postoperative examination prompt, filling of the gastric pouch is seen, which is approximately 3 to 4 cm in diameter and 20 to 30 cc in volume.[1,2] Because estimation of size and volume can be challenging on fluoroscopy, as a rule of thumb, the size of the gastric pouch should not be larger than the adjacent L1 vertebral body (which averages 2.3 x 4.8 x 3.4 cm CC x trans x AP and approximately 30 cc).[3] Contrast then flows through the 1- to 2-cm outflow channel and opacifies the 75- to 150-cm long Roux limb. The gastrojejunal end-to-side anastomosis creates a short blind ending shepherd's crook of the jejunum, also called Baker's pouch, not to be mistaken for leak (Figure 24-2). Adequate contrast opacification of the gastrojejunal and subsequently the end-to-side enteroenteric anastomosis needs to be achieved with water-soluble contrast before the swallow exam can be repeated with thin barium. The high-density barium is more sensitive to reveal occult small leaks that may not be evident with water-soluble contrast alone.

Expected postoperative findings are delayed esophageal or gastric emptying due to anastomotic edema and slow contrast passage through the Roux limb secondary to adynamic ileus. Staple lines mark the area of the gastrojejunal and eneteroenteric anastomosis between the Roux and

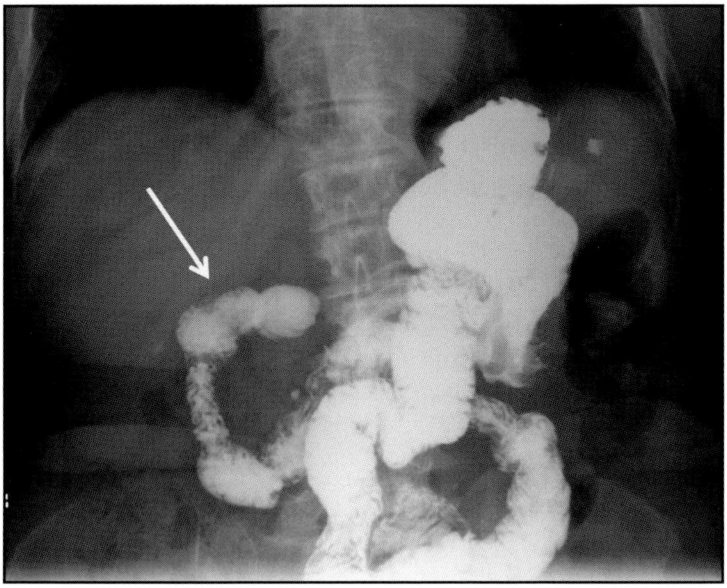

Figure 24-3. Single contrast barium UGI with small bowel follow through showing contrast refluxing back into the normal caliber biliopancreatic limb—normal finding.

biliopancreatic limb, which should not be mistaken for small contrast leak. The common channel is not routinely evaluated in the immediate postoperative period. Reflux into the biliopancreatic limb may occur, which is not necessarily abnormal unless distension or distal obstruction is observed (Figure 24-3).

Imaging of Early Complications

Anastomotic Leak

The most common immediate complication is a leak of the gastrojejunal anastomosis or less frequently of the enteroenteric anastomosis, which needs to be excluded before the patient can resume his or her diet after surgery. The incidence of anastomotic leak is approximately 2% to 5%[2,4] (Table 24-2). If UGI images do not show extra luminal contrast pooling adjacent to the anastomotic sites but the patient shows clinical signs and symptoms of a leak, such as pain, fever, and tachycardia, further investigation with CT scan can be performed. CT images may demonstrate a walled-off fluid collection adjacent to the anastomosis or oral contrast outside the confines of the gastrointestines in the peritoneal cavity (Figure 24-4). Extraluminal oral contrast may layer at dependent portions of the abdomen or pelvis, under the diaphragm, or flow along the surgical drains. Large leaks need immediate surgical attention and revision, while smaller leaks may seal off if adequate drainage of the collection is provided. This can be achieved via CT-guided percutaneous drain placement under moderate sedation to spare the patient from an undesirable reoperation. CT-guided drain placement can be challenging due to the location and size of the collection. Adequate drain care and revisualization of the collection is necessary before the drain can be removed.

Anastomotic Stricture/Edema

Anastomotic edema is commonly seen as transient delay of contrast passage through the gastroesophageal junction or at the level of the gastrojejunal anastomosis. This may present as contrast pooling in the esophagus or pooling and air-fluid level in the gastric pouch with a slow trickle of flow into the jejunum. The presumed edema is self-limiting and is treated conservatively, unless the patient's symptoms of post-prandial pain, reflux, or vomiting persist beyond 2 weeks, requiring reimaging (see Late Complications) (Figure 24-5).

Table 24-2

Imaging of Roux-en-Y Gastric Bypass Complications

COMPLICATION	INCIDENCE (%)	TIMELINE	IMAGING OF CHOICE
Anastomotic leak	2 to 5	Immediate	Fluoroscopy, CT
Obstruction due to edema		Immediate	Fluoroscopy
Pulmonary embolism	0.3 to 1	Early	CT
Wound infection	1 to 10	Early	CT
Obstruction	1 to 5	Late > early	CT, fluoroscopy
Gastrojejunostomy stricture	3 to 9		CT, fluoroscopy
Jejunojejunal stricture	< 1	Late > early	CT, fluoroscopy
Staple line dehiscence	0.7 to 8	Late > early	Fluoroscopy, CT
Internal or incisional hernia	3 to 14	Late	CT
Marginal ulcer	0.5 to 4	Late	Endoscopy, fluoroscopy
Gallstones	28	Late	Ultrasound, HIDA scan
Gastroesophageal reflux			Fluoroscopy
Blind pouch syndrome	Rare	Late	Fluoroscopy

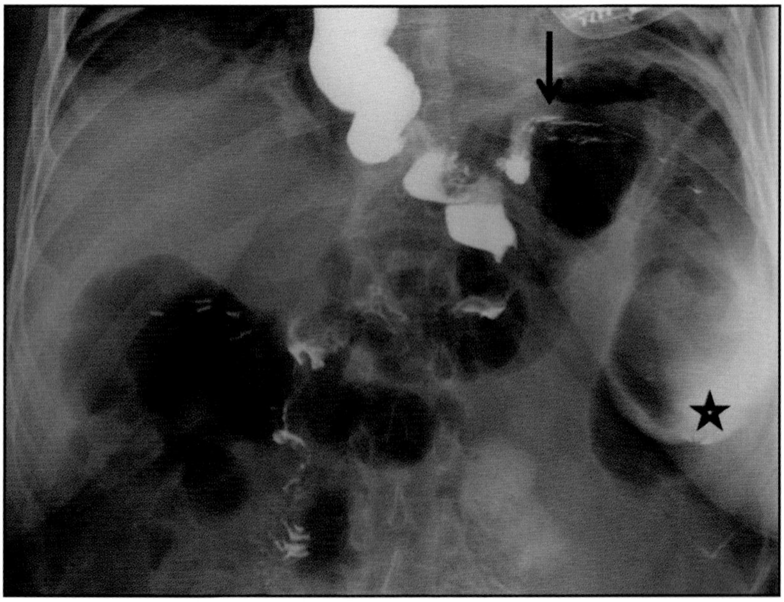

Figure 24-4. Water soluble UGI on postoperative day 1 demonstrating contrast leak from the stomach pouch (arrow) and contrast freely distributing in the peritoneum (star).

Infection

Wound infection can develop at the anastomotic sites, trocar sites, and at postoperative seromas and hematomas. Superficial collections may be evaluated with sonography, while deeper intra-abdominal collections can be diagnosed with CT. The typical CT appearance of abscess is a rim enhancing fluid collection (Figure 24-6).

If the abscess is related to anastomotic leak the cavity may contain gas or fill with oral contrast through the anastomotic breakdown. Treatment is CT-guided percutaneous drainage catheter

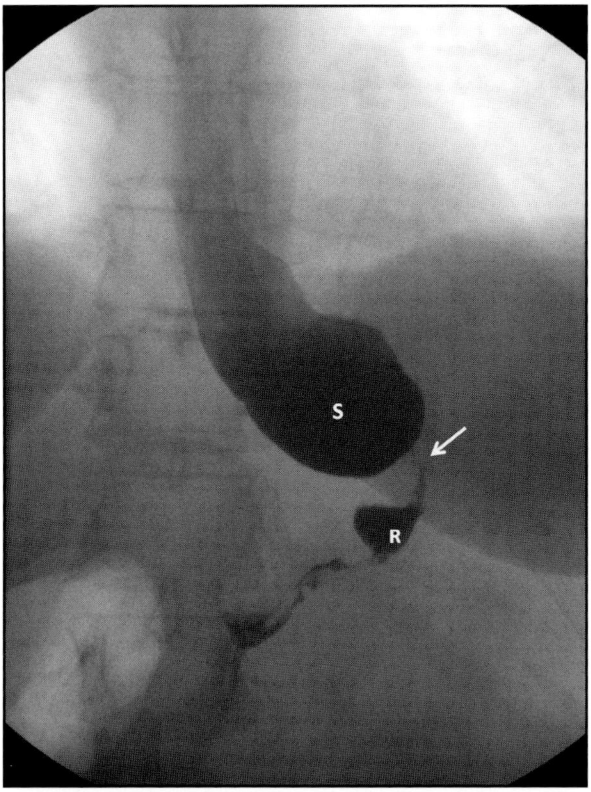

Figure 24-5. UGI showing postoperative edema. Narrow gastrojejunostomy (arrow) limiting flow from the stomach pouch (S) into the Roux limb (R).

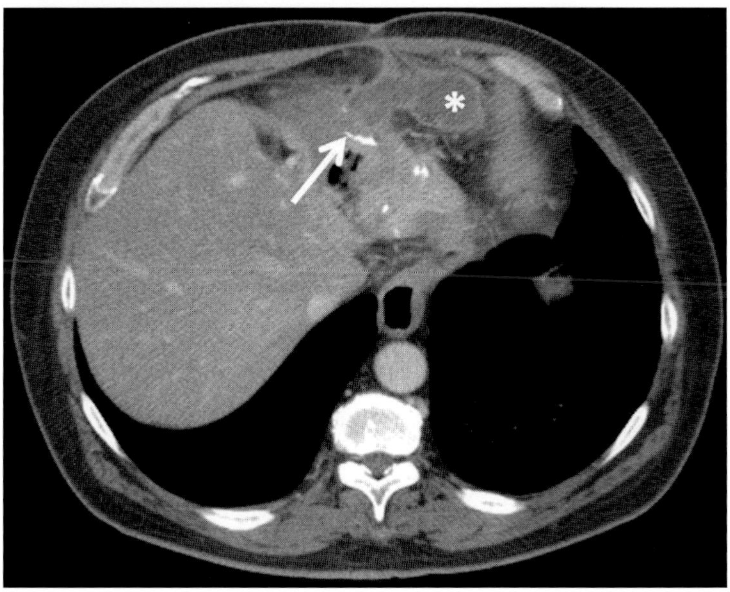

Figure 24-6. Intravenous contrast-enhanced CT scan of the abdomen showing small rim enhancing fluid collection (star) adjacent to the gastrojejunostomy staples (arrow), consistent with abscess due to a small anastomotic leak.

placement and antibiotic therapy. Because the collection contains a mixture of debris, fluid, and pus, large-bore 12 to 16 Fr. pigtail catheters are recommended for adequate drainage. The drain then needs to be flushed every 8 hours with normal saline to maintain patency (clean the side holes on the pigtail loop). The drain is attached either to a bag or a Jackson Pratt suction container. When the daily drain output falls below 15 to 20 cc reimaging or drain study is indicated to evaluate whether the drain can be removed.

Table 24-3

Presentation and Suggested Imaging Evaluation of Roux-en-Y Gastric Bypass Complications

SYMPTOMS	SUSPECTED COMPLICATION	IMAGING
Tachycardia, fever	Anastomotic leak	UGI water soluble, CT
Persistent vomiting	Gastrojejunal anastomotic stricture	UGI
Insufficient weight loss	Staple dehiscence	UGI, CT
	Pouch overdistension	UGI
Colicky pain, distension	Obstruction	UGI, CT
Epigastric pain, vomiting	Marginal ulcer	Endoscopy, UGI
Retrosternal burning	Gastroesophageal reflux	Endoscopy, esophagram
Lack of satiety	Pouch restriction degradation-wide gastrojejunal anastomosis	UGI

Bowel Obstruction

Adynamic ileus is commonly seen in the immediate postoperative period, which resolves spontaneously. Although adhesions start to develop as early 2 weeks postoperatively, mechanical bowel obstruction is typically a later concern.

Imaging of Late Complications

No routine imaging follow-up is indicated status post RYGB procedure. Symptomatic patients are evaluated by their bariatric surgeon, and specific imaging is requested based on the clinical symptoms (Table 24-3).

Anastomotic Stricture

Persistent narrowing at the gastrojejunostomy site beyond 2 weeks post surgery occurs in approximately 3% to 9% of cases[2,4] and is due to fibrosis or ischemia. Patients present with persistent nausea, vomiting, dehydration, and excessive weight loss. UGI is the first line of evaluation, which shows delayed passage of contrast through the anastomosis, gastroesophagel reflux, distended stomach pouch, and narrowing of the gastrojejunal anastomosis (Figure 24-7). Treatment with endoscopic balloon dilation is successful in the majority of cases.[4]

Bezoar

Bezoar is a ball of undigested food in the stomach, which may cause vomiting and intermittent obstruction of the stomach pouch. Bezoar may be visible on plain film as a collection of dense amorphous material projecting over the stomach. UGI shows barium outlining a variable size irregular filling defect in the stomach despite nothing-by-mouth status and obstruction or narrowing at the gastrojejunal anastomosis (Figure 24-8). Nuclear gastric emptying exam may show marked delay in liquid and solid gastric emptying.

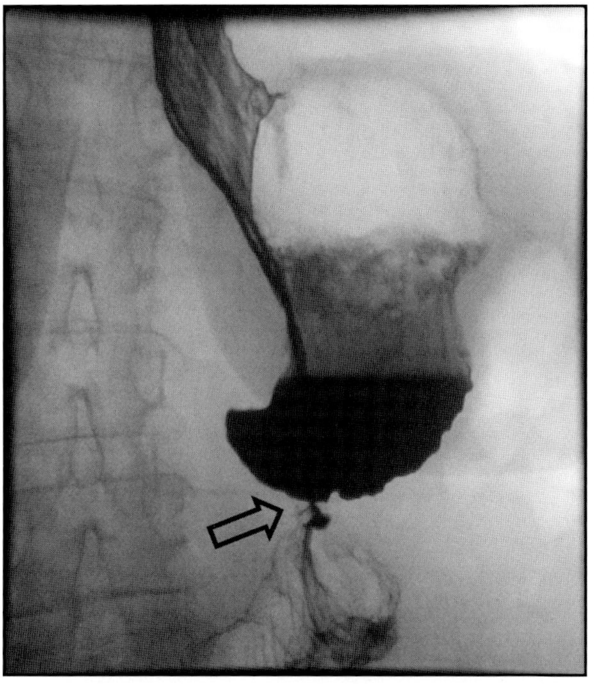

Figure 24-7. Single contrast barium UGI shows marked distention of the stomach pouch with air-debris-contrast level due to severe narrowing at the gastrojejunostomy site (hollow arrow).

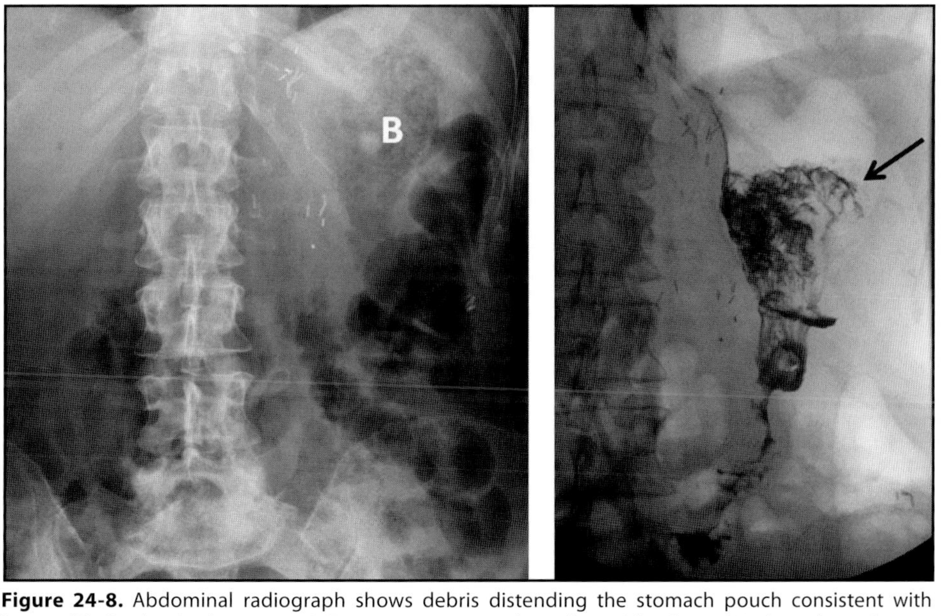

Figure 24-8. Abdominal radiograph shows debris distending the stomach pouch consistent with bezoar (B). On the single contrast UGI exam contrast outlines the residue (arrow) in the enlarged stomach pouch.

Degradation of Pouch Restriction

Patients presenting with lack of satiety, bloating after eating, and suboptimal weight loss may suffer from rapid passage of food through the stomach pouch. This lack of restriction may occur if the gastrojejunal anastomosis is widened, which is best evaluated with a double-contrast UGI exam, as real time fluoroscopy is able to well estimate the restrictive function. First the stomach pouch and jejunum are distended with effervescent crystals, followed by thick barium swallow to

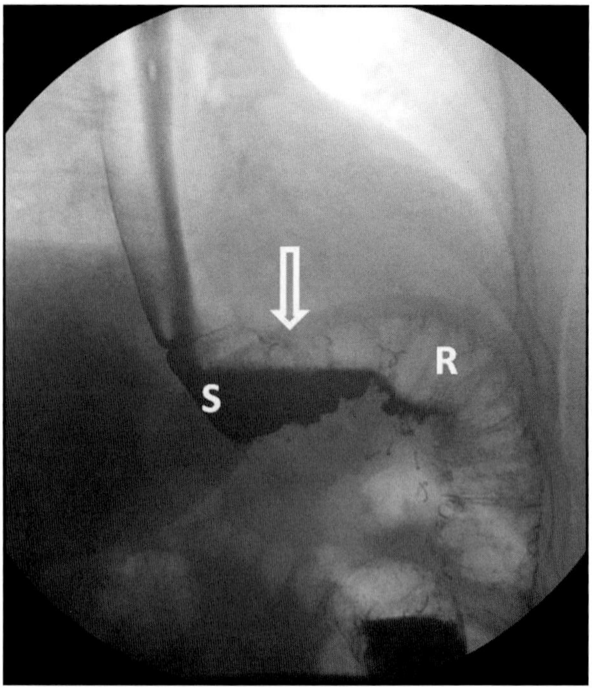

Figure 24-9. UGI exam shows a widely open gastrojejunal anastomosis (hollow arrow) allowing both liquid and solid substances to immediately empty from the stomach pouch (S) into the Roux limb (R).

coat the mucosal lining. This method allows for estimation of the gastric pouch volume and the width of the gastrojejunal anastomosis. Barium-coated burger or cracker can be also administered to evaluate passage of solid food in real time. Findings are widened proximal anastomosis and immediate passage of contrast into the jejunum without delay in the stomach pouch, leading to lack of satiety (Figure 24-9).

Dehiscence

Staple line failure or dehiscence typically presents as insufficient weight loss in the first year after surgery in 1% to 8% of patients.[2] This can be due to ischemic or mechanical stress on the staple line, such as overdistension of the stomach pouch. Overdistension is either secondary to stricture at the gastrojejunal anastomosis leading to gastric outlet obstruction or due to poor patient compliance and consumption of large volumes of not-well-chewed food. When weight gain is the clinical question and no radiographic or endoscopic abnormality can be found, behavioral causes must be also considered, such as overconsumption of high-calorie liquid or semisolid food.

With dehiscence of the staple line the 2 gastric chambers regain communication, leading to failing bypass results and antegrade filling of the biliary limb. This can be demonstrated on UGI exam, which can not only identify the dehiscence but well estimate the size and site of it. Under fluoroscopy contrast and air can be seen filling the alimentary gastric pouch and the excluded remnant stomach with subsequent filling of the duodenum and afferent limb (Figure 24-10). UGI exam is more specific in the diagnosis of dehiscence than CT, as retrograde contrast filling of the afferent limb may be normally seen on delayed imaging and mistaken for dehiscence or fistula.

Marginal Ulcer

Ulceration at the anastomosis site or proximal jejunum presents as epigastric pain, vomiting, and dyspepsia and occurs in approximately 0.5% to 4% of the patients.[2] The first line of diagnostic evaluation for marginal ulcer is endoscopy, as it often remains occult on UGI exam. It may show as a focal small outpouching of contrast material on typically the jejunal side of the gastrojejunal anastomosis (Figure 24-11) due to exposure to gastric secretions.

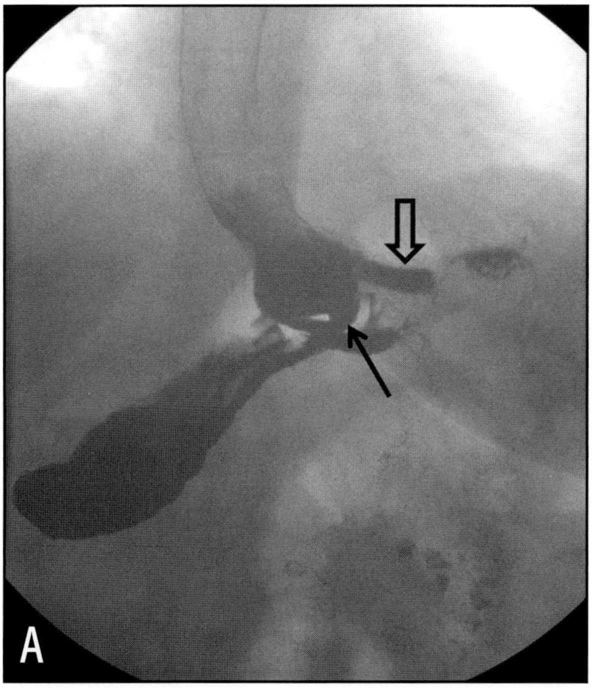

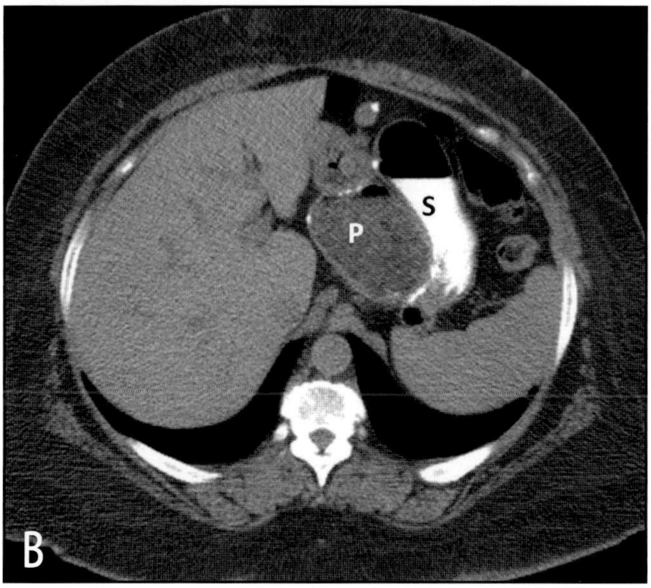

Figure 24-10. (A) Single contrast UGI exam shows contrast opacifying the stomach pouch, the jejunum through the gastrojejunal anastomosis (hollow arrow), and the stomach remnant through a dehiscence of the gastric staple line (arrow). (B) CT of the abdomen after administration of oral contrast shows contrast filling the excluded stomach remnant(s) consistent with a gastrogastric fistula.

Bowel Obstruction

Bowel obstruction can present as early as 2 weeks after surgery to up to many years due to adhesions, mesocolic window stenosis, anastomotic stricture, internal hernia (more common in transmesocolic pull through), incisional hernia, or intussusception.[4] The incidence of bowel obstruction is reported between 1% and 5%.[2] Patients present with colici abdominal pain, distention, and vomiting. The first line of imaging is plain abdominal radiography, which may show dilated loops of bowel with stair-stepping air-fluid levels prompting further investigation with oral

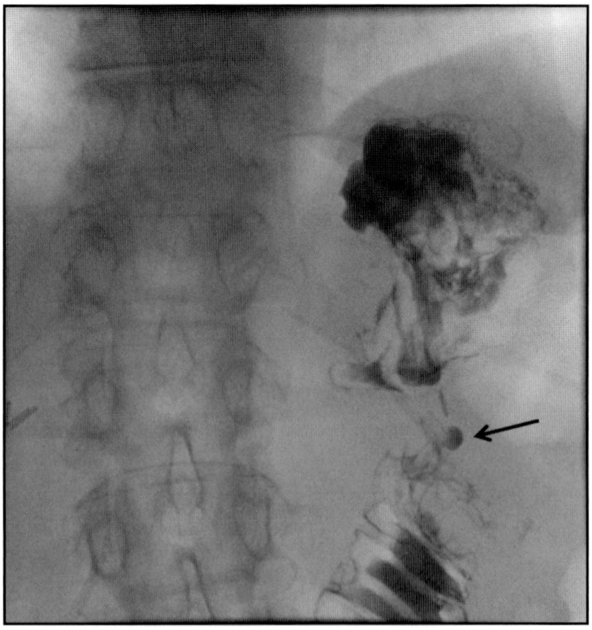

Figure 24-11. UGI exam demonstrates a persistent contrast filled pouch at the proximal jejunum (arrow), directly distal to the gastrojejunal anastomosis, consistent with an ulcer.

contrast-enhanced CT or UGI fluoroscopy with small bowel follow-through. CT is the preferred method of evaluation as it can readily demonstrate the site and degree of the obstruction, and it is particularly useful in closed-loop obstruction that may stay occult on UGI. While UGI can only show the level of obstruction in the alimentary limb or common loop, CT can demonstrate biliary limb pathology and the cause of the obstruction, such as incisional hernia, volvulus, or intussusception. CT may also provide additional information about other possible etiologies of the patient's complaint. The cause of obstruction is most commonly adhesions or stricture at the anastomosis sites. Findings are dilated proximal bowel loops with a beaked loop at the site of obstruction representing the transition point between dilated and decompressed bowel loops.

Afferent loop syndrome is dilation of the biliopancreatic limb due to adhesions, stenosis at the enteroenteric anastomosis, or internal hernia. This is a true closed-loop obstruction requiring immediate surgical attention, which if goes unrecognized can lead to bowel/stomach perforation. CT can readily demonstrate dilation of the stomach and duodenum and dilation of the biliary ductal system. On UGI the pancreaticobiliary limb cannot be evaluated; however, dilation and air-fluid levels in nonopacified small bowel loops in the background of the normal caliber opacified alimentary limb can give away the diagnosis (Figure 24-12).

Hernia

Hernia may occur after RYGB procedure in approximately 3% to 14% of patients[2] and present with signs of bowel obstruction.[4] If the Roux limb was brought up to the stomach in a retrocolic fashion, internal hernia can occur through the surgically created defect of the transverse mesocolon. With the antecolic approach a potential space is created between the alimentary jejunal limb and the transverse colon that may lead to the so-called Petersen's hernia. Herniation of bowel or omentum can also occur at the trocar or incision sites.

Transmesocolic hernia presents as a redundant Roux limb and its mesentery extending through the mesocolic defect with twisted swirling mesentery and possible small bowel volvulus.[4] Due to the resultant lymphatic and venous stasis the mesentery is engorged and edematous and the bowel wall is thickened, which are readily visible findings at CT.[2,5] As internal hernias may also result in a closed-loop obstruction it necessitates emergent surgical repair to avoid the threatening bowel ischemia, perforation, and possible death.

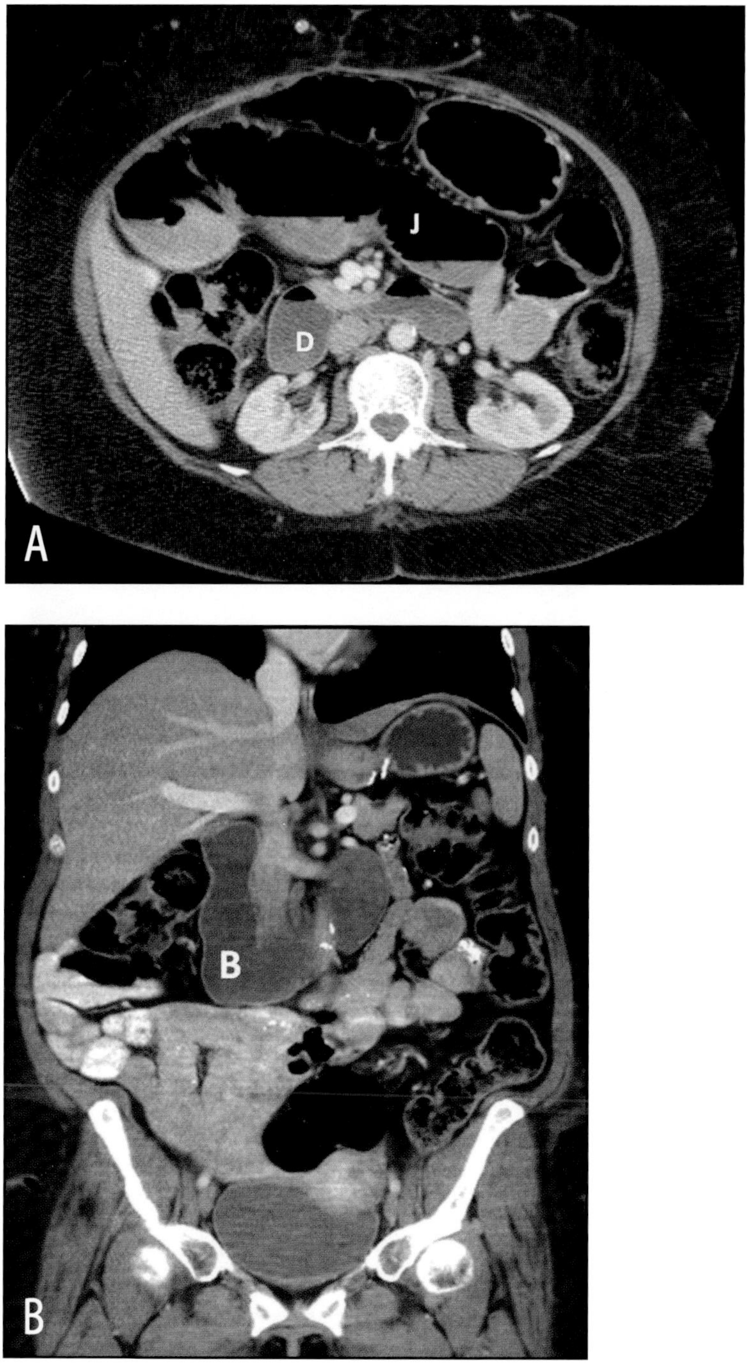

Figure 24-12. Obstruction of the biliopancreatic limb (B) on contrast enhanced CT. Note dilated loops of duodenum (D) and jejunum (J).

Gastroesophageal Reflux

Gastroesophageal reflux presents as pain, vomiting, and retrosternal burning sensation. On UGI exam contrast regurgitation from the stomach pouch into the esophagus is observed, or secondary signs may be seen, such as esophageal mucosal erosions. The diagnosis of reflux remains clinical because it often remains occult during the UGI exam.

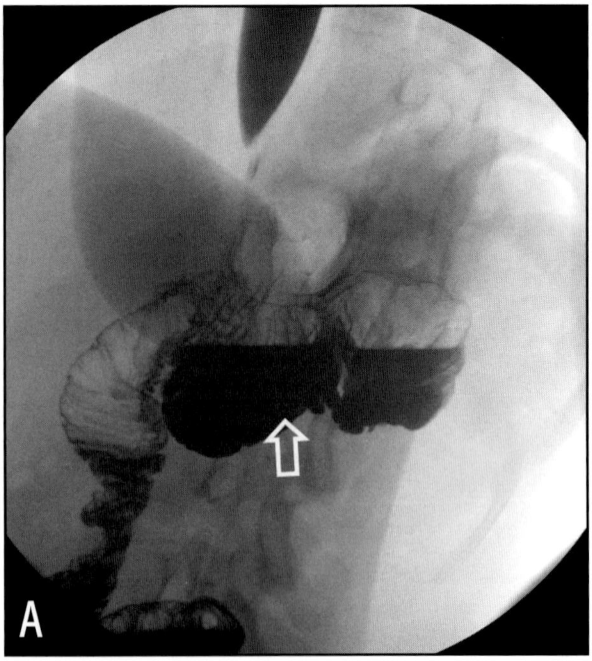

Figure 24-13A. Single contrast UGI exam demonstrates markedly dilated Baker's pouch (hollow arrow) with air-fluid level. On fluoroscopic imaging contrast was seen preferentially filling the jejunal pouch which then passively overflowed into the Roux limb. The gastrojejunal anastomosis is wide with loss of the restrictive function. *(continued)*

Gallstones

The gallbladder is not routinely removed during surgery unless the preoperative sonographic evaluation shows gallbladder pathology; therefore, in our institution, all patients are evaluated with right upper quadrant sonography in the month preceding the surgery.

Gallstones occur in up to one-third of postoperative bariatric patients due to mobilization of cholesterol during weight loss.[6] Patients may present with biliary colic and sonographic evidence of cholelithiasis. Clinical signs of acute cholecystitis are accompanied by additional sonographic findings, such as gallbladder wall thickening, pericholecystic fluid, sonographic Murphy sign, and dilated extra- and intrahepatic bile ducts.

Blind Pouch Syndrome

The development of a blind pouch is related to the creation of side-to-side or end-to-side enterostomies, where peristalsis fills rather than empties a small blind ending bowel pouch[7] (Figure 24-13). Consequently this loop may dilate over time, and although it may remain uncomplicated, it can lead to bacterial overgrowth, ulceration, and bleeding.

Duodenal Switch With Pancreaticobiliary Diversion

Due to its greater technical complexity and higher complication rate (approximately 20%), duodenal switch with pancreaticobiliary diversion is a less commonly used surgical weight loss solution.

The procedure consists of a pylorus-spearing sleeve gastrectomy that excludes approximately 70% of the stomach (restrictive component) and anastomosis of a 350-cm long segment of the ileum to the intact gastric pylorus (malabsorptive component). The excluded duodenum, jejunum, and proximal ileum form the biliary limb, anastomosed to the ileum approximately 75 cm from the ileocecal valve.[8]

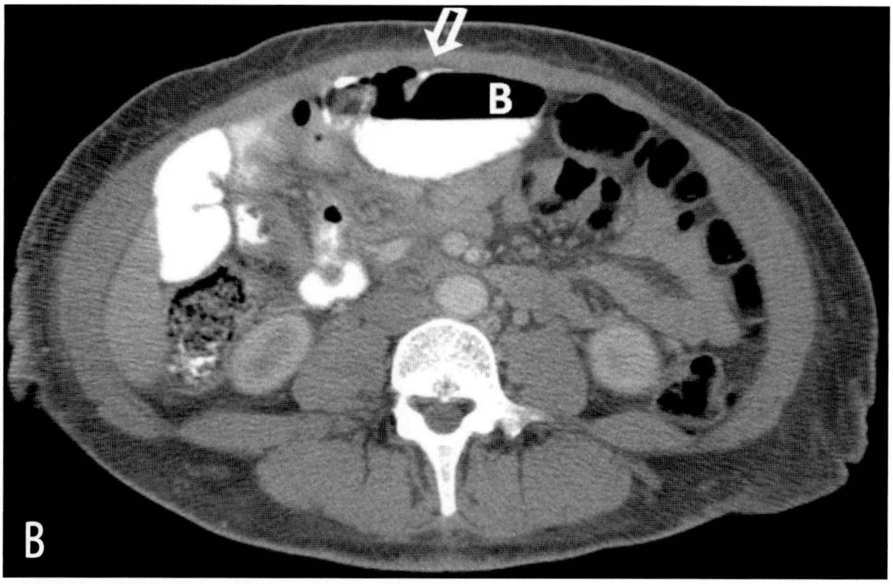

Figure 24-13B (continued). Dilated jejunal blind loop at the enteroenteric anastomosis.

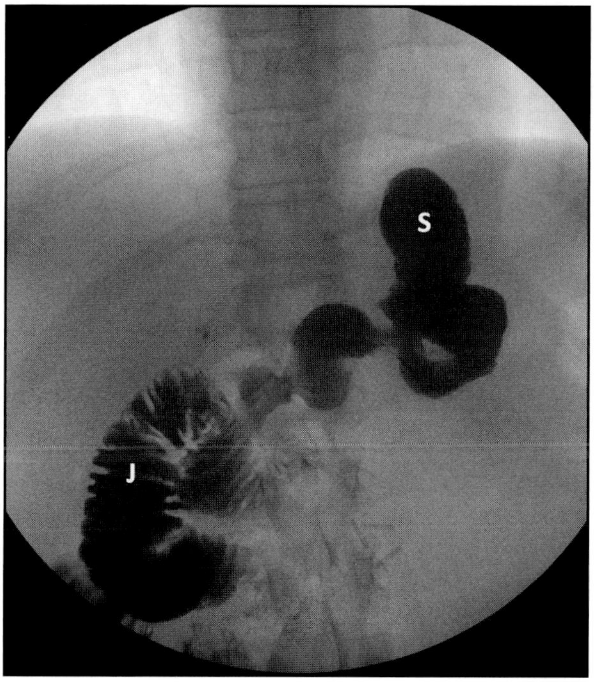

Figure 24-14. Normal postoperative anatomy on upper GI after duodenal switch and sleeve gastrectomy. Contrast opacifies the narrow lesser curvature of the stomach remnant (S) and end-to-side anastomosed jejunum (J). Complications and the imaging evaluation of them are similar to the Roux-en-Y procedure; therefore, they are not discussed here in further detail.

On UGI fluoroscopy a tubular-shaped elongated gastric pouch is seen in normal anatomic position representing the lesser curvature, with a staple line along its left lateral border. At the end-to-side gastro-ileal anastomosis, a small blind ending Baker's pouch of the ileum may be seen. The alimentary limb has an ileal mucosal fold pattern and courses through the right lower quadrant where the common channel enters the cecum (Figure 24-14).

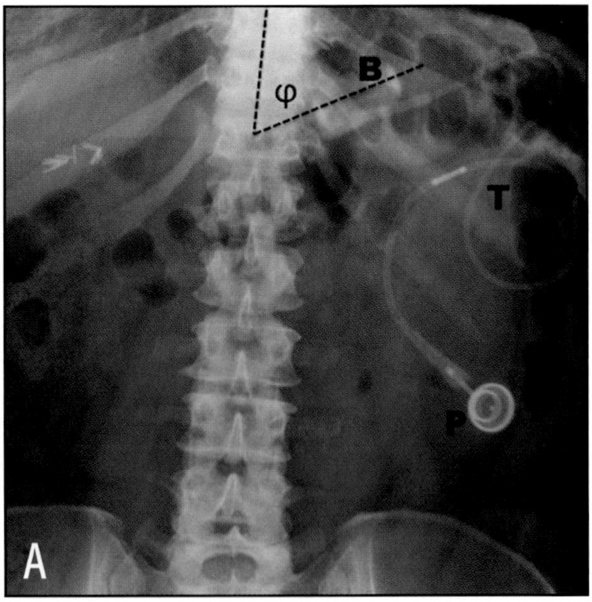

Figure 24-15A. Normal gastric band position (B) with intact tubing (T) and port (P). The angle between the line drawn tangential to the spine and the band represents the phi angle. *(continued)*

Laparoscopic Gastric Banding

Laparoscopically placed adjustable gastric banding is the least invasive restrictive weight loss procedure adequate for moderately obese patients. The adjustable silicone band is placed laparoscopically around the upper stomach, approximately 2 to 3 cm from the gastroesophageal junction. The band constricts the stomach and forms a small gastric pouch, limiting the amount of food available for absorption. The inflatable band is tightened with injection of saline solution via tubing that is attached to a subcutaneously placed port. The port is easily accessible with a special noncoring needle to adjust the diameter of the stoma.

On radiography the band is visualized 4 to 5 cm below the diaphragm at 4 to 58 degree angle (phi angle),[2,9] which is routinely seen on the postoperative chest or abdominal imaging. The phi angle is measured on an AP radiograph by intersecting a line drawn parallel to the spinal column with a line drawn parallel to the gastric band[2,9] (Figure 24-15A). Plain radiographs can be also useful in evaluating the position of the port, intactness of the tubing, and to guide for port access. If malposition or malfunction is suspected UGI fluoroscopy with water-soluble contrast or diluted barium is the modality of choice to investigate the cause. The patient swallows a few sips of contrast while the esophageal motility, gastric pouch size, and band position are evaluated under fluoroscopy. On a normal fluoroscopic exam a concentric 3- to 4-cm^2 gastric pouch is seen above the silicone band corresponding to a volume of approximately 20 to 30 mL. As previously discussed, the size of the adjacent vertebral body can be used for correlation to estimate the pouch size, as the average width of the L1 vertebral body is around 4.8 cm. The gastric stoma at the level of the band is between 5 to 10 mm, depending on the desired rate of weight loss and the patient's preference. Liquid contrast should begin emptying from the pouch immediately, and both liquid and solid substances should complete emptying within 15 to 20 minutes[2] (Figure 24-15B).

CT imaging is reserved for evaluation of nonspecific abdominal symptoms or if UGI exams fail to answer the clinical question (Table 24-4).

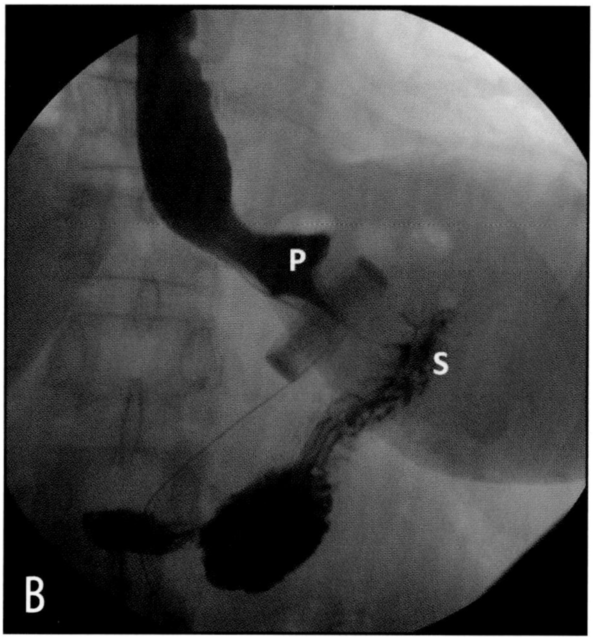

Figure 24-15B (continued). UGI after gastric banding showing normal size stomach pouch (P) and appropriate flow through the gastric band into the body of the stomach (S).

Table 24-4

Laparoscopic Gastric Banding Complications

COMPLICATION	INCIDENCE (%)	SYMPTOMS	RADIOLOGIC PRESENTATION
Band slippage too high	2.3 to 13	Lack of satiety	X-ray: Band at gastro-esophageal junction
Band slippage too low		Lack of satiety	UGI: Large gastric pouch
Band too tight	8 to 11	Reflux, vomiting	UGI: Dilated gastric pouch
Band too loose		Failure to lose weight	UGI: Inappropriate restriction
Band erosion into stomach	Rare	Pain, port infection, weight gain	UGI: Double gastric channel
Port rotation or inversion	1 to 5	Inaccessible port	X-ray: Tilted port
Tube disconnection/leak	1 to 5	Detected during inflation under fluoroscopy	X-ray: Discontinuity of tubing Port injection: Contrast leak
Paragastric herniation of gastric cardia	Rare	Pain after swallowing	UGI: Herniation adjacent to the stoma
Port infection	< 1	Fever, erythema, leukocytosis	Ultrasound/CT: Abscess
Gastric perforation	0.1 to 0.8	Fever, leukocytosis	UGI: Leak

Infection

Infection presents usually in the immediate postoperative period in less than 1% of the patients[2] and can occur anywhere along the port, tubing, or silicone band. Superficial infections can be diagnosed with ultrasound; deep abdominal abscesses are best evaluated with CT, which can be also used to guide abscess drainage if necessary.

Leak

Routine postoperative water-soluble UGI exam is often performed on postoperative day 1 to verify adequate positioning of the gastric band and to rule out perforation due to surgical trauma to the stomach wall. Water-soluble exam is preferred over barium study to avoid the possibility of inflammation and fibrosis caused by barium leaked into the peritoneum or aspirated due to stomal edema and obstruction. If fever, pain, or leukocytosis persists despite a negative fluoroscopic exam, occult small leaks can be diagnosed on CT by demonstration of extraluminal gas or contrast and abscess in the surgical bed or subphrenic region.

Stomal Stenosis

Stenosis at the stoma in the immediate postoperative period is usually due to self-limiting edema, requiring no treatment. Nonresolving stenosis may be the result of overinflation of the band or inflammation of the gastric mucosa and mucosal thickening, which can be treated conservatively if band slippage is not concurrently present. Long-standing stenosis results in delayed gastric emptying, overdistention of the gastric pouch, gastroesophageal reflux, and esophagitis, all readily visible on UGI fluoroscopy (Figure 24-16).

Band Slippage

With horizontal slippage of the band (> 55-degree phi angle) there is posterior herniation of the distal stomach superiorly through the band resulting in laterally eccentric gastric pouch (Figure 24-17). If the band tilts to a vertical position, anterior herniation of the distal stomach occurs with medial eccentric enlargement of the stomach pouch. If concurrent stomal stenosis develops, surgical correction is necessary, while mild nonobstructive slippage can be managed by deflation and observation to await spontaneous reposition.[10] UGI fluoroscopy can estimate the degree of stenosis, the size of the gastric pouch, the presence of gastroesophageal reflux, and the position of the band.

If the band slips to the level of the gastroesophageal junction, the restrictive function is lost and patients present with lack of satiety and insufficient weight loss. In this case the band is in an immediate subdiaphragmatic position with no gastric fold seen above the band on UGI exam.

Paragastric Herniation of the Gastric Cardia

Paragastric herniation of the gastric cardia presents as intermittent epigastric pain during swallowing. As this is an unusual but potentially emergent complication of laparoscopic gastric banding, awareness of this entity is important. UGI exam shows a small gastric segment herniating through the band along the normal stoma. During swallowing and distention of the stoma, this small herniated segment can get obstructed and strangulated (Figure 24-18).

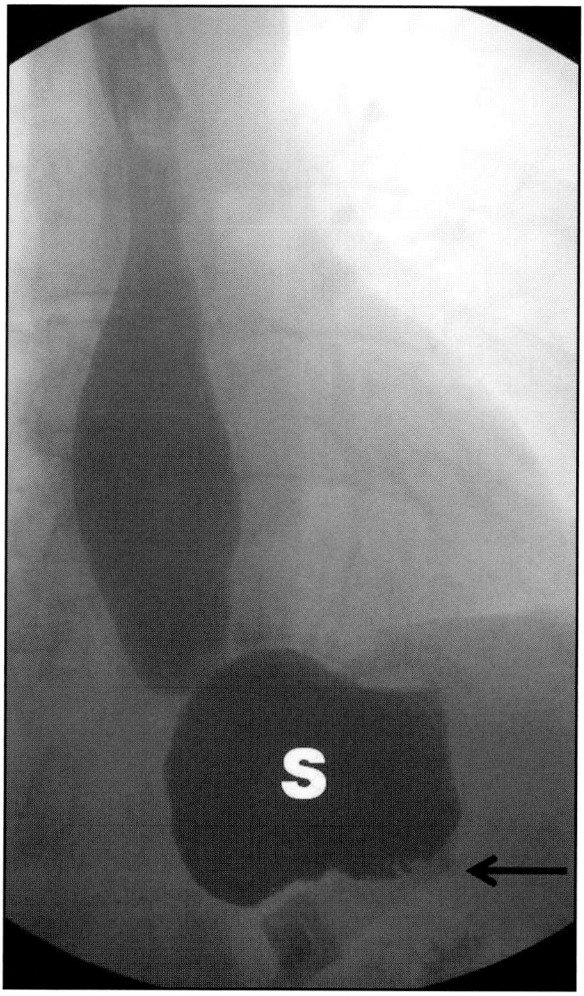

Figure 24-16. Single contrast UGI exam demonstrates overdistended stomach pouch with contrast pooling in the pouch and the esophagus and only minimal amount of contrast trickling through the obstructing band (arrow). This was due to an overinflated band.

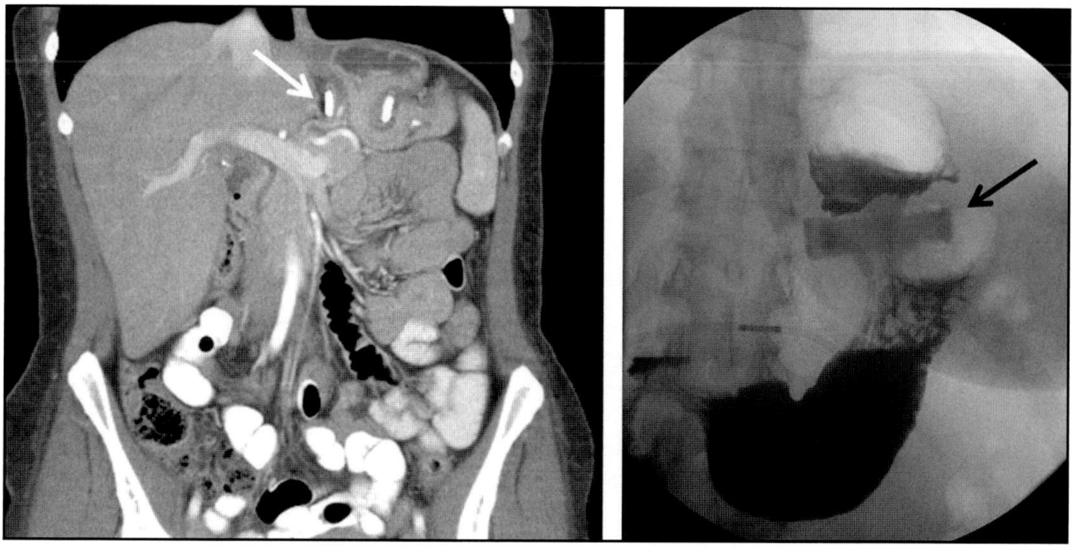

Figure 24-17. CT and UGI exam showing horizontally positioned slipped gastric band with enlarged gastric pouch.

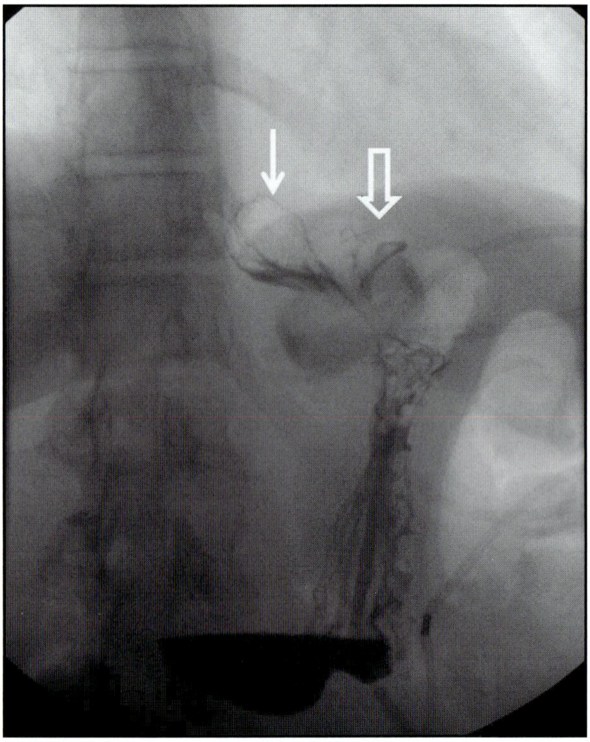

Figure 24-18. Single contrast UGI demonstrates the distal stomach (hollow arrow) herniating through the gastric band adjacent to the normal stomach pouch (arrow).

Erosion

Erosion of the band into the stomach lumen may present as an occult chronic condition due to inflammatory foreign body reaction or infection.[11] UGI shows contrast flowing both inside and outside of the band filling the distal stomach. If the erosion occurs acutely the contrast may freely enter the peritoneum.

Port System Malfunction

Possible complications involving the access port system include rotation of the access port, disconnected tubing, leakage of the banding system, and infection.

Rotation of the port can be suspected on manual evaluation and diagnosed on anterior and lateral abdominal radiographs. Disconnection of the radio-opaque connector tubing is also readily visible on radiographs and requires surgical revision. Leakage of the banding system is suspected if the band inflation is insufficient and the expected flow restriction does not occur. Leakage can occur anywhere from the band, along the connector tubing to the port site, and can be evaluated under fluoroscopy by administration of intravenous contrast via the access port.[10]

Summary

Morbid obesity has an increasing incidence in the Western industrialized nations with surgical solutions such as laparoscopic adjustable gastric banding and laparoscopic RYGB becoming more successful and popular weight loss procedures, necessitating the understanding of the procedures and possible complications at all provider levels. Imaging plays an important role in the follow-up and diagnosis of postoperative complications and may sometimes be the first to suggest the diagnosis of a postoperative complication to clinicians.

References

1. Blachar A, Federle MP, Pealer KM, Abu Abeid S, Graif M. Radiographic manifestations of normal postoperative anatomy and gastrointestinal complications of bariatric surgery, with emphasis on CT imaging findings. *Semin Ultrasound CT MR.* 2004;25(3):239-251.
2. Chandler RC, Srinivas G, Chintapalli KN, Schwesinger WH, Prasad SR. Imaging in bariatric surgery: a guide to postsurgical anatomy and common complications. *AJR Am J Roentgenol.* 2008;190(1):122-135.
3. Karabekir HS, Gocmen-Mas N, Edizer M, Ertekin T, Yazici C, Atamturk D. Lumbar vertebra morphometry and stereological assesment of intervertebral space volumetry: a methodological study. *Ann Anat.* 2011;193(3):231-236.
4. Blachar A, Federle MP. Gastrointestinal complications of laparoscopic roux-en-Y gastric bypass surgery in patients who are morbidly obese: findings on radiography and CT. *AJR Am J Roentgenol.* 2002;179(6):1437-1442.
5. Scheirey CD, Scholz FJ, Shah PC, Brams DM, Wong BB, Pedrosa M. Radiology of the laparoscopic roux-en-Y gastric bypass procedure: conceptualization and precise interpretation of results. *Radiographics.* 2006;26(5):1355-1371.
6. Nagem R, Lazaro-da-Silva A. Cholecystolithiasis after gastric bypass: a clinical, biochemical, and ultrasonographic 3-year follow-up study. *Obes Surg.* 2012;22(10):1594-1599.
7. Sandrasegaran K, Maglinte DD, Rajesh A, Tann M, Kopecky KK. CT findings for postsurgical blind pouch of small bowel. *AJR Am J Roentgenol.* 2006;186(1):110-113.
8. Mitchell MT, Carabetta JM, Shah RN, O'Riordan MA, Gasparaitis AE, Alverdy JC. Duodenal switch gastric bypass surgery for morbid obesity: imaging of postsurgical anatomy and postoperative gastrointestinal complications. *AJR Am J Roentgenol.* 2009;193(6):1576-1580.
9. Sonavane SK, Menias CO, Kantawala KP, et al. Laparoscopic adjustable gastric banding: what radiologists need to know. *Radiographics.* 2012;32(4):1161-1178.
10. Mehanna MJ, Birjawi G, Moukaddam HA, Khoury G, Hussein M, Al-Kutoubi A. Complications of adjustable gastric banding, a radiological pictorial review. *AJR Am J Roentgenol.* 2006;186(2):522-534.
11. Yoon CI, Pak KH, Kim SM. Early experience with diagnosis and management of eroded gastric bands. *J Korean Surg Soc.* 2012;82(1):18-27.

25

The Esophagus, Gastroesophageal Reflux Disease, and Bariatric Surgery

Tommy H. Lee, MD and Kalyana Nandipati, MD

With the rising prevalence of obesity in recent years, patient body mass index (BMI) has become an increasingly important consideration in the management of reflux. Although obesity would appear to be a natural risk factor for gastroesophageal reflux disease (GERD), the association has not been conclusively demonstrated in the literature. A recent meta-analysis found an association between BMI and GERD only when stratifying by country.[1] Even when there is an association, it is far from being 100%, with reported GERD rates as low as approximately 50% even in the superobese.[2] In the morbidly obese, excess body fat, particularly in a visceral distribution, is a risk factor for reflux, but not necessarily a cause of GERD on its own. The traditional gold-standard fundoplication in this population of patients may be doomed to long-term failure as the chronic condition of obesity over time wears at the hiatal hernia repair and reconstructed antireflux valve.

Bariatric surgery, similarly, can affect reflux. All currently commonly performed bariatric operations involve manipulation and alteration of gastroesophageal anatomy, resulting in change of multiple physiologic parameters, many of which are poorly understood, such as gastric emptying and even the function of the lower esophageal sphincter (LES) itself. Reflux control involves a complex interplay of LES function, esophageal function, and gastric emptying. While all 3 can be affected by any foregut procedure, LES function and gastric emptying are most directly altered in bariatric surgery, and hence the wider scale physiologic impact of these changes are an important consideration.

Reflux in this population of patients, therefore, presents an additional level of complexity to be considered. Obesity and reflux are tied closely enough together that effective management of reflux requires careful consideration of the relative contribution of obesity to the patient's reflux, and then failing conservative measures such as diet changes and weight loss without surgery, carefully planning a surgical procedure that will have excellent early and long-term outcomes.

Forse RA, Apovian CM, eds.
Bariatric Surgery: What Every Provider Needs to Know (pp 301-309).

Pathophysiology of Reflux Disease

In the past decade, the prevalence of GERD and morbid obesity has been on the rise. The following factors have been implicated in the pathophysiology of reflux disease: transient lower esophageal sphincter relaxation (TLESR) and/or weak LES, the presence of hiatal hernia, altered gastroesophageal pressure gradient, and esophageal body factors (poor esophageal clearance and altered esophageal motility). Recently, alteration in TLESR has been implicated as the most important factor. In addition, changes in LES pressure dynamics because of an increase in visceral fat and alterations in gastric motility secondary to hormonal and dietary habits have also been implicated in the pathophysiology of GERD in morbidly obese patients. Pathophysiology can therefore be broadly categorized as LES-related, gastric, and esophageal motility issues.

The temporal association between obesity and GERD has been investigated in numerous large population-based trials. A study performed in volunteers (VA employees)[3] and also a large database study in nurses identified BMI as an independent risk factor in the pathophysiology of GERD. Other factors that are implicated in pathophysiology by several other investigators include body weight, waist circumference, and visceral fat.[4]

Lower Esophageal Sphincter and Gastroesophageal Junction

LES pressure, TLESRs, altered LES gradient, and diaphragmatic factors (hiatal hernia) have been implicated in the pathogenesis of GERD. A normal LES pressure is important in preventing reflux and a hypotensive LES can predispose to GERD. Decreased LES pressure has been observed in patients with high BMI. Manometric studies comparing LES measurements between the normal and obese populations (BMI > 30 kg/m^2) reported an inverse correlation and also that increasing severity of reflux is higher in patients with higher BMI.

TLESRs are complete relaxations of the LES in the absence of swallowing and can allow acid reflux irrespective of the LES resting pressure. An increased number of TLESRs has been reported in overweight and obese patients, which is associated with increased acid reflux.[5]

Manometric studies showed a significant correlation between BMI, waist circumference, and visceral fat with intragastric pressure and gastroesophageal pressure gradient. This has been implicated in esophago-gastric junction disruption in patients with higher BMIs compared to the normal BMI population, which can predispose to development of hiatal hernia. Pandolfino et al, who reported that both intragastric pressure and the gastroesophageal pressure gradient strongly correlated with increasing levels of BMI, support this hypothesis.[6] It also evident from the literature that greater than 50% of patients undergoing bariatric procedure have hiatal hernia, and the incidence of reflux esophagitis is more than double in this subgroup of patients with hiatal hernia compared to the patients without hiatal hernia.

The LES complex in morbidly obese patients has an increased incidence of TLESRs, a higher incidence of hiatal hernias, and a lower LES pressure. The high number of TLESRs and lower LES pressures were reported to be consistently associated with a high incidence of reflux disease.

Esophageal Body and Gastric Motor Abnormalities

Esophageal body function has been implicated in reflux disease for several years in normal patients. Functional abnormalities in the esophageal body are also documented to predispose to the development of reflux in morbidly obese patients. The most common esophageal body abnormalities identified include nonspecific motility disorder and nutcracker esophagus. The frequency of esophageal motor abnormalities reported are higher than expected relative to nonobese, non-GERD individuals (overall, for all motor disorders approximately 10% to 15%). However, all these patients are not symptomatic. Interestingly the overall incidence of abnormal manometric findings are similar in nonobese GERD patients and obese GERD patients.[7] Studies comparing the obese and nonobese GERD population identified that patients with obesity have a higher chance of impaired esophageal clearance leading to a high incidence of esophagitis.

Reflux Monitoring

Any antireflux procedure requires careful patient selection. Objective measures of both reflux severity and esophageal function are key components of preoperative patient evaluation. Patients' subjective description of esophageal pathology is notoriously unreliable, particularly as words such as *reflux, GERD,* and *heartburn* have entered the common lexicon, with many people not truly understanding what the words mean.

Ambulatory pH Monitoring

Objective documentation of reflux is most often achieved by some form of ambulatory monitoring. Such monitoring, however, can be considered unnecessary in the presence of either erosive esophagitis or Barrett's esophagus on evaluation with upper endoscopy. These findings can be considered pathognomonic for GERD in most cases. Exceptions such as pill erosions from medications such as bisphosphonates or acetylsalicylic acid or Barrett's that may have developed prior to significant patient weight loss can usually be differentiated on history. If there is uncertainty, ambulatory monitoring can provide important information.

Single-Channel pH Monitoring

Single-channel pH monitoring can be achieved using either a catheter-based system or a wireless capsule-based system (Bravo, Given Imaging). Both systems are positioned 5 cm above the gastroesophageal junction so that data can be collected that conform to the currently known standards. With catheter-based systems, the sensor is positioned most accurately using the manometric LES, as both the pH and manometry catheters are passed transnasally. The Bravo capsule system is typically placed transorally, and hence an endoscopic LES measurement is used to position it.

Data are typically calculated over a 24-hour period for the catheter-based system and over 48 hours for the Bravo system. The system then measures the pH at the level of the sensor, with falls below a pH of 4 considered to be indicative of a reflux event. Analysis involves correlation of reflux events to meals, supine vs upright positioning, and symptoms. Interpretation typically involves calculation of either the percentage time of pH < 4 or the well-established composite DeMeester score. In calculating a DeMeester score, the parameters collected are (1) the percentage of time the pH was < 4 for the total 24 hours, (2) the percentage of time the pH was < 4 when the patient was upright, (3) the same for the supine position, (4) total number of reflux episodes, (5) the number of episodes lasting 5 minutes or longer, and (6) the duration of the longest episode. From these a composite score is calculated, and individuals with a score more than 2 standard deviations from the established control mean are considered abnormal.[8]

Dual-Channel pH Monitoring

Double-channel systems add a proximal sensor located 15 cm above the LES. This second sensor measures acid exposure in the proximal esophagus, and may be useful in the establishment of a diagnosis of laryngopharyngeal reflux. Data at the proximal sensor are often of limited additional benefit. Normal ranges are available only for rudimentary parameters, such as the number of reflux episodes, and hence measurements at this channel are useful as confirmatory testing at best. Correlation to symptoms is often poor since laryngopharyngeal reflux manifestations, such as cough and globus, are as much a result of chronic irritation as they are acute reflux events.

Impedance pH Monitoring

Impedance pH monitoring adds intralumenal impedance sensors at 3, 5, 7, 9, 15, and 17 cm above the LES. This permits the detection of nonacid reflux. Measured parameters are once again relatively basic and analysis focuses primarily on the number of nonacid and weakly acidic events. This information may be particularly useful in assessing breakthrough symptoms in patients with an incomplete response to proton pump inhibitor therapy.

Recommendations

Assessment of reflux symptoms in the morbidly obese requires the same basic elements as that of nonobese patients. Reflux testing should be reserved for symptomatic patients, as those without testing are unlikely to have positive findings.[9] Objective measurement and documentation of both reflux and esophageal function are important prior to any antireflux procedure, both to confirm the diagnosis, as well as to ensure that there is no underlying esophageal motility disorder that would be an absolute or relative contraindication to traditional antireflux surgery.

Treatment Options: Fundoplication

Results and Factors Predicting Success

Fundoplication is the gold-standard surgical management of GERD. Long-term outcomes of laparoscopic fundoplication demonstrate durable excellent results. Dallemagne et al[10] reported 89.5% symptom resolution at 10 years, while 79.7% of patients had good or excellent symptom control in a 20-year follow-up study by Salminen et al.[11] However, failures do occur, with patterns usually exhibiting a combination of crus failure (recurrent hiatal hernia) and fundoplication distortion.[12] Assuming the fundoplication was correctly constructed to begin with, when failures occur, there is often a history of elevated diaphragm stressors such as gagging, retching, or heavy lifting. In the morbidly obese, in particular, intact fundoplication herniation is relatively low, and fundoplication disruption is relatively high.[13] A mechanism for this differing failure pattern has not been firmly established, but possibilities include the chronically elevated intra-abdominal pressure of the obese, the tendency to overeat, and technical difficulties at the first operation.

Care must be taken when reviewing the literature of fundoplication in morbidly obese patients, because the follow-up in the majority of these studies is short, while the pertinent concerns are in long-term outcomes. Poor long-term outcomes are reflected in the reported literature, where morbid obesity with a BMI > 35 has been found to be a risk factor for failure. Interestingly, a lesser degree of obesity (BMI < 35) was not associated with a higher probability of failure in this study.[14]

With fundoplication at higher risk of long-term failure in the morbidly obese, alternative options need to be considered. The ideal option will address both the obesity of the patient and GERD, and is robust in the face of the elevated intra-abdominal pressures of the morbidly obese.

Alternative Options

Mechanical reconstructions of the LES are all subject to the chronic stressors described previously, and hence are at relatively high risk of failure. This would include all varieties of fundoplications (Nissen complete, Toupet or Dor partial), as well as the Hill procedure to augment the LES with a gastropexy.

Alternative procedures that do not attempt augmentation of the LES, but instead divert acid and bile away from the esophagus, are excellent options. Roux-en-Y gastric bypass (RYGB) is an excellent antireflux operation, and its benefits and results will be discussed in the next section.

In the setting of a reoperation, other operations can be considered, mostly for salvage. End-stage esophageal disease, where there is a dilated, tortuous, aperistaltic esophagus, resulting in significant esophago-esophageal reflux, in many cases would benefit most from esophageal resection. Augmentation of the LES or acid/bile diversion is usually inadequate in this population of patients as there will continue to be esophago-esophageal reflux, although it may be improved somewhat by the reduction of refluxate into the esophagus, or the improvement of esophago-gatsric emptying if there is outflow obstruction from either a distorted fundoplication or recurrent hiatal hernia.

Esophagectomy is also a salvage option in patients in whom during a remedial foregut operation the esophagus is irreparably damaged, either by inadvertent surgical trauma or in the setting of mesh or pledget erosion into the esophagus.

Other salvage operations include total or near-total gastrectomy with esophagojejunostomy, which may need to be considered in patients with damage to the proximal stomach near the gastroesophageal junction that is not amenable to repair or again in the presence of mesh erosion.

Weight Loss Procedures and Role in Gastroesophageal Reflux Disease

The pathophysiology and increasing evidence of failure of primary antireflux procedures like fundoplication in morbidly obese patients has led investigators to look for alternative procedures. Since the mid-1990s, there has been a growing body of literature on the impact of surgical techniques for weight loss on GERD. Gastric banding, sleeve gastrectomy, and gastric bypass are the most commonly performed weight loss procedures. The other less commonly performed procedures include biliopancreatic diversion and vertical banded gastroplasty ([VBG] no longer performed as a primary treatment option). These procedures have been reported to be effective in weight reduction (primary goal), but they also have shown to influence the gastroesophageal reflux in various ways.

Laparoscopic Adjustable Gastric Banding

Since its introduction in the mid-1990s, laparoscopic adjustable gastric banding (LAGB) has rapidly become one of the commonly performed surgical options. It is the least invasive of the commonly performed procedures and is associated with fewer complications, such as malnutrition and vitamin deficiencies. The procedure involves placing an adjustable band around the proximal stomach and placing a reservoir subcutaneously. This reservoir allows adjustment of the size of the band to appropriate restriction by filling it with fluid. Literature reports regarding the association of LAGB and GERD are still controversial. Conflicting results have been published with some studies showing improvement, some no difference, and some showing worsening of GERD.

The initial studies by Dixon and O'Brien reported that LAGB placement was associated with either resolution or marked improvement in the reflux symptoms. After follow-up of 2 years, the authors found that 76% of patients reported complete resolution of GERD symptoms, while the symptoms remained unchanged in 6% and worsened in 4%.[15] A later study by Tolonen et al[16] reported that after a median time of 19 months (range, 7 to 32 months), symptomatic patients decreased from 48.4% preoperatively to 16.1% postoperatively ($p=.01$); 24-hour pH monitoring also showed improvement in DeMeester score and reflux episodes postoperatively. In both studies, authors suggested that a reduction of meal size in the early postoperative period, weight reduction, and a small pouch might be the reasons for decreased reflux after LAGB. Meta-analysis reported decrease in the prevalence of reflux symptoms from 32.9% preoperatively to 7.7% postoperatively, and a decrease in the use of antireflux medication from 27.5% preoperatively to 9.5% postoperatively. On the other hand, authors also reported that 15% of patients reported a new development of reflux along with 22.9% of patients having new development of esophagitis after LAGB.[17]

LAGB has been shown to have mixed results in terms of development of reflux disease. The majority of the literature showed improvement or resolution of symptoms after LAGB. However, it is also important to note that a significant subset of the population reported either worsening or new development of reflux symptoms after the procedure. It is important to inform patients with GERD about the mixed results associated with LAGB and also discuss other weight loss options, such as gastric bypass.

Sleeve Gastrectomy

Laparoscopic sleeve gastrectomy (LSG) was originally intended as a first-stage procedure in high-risk patients; it has now become a stand-alone operation for many bariatric surgeons. The procedure has become a popular treatment option for morbid obesity over the past 10 years, with reported excess weight loss of up to 60%. Sleeve gastrectomy is performed by stapling the stomach over a dilator to create a tubular stomach. Although sleeve gastrectomy functions as a restrictive procedure, removal of a large part of the gastric fundus leads to decreased levels of ghrelin and possibly is a cause of appetite suppression.

The role of sleeve gastrectomy as a definitive procedure for the treatment of reflux disease has not been studied in the literature. Initial studies comparing LAGB with sleeve gastrectomy reported a higher incidence of reflux disease at 1 year and also a high incidence of the development of erosive esophagitis. On long-term follow-up of 3 years in the same cohort, authors reported that only 3.1% reported GERD in the sleeve gastrectomy population while 20.% reported it following LAGB. This benefit at 3 years was because of more weight loss in the sleeve gastrectomy population compared to LAGB.[18] Studies also compared sleeve gastrectomy with gastric bypass in morbidly obese patients with erosive esophagitis. One year following bariatric intervention, the percentage of patients with erosive esophagitis rose in the sleeve gastrectomy group to 45% from 18% preoperatively and decreased in the gastric bypass group to 6% from 28%. The prevalence of erosive esophagitis was significantly different in the post-sleeve vs post-bypass group ($p<.001$).[19]

The incidence of GERD after sleeve gastrectomy can be variable depending on the following factors: the degree of weight loss after sleeve gastrectomy and technical factors relating to the construct of the sleeve (affected by the shape and size of the bougie). Technical factors such as the shape of the sleeve gastrectomy have been implicated in numerous studies as an important factor for the development of reflux. The shape can be completely tubular or with either a superior or inferior pouch, usually demonstrated on a gastrograffin evaluation. It has been reported that the intensity of regurgitation and vomiting was higher in patients with either a tubular pattern or a superior pouch compared to patients with an inferior pouch.[20]

Sleeve gastrectomy is increasingly performed as a weight loss procedure. It has been well established that weight loss outcomes at 1 year are similar to RYGB. However, long-term outcomes are still not well established. Its role in the treatment of reflux disease is not well reported in the literature. Currently available data are conflicting and several studies even report an increased prevalence in esophageal erosions and GERD symptoms in patients undergoing sleeve gastrectomy. Uncertainty also exists regarding the size and shape of the sleeve gastrectomy and its impact in the development or resolution of reflux. Until these questions are answered with good mechanistic studies, the role of sleeve gastrectomy in reflux patients with morbid obesity is controversial, and these patients should be well informed about alternative options such as gastric bypass.

Roux-en-Y Gastric Bypass

Gastric bypass is the most commonly performed weight loss procedure. The procedure involves reducing gastric volume by creating a small pouch in the proximal stomach and anastomosing it with jejunum, bypassing the remainder of the stomach and duodenum. Gastric bypass produces weight loss secondary to both restrictive (small gastric pouch) and malabsorptive (intestinal bypass decreases the calorie absorption) mechanisms.

Gastric bypass has been shown to decrease reflux and is considered to be the treatment of choice for patients with reflux disease associated with morbid obesity. Several mechanisms have been implicated in reflux disease, including exclusion of the acid-producing part of the stomach, reduction in intra-abdominal pressure, and improvement in the diaphragm and LES complex.

A study investigating the effects of RYGB in 57 patients with recalcitrant GERD in morbidly obese patients (BMI > 35) reported that the incidence of reflux was reduced to 5% from 84% before the surgery.[21] Based on these results, the authors concluded that laparoscopic RYGB should be considered for treating GERD in morbidly obese patients. Similarly, patients who underwent RYGB had a significant improvement in postoperative GERD-related symptoms. Symptomatic improvement was significant in terms of heartburn, which decreased to 22% from 87% preoperatively, and the incidence of aspiration, which was decreased to 2% after the procedure. The study concluded that RYGB not only provided improvement in terms of the symptoms related to reflux, but also decreased the incidence of use of proton pump inhibitors and complications associated with reflux disease such as aspiration.[22] This benefit was seen in addition to the benefits commonly associated with gastric bypass in terms of metabolic syndrome. A study by Portmann et al included 606 patients, of which 259 reported reflux related symptoms before surgery. Within 3 months after surgery the majority of these patients showed a significant improvement in reflux-related symptoms and after long-term follow-up of 19 months, 94% of the patients available for follow-up reported symptomatic improvement compared to the preoperative assessment.[23] The literature suggests that patients with morbid obesity and reflux disease should consider RYGB because of a higher success rate in terms of symptomatic improvement and also overall quality of life.

RYGB has been shown to improve GERD immediately after the procedure secondary to the exclusion of the acid-producing portion of the stomach. However, weight loss and reduction of intra-abdominal pressure on a long-term basis are proposed to improve LES mechanisms and decrease the incidence of reflux disease.

Roux-en-Y Gastric Bypass for Revision

RYGB has also been increasingly performed as a salvage operation after failed weight loss procedures such as sleeve gastrectomy, LAGB, or VBG, as well as following a failed primary antireflux procedure such as fundoplication.

A study by Langer et al reported that patients who have reflux disease confirmed by pH monitoring before conversion to gastric bypass had complete resolution of reflux disease after the procedure.[24] The other patients who had symptoms of reflux disease and were on acid suppressive medication with a negative pH study reported resolution of symptoms and discontinuation of medications after the procedure. In addition, studies also published reported the success of converting VBG to RYGB. VBG was the primary weight loss operation in the mid 1980s and early 1990s. However, patients who underwent this procedure later increasingly presented with weight gain and worsening of reflux disease.[25] Gagne et al reported results of laparoscopic revision of VBG to RYGB in 105 patients. This study showed that 95% of patients reported marked improvement of reflux symptoms after conversion to gastric bypass with the additional benefit of weight loss and reversal of weight-related comorbidities.[26] These results showed that patients with failed VBG or complications associated with VBG can be converted to gastric bypass with good patient satisfaction. However, the literature has a mixed view in terms of complications associated with these revisional procedures. The current series reported a lower overall complications rate of less than 10%, compared to the other series, which reported complication rates greater than 30%, raising concerns associated with these revisions and reoperations.

The role of RYGB in patients with previous fundoplication has also been reported in the literature. Patients with multiple previous foregut procedures, associated morbid obesity, and complex anatomy can be a significant challenge in terms of symptomatic improvement. Long-term results in these patients have shown significant improvement in reflux-related symptoms and patient satisfaction with takedown of fundoplication and conversion to a Roux-en-Y gastrojejunostomy.[12] However, controversy exists regarding the size of the gastric pouch and the long-term metabolic complications associated with these procedures. If a failed fundoplication is associated with morbid obesity and its related metabolic complications, conversion to gastric bypass is, though technically challenging, associated with good long-term success.[13]

With an aim to achieve successful weight loss and improvement of reflux-related symptoms, patients who have failed other weight loss procedures, such as gastric banding, sleeve gastrectomy, or VBG, with reflux disease can be safely converted to an RYGB with significant improvement in both reflux-related symptoms and weight loss.

Summary

While the workup of reflux in the morbidly obese is the same as in patients of normal body mass, the management of GERD in the morbidly obese population requires an understanding of how the 2 disease processes and their surgical treatments are intertwined. In particular, typical procedures aimed at augmenting the LES and the angle of His are prone to failure in the morbidly obese population due to the chronic wear and tear at the augmented LES. A gastric bypass is an excellent acid/bile diversionary procedure that treats both reflux and morbid obesity.

In less than ideal situations, other resectional procedures such as esophagectomy or gastrectomy with gastrojejunostomy may need to be considered.

References

1. Corley DA, Kubo AI. Body mass index and gastroesophageal reflux disease: a systematic review and meta-analysis. *Am J Gastroenterol.* 2006;108:2619-2628.
2. Prachand VN, Ward M, Alverdy JC. Duodenal switch provides superior resolution of metabolic comorbidities independent of weight loss in the super-obese (BMI > or = 50 kg/m2) compared with gastric bypass. *J Gastrointest Surg.* 2010;14:211-220.
3. El-Serag HB. Obesity and disease of the esophagus and colon. Gastroenterol Clin North Am. 2005;34:63-82.
4. El-Serag HB, Tran T, Richardson P, et al. Anthropometric correlates of intragastric pressure. *Scand J Gastroenterol.* 2006;41:881-891.
5. Kahrilas PJ. Clinical practice gastroesophageal reflux disease. *N Engl J Med.* 2008;359:1700-1707.
6. El-Serag HB, Ergun GA, Pandolfino J, et al. Obesity increases esophageal acid exposure. *Gut.* 2007;56:749-755.
7. Jaffin BW, Knoepflmacher P, Greenstein R. High prevalence of asymptomatic esophageal motility disorders among morbidly obese patients. *Obes Surg.* 1999;9:390-395.
8. Johnson LF, DeMeester TR. Development of the 24-hour intra-esophageal pH monitoring composite scoring system. In: DeMeester TR, Skinner DB, eds. *Esophageal Disorders: Pathophysiology and Therapy.* New York, NY: Raven Press; 1985:561-570.
9. Tolone S, Limongelli P, del Genio G, et al. Gastroesophageal reflux and obesity: do we need to perform reflux testing in all candidates to bariatric surgery? *Inter J Surg.* 2014;12(Suppl 1):S173-S177.

10. Dallemagne B, Weerts J, Markiewicz S, et al. Clinical results of laparoscopic fundoplication at ten years after surgery. *Surg Endosc.* 2006;20:159-165.
11. Salminen P, Hurme S, Ovaska J. Fifteen-year outcome of laparoscopic and open Nissen fundoplication: a randomized clinical trial. *Ann Thorac Surg.* 2012;93:228-233.
12. Juhasz A, Sundaram A, Hoshino M, Lee T, Filipi C, Mittal S. Endoscopic assessment of failed fundoplication: a case for standardization. *Surg Endosc.* 2011;25:3761-3766.
13. Kellogg T, Andrade R, Maddaus M, Slusark S, Buchwald H, Ikramuddin S. Anatomic findings and outcomes after antireflux procedures in morbidly obese patients undergoing laparoscopic conversion to Roux-en-Y gastric bypass. *Surg Obes Relat Dis.* 2007;3:52-57.
14. Morgenthal C, Lin E, Shane M, Hunter J, Smith C. Who will fail laparoscopic Nissen fundoplication? Preoperative prediction of long-term outcomes. *Surg Endosc.* 2007;21:1978-1984.
15. Dixon JB, O'Brien PE. Gastroesophageal reflux in obesity: the effect of lap-band placement. *Obes Surg.* 1999;9:527-531.
16. Tolonen P, Victorzon M, Niemi R, Mäkelä J. Does gastric banding for morbid obesity reduce or increase gastroesophageal reflux? *Obes Surg.* 2006;16:1469-1474.
17. de Jong JR, Besselink MG, van Ramshorst B, et al. Effects of adjustable gastric banding on gastroesophageal reflux and esophageal motility: a systematic review. *Obes Rev.* 2010;11:297-305.
18. Himpens J, Dapri G, Cadière GB. A prospective randomized study between laparoscopic gastric banding and laparoscopic isolated sleeve gastrectomy: results after 1 and 3 years. *Obes Surg.* 2006;16:1450-1456.
19. Miguel GP, Azevedo JL, de Souza PH, et al. Erosive esophagitis after bariatric surgery: banded vertical gastrectomy versus banded Roux-en-Y gastric bypass. *Obes Surg.* 2011;21:167-172.
20. Lazoura O, Zacharoulis D, Triantafyllidis G, et al. Symptoms of gastroesophageal reflux following laparoscopic sleeve gastrectomy are related to the final shape of the sleeve as depicted by radiology. *Obes Surg.* 2011;21:295-299.
21. Perry Y, Courcoulas AP, Fernando HC, et al. Laparoscopic Roux en-Y gastric bypass for recalcitrant gastroesophageal reflux disease in morbidly obese patients. *JSLS.* 2004;8:19-23.
22. Smith SC, Edwards CB, Goodman GN. Symptomatic and clinical improvement in morbidly obese patients with gastroesophageal reflux disease following Roux-en-Y gastric bypass. *Obes Surg.* 1997;7:479-484.
23. Clements RH, Gonzalez QH, Foster A, et al. Gastrointestinal symptoms are more intense in morbidly obese patients and are improved with laparoscopic Roux-en-Y gastric bypass. *Obes Surg.* 2003;13:610-614.
24. Langer FB, Bohdjalian A, Shakeri-Leidenmühler S, et al. Conversion from sleeve gastrectomy to Roux-en-Y gastric bypass–indications and outcome. *Obes Surg.* 2010;20:835-840.
25. Rebecchi F, Rocchietto S, Giaccone C, et al. Gastroesophageal reflux disease and esophageal motility in morbidly obese patients submitted to laparoscopic adjustable silicone gastric banding or laparoscopic vertical banded gastroplasty. *Surg Endosc.* 2011;25:795-803.
26. Gagné DJ, Dovec E, Urbandt JE. Laparoscopic revision of vertical banded gastroplasty to Roux-en-Y gastric bypass: outcomes of 105 patients. *Surg Obes Relat Dis.* 2011;7:493-499.

26

Psychological Issues in the Bariatric Surgery Patient

Stephanie Sogg, PhD and Kelli E. Friedman, PhD

Few other medical treatments are as intricately intertwined with psychological and behavioral factors as weight loss surgery (WLS).[1] In WLS, successful outcomes are not purely related to the surgical procedures themselves; optimal long-term surgical outcomes require significant and life-long behavioral and dietary changes, and surgery often has wide-ranging and profound psychosocial effects. It is important for physicians working with the WLS population to have some familiarity with the psychosocial aspects of obesity and WLS to best assist their patients with the many changes and potential challenges associated with surgery.

Presurgical Considerations

Psychiatric Comorbidities of Obesity

Severe obesity is often associated with psychiatric comorbidities, and there seems to be a high rate of psychopathology in patients who are evaluated for WLS.[1] The prevalence of psychiatric comorbidity in obesity is likely related to numerous factors, including weight-based stigmatization, impaired health-related quality of life, functional impairment, and the chronic medical conditions that often accompany obesity.

Studies of both community-based samples and patients seeking obesity treatment find elevated rates of affective, anxiety, and eating disorders in individuals with obesity, compared to average-weight individuals. This association seems to be even stronger at severe levels of obesity,[2] particularly for depression. Research suggests that the association between obesity and depression is likely bidirectional, with individuals who have obesity being at higher risk of developing depression over time and those with depression at an increased risk of developing obesity.[3]

Anxiety disorders have also been found to be more prevalent both in individuals with obesity and in patients presenting for WLS than they are in the general population; one well-designed study of patients seeking WLS found that anxiety disorders were the most common psychiatric

Forse RA, Apovian CM, eds.
Bariatric Surgery: What Every Provider Needs to Know (pp 311-318).

disorder observed in this population.[4] For some, anxiety may be related to embarrassment about weight, which sometimes engenders both social distress and associated avoidant behaviors, while for others, anxiety symptoms are unrelated to the obesity but may represent barriers to maintaining behaviors that would promote a healthier weight.

Rates of eating pathology have been found to be higher in individuals with obesity than in the general population[5]; however, while many individuals with obesity may report unhealthy or unstructured eating habits, only a subset of individuals with obesity will also meet criteria for an eating disorder. Binge eating disorder is the eating disorder most commonly observed among bariatric surgery patients, with prevalence estimates ranging from 2% to 49% depending on mode of assessment.[5] As is the case with depression, the relationship between binge eating disorder and obesity may be bidirectional. Binge eating disorder may contribute to an individual's obesity, but obesity also may contribute to binge eating through factors such as body image dissatisfaction and frustration with the ineffectiveness of behavioral weight loss efforts, which may exacerbate an eating style characterized by restriction and deprivation alternating with loss of control and overeating.

Given the elevated rates of psychopathology observed in patients presenting for surgery, it is not surprising that a significant percentage of these patients are engaged in mental health treatment at the time of their presurgical psychological evaluation. Data indicate the most common mode of mental health treatment for these patients is psychotropic medication, with a much smaller percentage of patients enrolled in treatment with a mental health provider.[6]

It should be noted that bariatric behavioral health providers do not necessarily consider existing psychopathology, even when relatively severe, to be a definitive contraindication for surgery.[1] Mediating factors, such as how well managed the patient's symptoms are, and whether the patient is in adequate treatment for these symptoms, are important to consider; one of the roles of the bariatric behavioral health provider is to assist the patient in optimizing treatment for his or her symptoms in preparation for WLS.

Other Relevant Psychosocial Issues

In addition to psychopathology, individuals with obesity experience other psychosocial challenges. Weight-based stigmatization has been argued to be "the last socially acceptable form of prejudice,"[7] and remains quite common. This type of stigmatization can affect numerous aspects of life for the individual with obesity, including social, educational, and occupational functioning, as well as the quality of and access to medical care.[8] Weight bias has been found to be common even in medical professionals who specialize in obesity.[9] This type of stigmatization is important to consider because it likely contributes to a variety of other psychological concerns, including poor weight-related and general quality of life, mood and anxiety symptoms, and other psychosocial issues.

Generally, it appears that quality of life in patients seeking WLS is lower than that observed in the general population, and quality of life seems to worsen with increasing severity of obesity. Among individuals with obesity, WLS patients present with the most significantly impaired quality of life.[10] This should not be surprising, given that the decision to seek surgery is often motivated in large part by the impact that weight is having on many aspects of the patient's day-to-day functioning (eg, hygiene, mobility, health, social relationships, activity level).

The negative health effects of obesity are well documented, and many patients who present for surgery have multiple chronic medical comorbidities that require daily treatment and regular monitoring. Thus, not only does obesity impact an individual's functioning directly, but it also exerts indirect effects through impaired health and many of the aforementioned issues.

Although bariatric surgery has been demonstrated to be the most effective, durable treatment for obesity currently available, it often takes patients months, years, or even decades to decide to pursue surgery. For most patients, this is not a decision that is made lightly, and is only sought after multiple behavioral attempts have proven to be ineffective.[11] Although it has been clearly demonstrated that weight is strongly biologically determined, many patients experience their inability to lose weight through nonsurgical means as a "failure"; these patients often express a desire to make more attempts to "do it on my own" before pursuing WLS, which some patients conceptualize as "giving up."

Although patients have often devoted a good deal of thought and research to the decision to undergo WLS, the members of their social support network may not be supportive of this decision. This can be problematic, as WLS entails a significant life change not only for patients themselves, but also for their significant others. The patient's decision to undergo WLS may be met with resistance from friends and family, often related to misinformation about surgery or concerns with how surgery will negatively impact their own lives. Surgery should be undertaken at a time when the patient has at least some support for surgery from friends and family, as social support is needed both before and after a life-changing procedure like bariatric surgery.

Education, Preparation, and Informed Consent

Bariatric surgery not only affects but is also greatly affected by psychological and behavioral factors.[1] Unlike most other surgical procedures, WLS entails significant behavioral changes that must be sustained throughout one's life to ensure optimal surgical safety and success. Thus, it is essential that WLS patients are well informed about the procedure they plan to undergo; this is also a necessary component of the informed consent process. Education about surgery is typically obtained through both formal and informal means (eg, most programs require patients to attend an information session about surgery, and patients often peruse various websites or talk to people they know who have had WLS for information). Education should also be incorporated at several points during the various presurgical assessments with providers of relevant disciplines (eg, dietician, surgeon, behavioral health provider) that are typically required. However, for many patients, the first formal discussion about WLS takes place with their primary care or specialist physician, so it is important that all providers working with patients with obesity be prepared to provide basic information and education about WLS.

Prior to surgery, it can be useful to help the patient to prepare by proactively working to change relevant behaviors, which may be done during the various presurgical assessments. These behaviors include not only eating patterns and physical activity, but also may include addressing substance use (eg, tobacco, drug, or alcohol use), caffeine consumption, organizational strategies, communication patterns, etc. When done well, the presurgical psychological evaluation can be used as an intervention in its own right to promote this type of change.[1] Ideally, the psychological evaluation is not only a time to gather information about the patient, but also represents an ideal opportunity to provide education, as well as interventions that may assist with the transition to post-surgery life, which requires profound behavioral changes for all patients.

Post-Surgical Issues

Most patients report a host of positive changes after WLS, including improvements in health, mobility, self-image, and interpersonal relationships. However, a wide variety of psychosocial issues may arise after WLS, which can be broadly grouped into 3 different domains: psychological, interpersonal, and behavioral. Each domain will be considered separately below.

Psychological Issues

As noted above, individuals with severe obesity are at increased risk for psychiatric comorbidities, such as mood, anxiety, and eating disorders. Research has shown that, particularly in the case of depression, psychiatric functioning tends to improve significantly with weight loss after WLS.[12] However, several studies have found that these improvements tend to deteriorate somewhat 1 to 2 years after surgery,[13] when weight loss slows or regains may begin, appetite and capacity for eating increase, and the post-surgical changes feel less new and exciting. Further, it has been found that though presurgical psychopathology does not predict postoperative weight loss (at least in the relatively short term), when psychopathology is present after surgery, weight loss outcomes may be compromised.[12] Additionally, practitioners must be aware that certain medications, including some psychotropic medications, may require adjustment after WLS procedures such as Roux-en-Y gastric bypass (RYGB), biliopancreatic diversion with duodenal switch (BPD-DS), and laparoscopic sleeve gastrectomy (LSG) because of changes in absorptive process along the digestive tract,[14] with potential for decreased effectiveness of certain medications. While the use of many types of medications (eg, antidiabetic, antihypertensive) is often decreased after surgery, this has not been found to be the case for antidepressants,[15] suggesting that depression may continue in the postoperative period and likely was not solely related to weight for a portion of WLS patients. Although it is rare for patients to experience significant psychiatric decompensation after surgery, it should be noted that a few epidemiological studies have found evidence suggesting that risk for suicide may be elevated after WLS,[16] though the reasons for an association between WLS and suicide remain uncertain.

Certain psychological challenges may arise after surgery as a consequence of the significant changes that take place in patients' eating behaviors. Although typically patients report that their preference for unhealthy foods decreases and their preference for healthy foods increases after surgery, occasionally patients struggle with the required dietary changes. Most often, patients report that they do not tend to crave or be as interested in the same types of food as before surgery, and that when they do eat a less-healthy food, they find that they are satisfied with moderate amounts. Patients often describe feeling quite freed from constant thoughts about food and dieting after surgery. However, because the suggested life-long postoperative eating regimen emphasizes healthy eating and avoidance of high-fat, high-calorie foods, and because patients' eating is also limited by pouch size and, occasionally, various food intolerances, WLS patients may report feelings of loss or deprivation after surgery.

For some patients, post-WLS eating changes present a different dilemma. Patients who tended to rely heavily on eating as their primary means of coping with emotions before surgery may find themselves more vulnerable to emotional dysregulation after surgery. Many of these patients report that they were not even aware of their presurgical tendency to use eating as a coping mechanism until after surgery, when they were left to deal with emotions without food as a resource.

Some postoperative psychological issues revolve around the weight loss itself. Similar to patients in behavioral weight loss programs, WLS patients almost universally hold unrealistic weight loss expectations before treatment, which tend to be highly resistant to modification, even in the face of information about typical surgical weight loss outcomes.[17] Thus, a number of patients express disappointment with their weight loss results, despite achieving medically beneficial and statistically typical or even better-than-typical weight loss; this disappointment is magnified in cases in which some of the lost weight is regained over time, which is not an unusual occurrence. Still other patients appreciate their significant weight loss, but may be disappointed to find that some of their preexisting problems were not ameliorated by the weight loss alone (eg, depression, relationship issues).

Even when post-WLS weight loss is significant, it is quite common for patients to report a powerful fear of regaining the weight that was lost. The nearly universal nature of this phenomenon is related, at least in part, to the fact that, given the limited effectiveness of behavioral weight loss interventions for those with severe obesity, WLS patients typically have a history of losing weight only to gain it back, often multiple times. Patients frequently report that they fear another "failure," or appearing to fail in the eyes of others. This fear of weight regain can, in rare cases, lead patients to adopt a hypervigilant approach to eating and weight, which, in more severe cases, can be manifested in the form of overly restrictive eating patterns or even compensatory behaviors such as inducing vomiting or chewing food and then spitting it out to avoid gaining weight.[18]

Because most WLS patients lose a significant amount of weight after surgery, it is common for them to experience redundant, hanging, or "loose" skin. Reactions to loose skin after WLS vary—some patients are not distressed by it at all, or even experience it as a way of visually measuring their weight loss success, while a subset of patients find the excess skin to be extremely distressing, and experience significant body image dissatisfaction, sometimes to the extent that these patients will limit their social activities, wardrobe choices, and even sexual activities as a result. Overall, the majority of patients do express a certain degree of dissatisfaction with excess skin, but most do not seem to be impaired in their functioning by their distress.

Interpersonal Issues

After WLS, a variety of factors, including improved daily functioning, increased energy, dramatically changed appearance, and significant changes in eating habits, may lead to changes in the interpersonal realm. On the most basic level, some patients find it difficult to adjust to increased attention from other people, and may feel uncomfortable about receiving comments about their appearance, even when these comments are positive. In addition, some patients notice that other people, whether they were previously known to the patient or not, treat them with more courtesy, respect, and interest after surgery. Although this would be expected to be a positive change, some patients report experiencing anger and resentment that people are treating them more positively because of a change in their appearance. It is important to note that the perceived change in how others act toward the patient after surgery may be at least partly related to improvements in the patient's own level of confidence, which often leads him or her to interact with others in a way that elicits more positive responses.

For some patients, an increase in positive attention may actually feel threatening. Although research suggests that patients with a history of sexual abuse or trauma have equally good WLS outcomes as patients without such a history, significant weight loss may, for some patients, lead to a sense of increased vulnerability, particularly when weight loss is accompanied by an increase in romantic or sexual attention from others. For some patients with a trauma history, significant weight loss may lead to an exacerbation or recurrence of post-traumatic stress disorder symptoms.

WLS patients also occasionally contend with reactions from other people who may be insensitive, or may at least be perceived that way. For instance, some WLS patients report that they are frequently asked intrusive questions, such as inquiries about how much weight they have lost or how they lost it. It is also common to hear that patients' friends and loved ones are closely monitoring and commenting on their food intake; although this often reflects caring and concern, this "food policing" may be done or experienced in an intrusive or critical manner. At the other end of the spectrum, some patients report that friends or loved ones resent the loss of an "eating buddy," or that changes in their own eating habits lead to discomfort or conflict during social eating occasions. Friends and family members may continue to offer unhealthy foods, or encourage the patient to eat more, and the patient may find it difficult to set limits in a way that is both effective and respectful. Another significant issue is the feedback that some WLS patients report receiving from others that they have "taken the easy way out" in losing weight with surgery, rather than through nonsurgical means. This type of comment is rooted in a general misinformation among the lay population regarding the strong influence of biological/genetic factors on obesity, as well as the empirically demonstrated ineffectiveness of nonsurgical weight loss interventions. These comments are often the most hurtful to WLS patients, as they frequently share these mistaken beliefs about obesity themselves.

The significant weight loss after WLS may at times lead to disruptions in patients' relationships with friends and/or family. All relationships, whether healthy or otherwise, involve an established set of dynamics between the participants in that relationship, and when one of the individuals experiences a dramatic change in body shape or level of functioning, the relationship homeostasis that had long been established may become destabilized. In healthy, supportive relationships, this type of challenge is normally easily overcome through good communication and collaborative problem solving. However, some relationships are vulnerable to the deleterious effects of changing dynamics. For instance, patients sometimes note that before WLS, they played a role within their family or circle of friends as "the fat one," someone who might have been nonthreatening, posed little competition for attention, or made few demands. When the patient loses weight after surgery, he or she no longer fits into this role, and friends and family members may feel resentful or threatened. It is frequently observed that after WLS, as patients' self-regard and energy level increase significantly, they are more able to prioritize their own needs appropriately, and they often become less tolerant of unacceptable treatment by others and less willing to subjugate their own preferences. Although this is a healthy, desirable change, it may be disruptive in relationships in which the other participant has grown used to the patient doing most of the giving or tolerating various types of behavior on the part of friends or relatives. In extreme cases, patients choose to end relationships with individuals whom they realize were not treating them appropriately. In other cases, patients report that a friend or relative has avoided them or even cut ties with the patient since surgery, because of an inability to tolerate the changes that have occurred.

Research examining the effects of WLS on patients' romantic relationships suggests that strong relationships tend to get stronger, while unhealthy relationships often suffer.[19] Some patients report that as they lose weight, their spouses or partners experience jealousy or insecurity. In cases in which the patient's functioning was significantly limited by obesity and related comorbidities, the patient's partner may have become accustomed to the helping role. As the patient's health and functioning improve, his or her partner may feel threatened at the prospect of no longer being needed. Although this is not a common occurrence, there are some cases in which patients come to realize that, before surgery, they chose, or stayed with, a partner whom they did not really believe was right for them, because they worried that their romantic options were limited by their obesity, and as they lose weight, they become less willing to stay with that partner. In rare cases, patients choose to end their marriages or partnerships. Even in cases in which this represents a desirable and positive outcome, it can be a very disruptive one as well.

Challenges may also arise for patients who are starting romantic relationships after WLS. WLS patients who have reached adulthood with little or no history of dating or romantic relationships, or those for whom it has been many years since they participated in the world of dating, may find entering or reentering this world to be challenging, as their dating-related knowledge and skills may be lacking or rusty. Patients may also struggle with the question of whether and when to tell a new partner that they have had surgery, how to manage eating in social situations, etc.

Behavioral Issues

As time passes after WLS, a variety of behavioral issues may arise. Most commonly seen are difficulties with adhering to the post-WLS behavioral regimen, which includes multiple domains such as consuming adequate protein and fluids, eating in a structured way at intervals throughout the day, taking nutritional supplements, and engaging in consistent physical activity. Nonadherence to post-WLS behavioral guidelines may stem from one or more of a variety of underlying challenges. For some patients, there may be logistical barriers to adhering to the various behavioral guidelines, such as busy schedules, lack of support from significant others, environments that promote unhealthy and/or unstructured eating, or poor access to appropriate means of engaging in physical activity. For other patients, preexisting mental health conditions such as depression or anxiety may interfere through their effects on motivation, self-efficacy, or other factors. In many cases, nonadherence to post-WLS behavioral guidelines can be traced to simple "behavioral fatigue"[20]—in other words, it is challenging to consistently and permanently maintain multiple healthy behaviors every day, and behavioral deterioration may occur in even the most motivated patients.

Some patients experience symptoms of disordered eating after WLS. For many of these patients, some form of eating pathology was present before surgery (eg, binge or emotionally triggered eating, night eating syndrome). A great deal of research has examined whether presurgical eating pathology predicts behavioral or weight loss outcomes after surgery. Taken together, the results of these studies suggest that baseline eating pathology is not a reliable predictor of post-surgical weight loss.[5] Further, there is evidence that eating pathology tends to remit during the first 6 to 12 months after surgery.[21] However, some patients with baseline eating pathology will experience a recurrence of these symptoms in the long term after surgery, albeit often in somewhat different form. For instance, patients may not be able to consume objectively large amounts of food after surgery, and thus might not exhibit binge eating, but they may continue to use eating as a way of coping with negative emotions, or to experience eating episodes characterized by loss of control, a cardinal feature of a binge episode. Few studies have examined the emergence or recurrence of eating pathology after WLS, but those that do exist suggest that this does happen in some cases, and when it does, it tends to be associated with poorer weight loss and psychosocial outcomes in the long term.[5]

Although less commonly observed, on occasion patients develop symptoms that resemble anorexia or bulimia nervosa after WLS; however, most published literature on this topic consists of case reports. As noted, fear of weight regain is quite common among post-WLS patients, and in more severe cases, this fear may manifest in an overly restrictive eating style and preoccupation with weight that can reach clinical levels of severity and pose a threat to the patient's health.[22] It has also been observed that the involuntary vomiting that many patients experience after WLS may evolve into a pattern of deliberate vomiting due to weight or shape concerns for some patients.[18]

Another concerning issue that arises in a subset of patients after WLS is addictive behavior, which has received increased attention in the scientific and popular media in recent years. This is most commonly manifested in the misuse of alcohol, which may be due to the changed pharmacodynamics of alcohol after procedures such as RYGB and LSG, in which it has been observed in postoperative patients that after consuming alcohol, blood alcohol levels reach a higher peak more rapidly than in nonoperated individuals.[23] Although there is some risk of relapse for individuals who struggled with substance abuse before WLS, it has also been demonstrated that some individuals experience new-onset problem drinking after surgery.[23] Misuse of other drugs, such as opiate pain medications, as well as compulsive (ie, addictive) engagement in other behaviors, such as shopping, gambling, shoplifting, and sexual promiscuity, have also been reported.[24] Although the mechanisms underlying this type of complication have yet to be fully elucidated, there is some evidence that WLS promotes changes in brain reward pathways,[25] which may contribute to these behavioral phenomena. Again, it should be noted that the overwhelming majority of patients do not develop any addictive behaviors post surgery.

Summary

This chapter has reviewed numerous behavioral and psychological factors related to WLS. While it is important for practitioners to be aware of and alert to these factors, it is also important to keep in mind that the overwhelming majority of patients who undergo WLS have extremely positive experiences in both the short and long term. For most, surgery not only improves physical health, but also dramatically improves psychological functioning and quality of life. When asked whether they have any regrets about undergoing WLS, it is not uncommon for patients to indicate that their biggest regret about WLS is that they did not do so sooner.

References

1. Sogg S, Mori DL. Psychosocial evaluation for bariatric surgery: the Boston interview and opportunities for intervention. *Obes Surg.* 2009;19(3):369-377.
2. Wadden TA, Butryn ML, Sarwer DB, et al. Comparison of psychosocial status in treatment-seeking women with class III vs. class I-II obesity. *Obesity.* 2006;14(Suppl 2):90S-98S.
3. Luppino FS, de Wit LM, Bouvy PF, et al. Overweight, obesity, and depression: a systematic review and meta-analysis of longitudinal studies. *Arch Gen Psychiatry.* 2010;67(3):220-229.
4. Kalarchian MA, Marcus MD, Levine MD, et al. Psychiatric disorders among bariatric surgery candidates: relationship to obesity and functional health status. *Am J Psychiatry.* 2007;164(2):328-334.
5. Niego SH, Kofman MD, Weiss JJ, Geliebter A. Binge eating in the bariatric surgery population: a review of the literature. *Int J Eat Disord.* 2007;40(4):349-359.
6. Friedman KE, Applegate KL, Grant J. Who is adherent with preoperative psychological treatment recommendations among weight loss surgery candidates? *Surg Obes Relat Dis.* 2007;3(3):376-382.
7. Sobal J, Stunkard AJ. Socioeconomic status and obesity: a review of the literature. *Psychol Bull.* 1989;105(2):260-275.
8. Puhl RM, Heuer CA. The stigma of obesity: a review and update. *Obesity.* 2009;17(5):941-964.
9. Teachman BA, Brownell KD. Implicit anti-fat bias among health professionals: is anyone immune? *Int J Obes Relat Metab Disord.* 2001;25(10):1525-1531.
10. Kolotkin RL, Crosby RD, Pendleton R, Strong M, Gress RE, Adams T. Health-related quality of life in patients seeking gastric bypass surgery vs non-treatment-seeking controls. *Obes Surg.* 2003;13(3):371-377.
11. Gibbons LM, Sarwer DB, Crerand CE, et al. Previous weight loss experiences of bariatric surgery candidates: how much have patients dieted prior to surgery? *Surg Obes Relat Dis.* 2006;2(2):159-164.
12. de Zwaan M, Enderle J, Wagner S, et al. Anxiety and depression in bariatric surgery patients: a prospective, follow-up study using structured clinical interviews. *J Affect Disord.* 2011;133(1-2):61-68.
13. Bocchieri LE, Meana M, Fisher BL. A review of psychosocial outcomes of surgery for morbid obesity. *J Psychosom Res.* 2002;52(3):155-165.
14. Roerig JL, Steffen K, Zimmerman C, Mitchell JE, Crosby RD, Cao L. Preliminary comparison of sertraline levels in postbariatric surgery patients versus matched nonsurgical cohort. *Surg Obes Relat Dis.* 2012;8(1):62-66.
15. Steffen KJ, Roerig JL, Engel SG. Psychpharmacology pre- and postbariatric surgery. In: Mitchell J, De Zwaan M, eds. *Psychosocial Assessment and Treatment of Bariatric Surgery Patients.* New York, NY: Routledge; 2011:115-130.
16. Tindle HA, Omalu B, Courcoulas A, Marcus M, Hammers J, Kuller LH. Risk of suicide after long-term follow-up from bariatric surgery. *Am J Med.* 2010;123(11):1036-1042.
17. Bauchowitz A, Azarbad L, Day K, Gonder-Frederick L. Evaluation of expectations and knowledge in bariatric surgery patients. *Surg Obes Relat Dis.* 2007;3(5):554-558.
18. de Zwaan M, Hilbert A, Swan-Kremeier L, et al. Comprehensive interview assessment of eating behavior 18-35 months after gastric bypass surgery for morbid obesity. *Surg Obes Relat Dis.* 2010;6(1):79-85.
19. Wadden TA, Sarwer DB, Womble LG, Foster GD, McGuckin BG, Schimmel A. Psychosocial aspects of obesity and obesity surgery. *Surg Clin North Am.* 2001;81(5):1001-1024.
20. Wadden TA, Butryn ML, Byrne KJ. Efficacy of lifestyle modification for long-term weight control. *Obes Res.* 2004;12(Suppl):151S-162S.
21. Wadden TA, Faulconbridge LF, Jones-Corneille LR, et al. Binge eating disorder and the outcome of bariatric surgery at one year: a prospective, observational study. *Obesity.* 2011;19(6):1220-1228.
22. Rusch MD, Andris D. Maladaptive eating patterns after weight-loss surgery. *Nutr Clin Pract.* 2007;22(1):41-49.
23. King W, Chen J, Mitchell J, et al. Prevalence of alcohol use disorders before and after bariatric surgery. *JAMA.* 2012;307(23):2516-2525.
24. Conason A, Teixeira J, Hsu CH, Puma L, Knafo D, Geliebter A. Substance use following bariatric weight loss surgery. *JAMA Surg.* 2013;148(2):145-150.
25. Ochner CN, Kwok Y, Conceicao E, et al. Selective reduction in neural responses to high calorie foods following gastric bypass surgery. *Ann Surg.* 2011;253(3):502-507.

Financial Disclosures

Dr. Nadia N. Ahmad is a consultant for Johnson & Johnson.

Dr. Venkata M. Alla has no financial or proprietary interest in the materials presented herein.

Dr. Caroline M. Apovian has participated on advisory boards for Amylin, Merck, Johnson and Johnson, Arena, Nutrisystem, Zafgen, Sanofi-Aventis, Orexigen, EnteroMedics, GI Dynamics, Scientific Intake, Gelesis and Novo Nordisk. She has received research funding from Eli Lilly, Amylin, Aspire Bariatrics, GI Dynamics, Pfizer, Sanofi-Aventis, Orexigen, MetaProteomics, Takeda, the Dr. Robert C. and Veronica Atkins Foundation and MYOS Corporation. Dr. Apovian is currently on the Takeda Speakers Bureau for the medication Contrave. She has an ownership interest in Science-Smart LLC.

Dr. Dustin M. Bermudez has no financial or proprietary interest in the materials presented herein.

Dr. George L. Blackburn has no financial or proprietary interest in the materials presented herein.

Dr. Stacy A. Brethauer has no financial or proprietary interest in the materials presented herein.

Dr. W. Scott Butsch has no financial or proprietary interest in the materials presented herein.

Dr. Judy Y. R. Chen has no financial or proprietary interest in the materials presented herein.

Dr. Elizabeth Colsen has no financial or proprietary interest in the materials presented herein.

Dr. Yaniv Cozacov has no financial or proprietary interest in the materials presented herein.

Dr. Attila Csordas has no financial or proprietary interest in the materials presented herein.

Dr. Ashley Cuellar has no financial or proprietary interest in the materials presented herein.

Emily R. Cunningham has no financial or proprietary interest in the materials presented herein.

Dr. Dennis Esterbrooks has no financial or proprietary interest in the materials presented herein.

Dr. R. Armour Forse has no financial or proprietary interest in the materials presented herein.

Dr. Kelli E. Friedman has no financial or proprietary interest in the materials presented herein.

Dr. Daniel M. Herron is a consultant for Lexington Medical, Virtual Incision, and Covidien and receives travel and education support from Intuitive Surgical.

Kathleen B. Hrovat has no financial or proprietary interest in the materials presented herein.

Dr. Mustafa Hussain has no financial or proprietary interest in the materials presented herein.

Dr. Sayeed Ikramuddin lists the following financial disclosures: Novo Nordisk Bariatric Surgery Advisory Board, Medica Bariatric Surgery Advisory Board, OptumHealth Bariatric Expert Panel, USGI Medical Inc Advisory Board, Metamodix Inc Consultant, EnteroMedics Consultant, Grant: ESSENTIAL, Grant: ReCharge Trial, EnteroMedics Grant: EMPOWER, Covidien Grant: DSS Study, Diabetes Surgery Study, ReShape Medical Grant: REDUCE Study, Grant: ADA.

Dr. Thomas H. Inge has received bariatric research grant funding from Ethicon Endo-Surgery and has served as consultant for Sanofi Corp, both unrelated to this chapter.

Dr. Daniel B. Jones is a consultant for Allurion.

Dr. Stephanie B. Jones's spouse is a consultant for Allurion.

Dr. Sangeeta Rao Kashyap has received research funding and honoraria from Ethicon Endo-Surgery for presentation and has received research funding from Covidien.

Dr. Lalita Khaodhiar has not disclosed any relevant financial relationships.

Dr. Eugene Kim has no financial or proprietary interest in the materials presented herein.

Linda Kollar has no financial or proprietary interest in the materials presented herein.

Dr. Nitin Kumar has no financial or proprietary interest in the materials presented herein.

Dr. Tommy H. Lee has no financial or proprietary interest in the materials presented herein.

Dr. Daniel B. Leslie has a consulting agreement with Enteromedics and has a grant from the Minnesota Obesity Center.

Dr. Natalia Leva has no financial or proprietary interest in the materials presented herein.

Dr. Emanuele Lo Menzo has no financial or proprietary interest in the materials presented herein.

Dr. Karen C. McCowen has no financial or proprietary interest in the materials presented herein.

Dr. Lee E. Morrow has no financial or proprietary interest in the materials presented herein.

Dr. John Magaña Morton has no financial or proprietary interest in the materials presented herein.

Dr. Kalyana Nandipati has not disclosed any relevant financial relationships.

Dr. Jaisa Olasky has no financial or proprietary interest in the materials presented herein.

Dr. Pradeep K. Pallati has no financial or proprietary interest in the materials presented herein.

Dr. Alfons Pomp has no financial or proprietary interest in the materials presented herein.

Dr. Walter J. Pories receives grant support from the NIH and Johnson & Johnson.

Dr. Amanda Powell has no financial or proprietary interest in the materials presented herein.

Dr. Christine Ren Fielding is a consultant for Apollo Endosurgery.

Dr. Raul J. Rosenthal has no financial or proprietary interest in the materials presented herein.

Dr. Francesco Rubino has not disclosed any relevant financial relationships.

Dr. Philip R. Schauer has no financial or proprietary interest in the materials presented herein.

Dr. Johanna Schubert has no financial or proprietary interest in the materials presented herein.

Dr. Scott A. Shikora has no financial or proprietary interest in the materials presented herein.

Dr. Alpana Shukla has no financial or proprietary interest in the materials presented herein.

Dr. Stephanie Sogg has no financial or proprietary interest in the materials presented herein.

Dr. Ashwin Soni has not disclosed any relevant financial relationships.

Dr. Wendy Jo Svetanoff has no financial or proprietary interest in the materials presented herein.

Dr. Charles E. Thompson III has no financial or proprietary interest in the materials presented herein.

Dr. Christopher C. Thompson lists the following: Boston Scientific (consultant [consulting fees]), Covidien (consultant [consulting fees]/Endoluminal Advisory Board Member), USGI Medical (consultant [consulting fees]/Advisory Board Member [consulting fees]/research grant), Olympus (lab support [lab supplies/equipment], consultant), Apollo Endosurgery (consultant/research support [consulting fees/research grants]), GI Windows (ownership interest), and Aspire Bariatrics (research grant).

Dr. Oliver A. Varban has no financial or proprietary interest in the materials presented herein.

Dr. Bruce M. Wolfe has no financial or proprietary interest in the materials presented herein.

Dr. Andrew S. Wu has no financial or proprietary interest in the materials presented herein.

Index